REGENERATIVE TREATMENTS IN SPORTS AND ORTHOPEDIC MEDICINE

REGENERATIVE TREATMENTS IN SPORTS AND ORTHOPEDIC MEDICINE

EDITORS

Gerard A. Malanga, MD

Partner/Founder
New Jersey Sports Medicine, LLC
Partner/Founder
New Jersey Regenerative Institute
Cedar Knolls, New Jersey
Clinical Professor
Department of Physical Medicine and Rehabilitation
Rutgers School of Medicine—New Jersey Medical School
Newark, New Jersey

Victor Ibrahim, MD

Founding Partner
Regenerative Orthopedics and Sports Medicine
Washington, DC

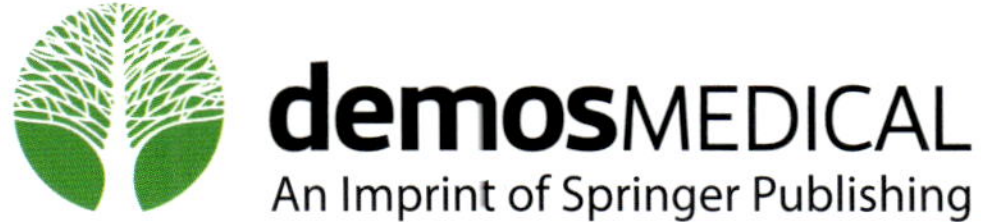

demosMEDICAL
An Imprint of Springer Publishing

Visit our website at www.demosmedical.com

ISBN: 9781620701126
ebook ISBN: 9781617052897

Acquisitions Editor: Beth Barry
Compositor: Newgen KnowledgeWorks

Medicine is an ever-changing science. Research and clinical experience are continually expanding our knowledge, in particular our understanding of proper treatment and drug therapy. The authors, editors, and publisher have made every effort to ensure that all information in this book is in accordance with the state of knowledge at the time of production of the book. Nevertheless, the authors, editors, and publisher are not responsible for errors or omissions or for any consequences from application of the information in this book and make no warranty, expressed or implied, with respect to the contents of the publication. Every reader should examine carefully the package inserts accompanying each drug and should carefully check whether the dosage schedules mentioned therein or the contraindications stated by the manufacturer differ from the statements made in this book. Such examination is particularly important with drugs that are either rarely used or have been newly released on the market.

Library of Congress Cataloging-in-Publication Data
Names: Malanga, Gerard A., editor. | Ibrahim, Victor, editor.
Title: Regenerative treatments in sports and orthopedic medicine / editors,
  Gerard A. Malanga, Victor Ibrahim.
Description: New York : Demos Medical Publishing, [2018] |
  Includes bibliographical references and index.
Identifiers: LCCN 2017024551| ISBN 9781620701126 (hardcover) |
  ISBN 9781617052897 (ebook)
Subjects: | MESH: Orthopedic Procedures | Regenerative Medicine |
  Stem Cell Transplantation | Sports Medicine | Athletic Injuries—surgery
Classification: LCC RD755 | NLM WE 168 | DDC 617.9—dc23
LC record available at https://lccn.loc.gov/2017024551

Printed in the United States of America by Bang Printing.
17 18 19 20 21/ 5 4 3 2 1

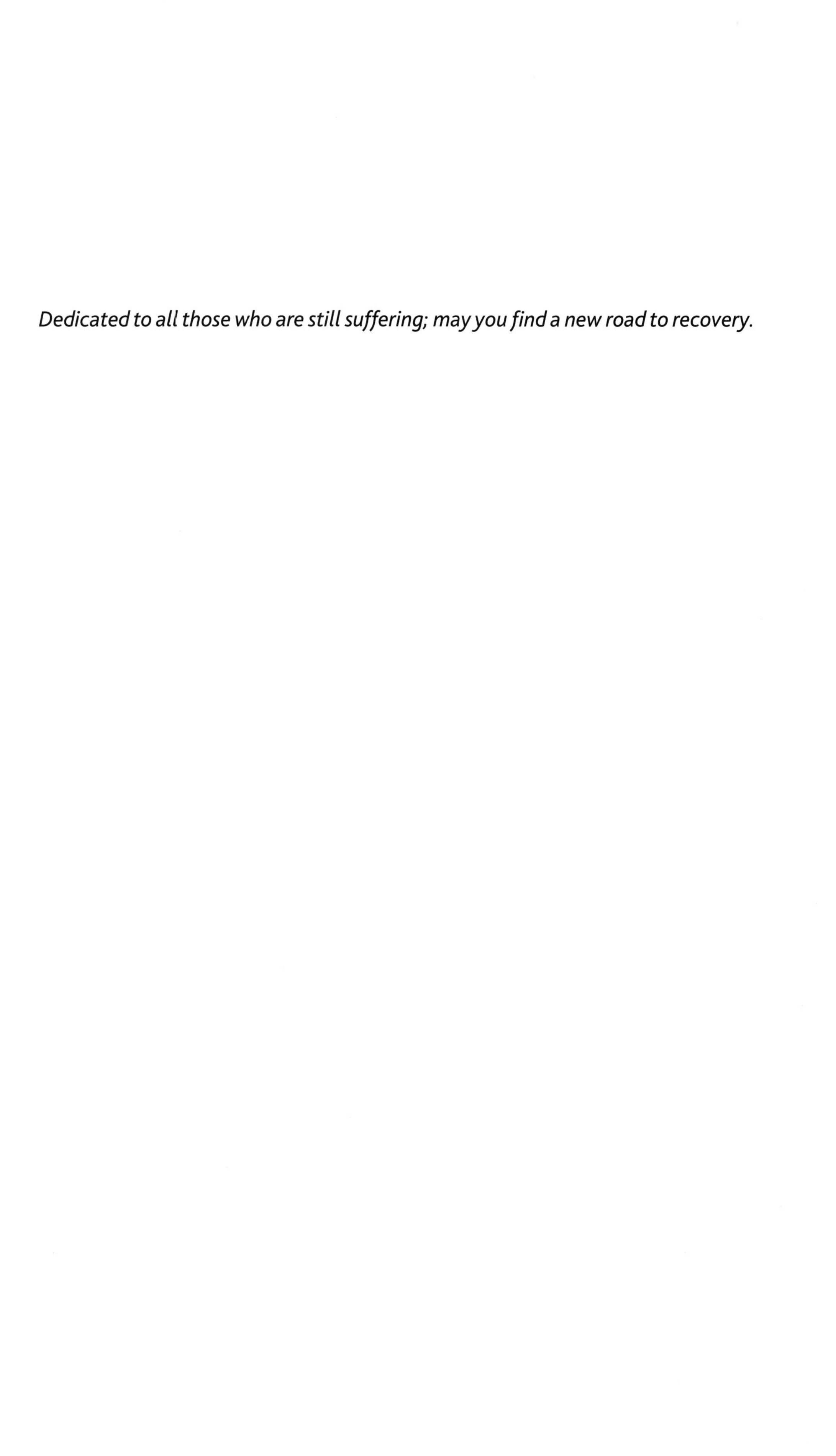

Dedicated to all those who are still suffering; may you find a new road to recovery.

Contents

Contributors

Raisa Bakshiyev, MD
Department of Physical Medicine and
    Rehabilitation
Northwell Health
Manhasset, New York

Marko Bodor, MD
Assistant Professor
Department of Physical Medicine and
    Rehabilitation
University of California at Davis
Sacramento,California;
Interventional Physiatrist
Department of Spine and Sports Medicine
Bodor Clinic
Napa, California

Joanne Borg-Stein, MD
Associate Professor/Associate Chair
Sports and Musculoskeletal Rehabilitation;
Associate Director, Harvard/Spaulding Sports
    Medicine Fellowship
Department of Physical Medicine and
    Rehabilitation
Harvard Medical School
Wellesley, Massachusetts

Jay E. Bowen, DO
New Jersey Regenerative Institute, LLC
Cedar Knolls, New Jersey

**Sherman O. Canapp, Jr., DVM, MS, CCRT,
    DACVS, DACVSMR**
Chief of Staff
Orthopedic Surgery, Sports Medicine, and
    Regenerative Medicine
Veterinary Orthopedic and Sports Medicine
    Group;
President and CEO
Orthobiologic Innovations
Annapolis Junction, Maryland

Brittany Jean Carr, DVM, CCRT
Canine Sports Medicine and Rehabilitation
    Veterinarian
Sports Medicine and Rehabilitation
Veterinary Orthopedic and Sports
    Medicine Group
Annapolis Junction, Maryland

Ricardo E. Colberg, MD, RMSK
Sports Medicine Physician
Andrews Sports Medicine and Orthopedic
    Center
American Sports Medicine Institute
Birmingham, Alabama

Sean Colio, MD
Clinical Assistant Professor
Department of Orthopedic Surgery
Stanford University
Redwood City, California

Robert Diaz, MD
Resident Physician
Department of Physical Medicine and
    Rehabilitation
Spaulding Rehabilitation Hospital/Harvard
    Medical School
Charlestown, Massachusetts

Ryan Dregalla, PhD
Regenerative Science Research and
    Development
Dregalla Medical Technologies, LLC
Scottsdale, Arizona

Robert W. Engelen, DO
Sports Medicine Physician
Department of Orthopedics
Comprehensive Orthopedics and Sports
    Medicine/Physician Group of Utah
Salt Lake City, Utah

Angela T. Gordon, PT, DSc, MPT, COMT, OCS, ATC, FMS
Co-Founder and Physical Therapist
Advanced Kinetics Physical Therapy and Sports Performance
Falls Church, Virginia

Kwang Han, PT, MPT
Co-Founder and Physical Therapist
Advanced Kinetics Physical Therapy and Sports Performance
Falls Church, Virginia

Zaid Hashim, MBBS, MRCS (Eng), PGCMedEd
Specialty Trainee in Trauma and Orthopedics
Department of Trauma and Orthopedics
York Teaching Hospitals
York, United Kingdom

Fadi Hassan, MBBS, BSc (Hons)
Junior Doctor
Good Hope Hospital
Heart of England NHS Foundation Trust
Birmingham, United Kingdom

Sony M. Issac, MD
Resident
Department of Physical Medicine and Rehabilitation
Nassau University Medical Center
East Meadow, New York

Wade Johnson, DO
Department of Physical Medicine and Rehabilitation
New York-Presbyterian Hospital
New York, New York

Leah M. Kujawski, RN, BSN
Clinical Operations Manager
Regenerative Orthopedics and Sports Medicine
Washington, DC

Ariane Maico, MD
Department of Physical Medicine and Rehabilitation
University of Alabama School of Medicine
Birmingham, Alabama

Kenneth R. Mautner, MD
Associate Professor
Departments of Physical Medicine and Rehabilitation and Orthopedics
Emory University;
Director, Primary Care Sports Medicine
Emory Sports Medicine Center
Atlanta, Georgia

Timothy J. Mazzola, MD
Non-Operative Orthopedic and Regenerative Medicine Specialist
Cornerstone Orthopedics and Sports Medicine
Louisville, Colorado;
Senior Clinical Instructor
Department of Family Medicine
University of Colorado School of Medicine
Aurora, Colorado

William D. Murrell, MD, MS
Chief Science Officer
Emirates Healthcare
CEO and Consultant
Orthopedic Sports Medicine
Emirates-Integra Medical and Surgical Centre
Dubai, UAE;
Orthopedics, Rehabilitation, and Podiatry Department
Fort Belvoir Community Hospital
Fort Belvoir, Virginia

Karl M. Nobert, Esq.
FDA Regulatory Attorney
Principal
The Nobert Group, LLC
Sterling, Virginia;
President
ReCellerate Inc.
Middleburg, Virginia

José A. Ramírez-Del Toro, MD
Director of Sports Medicine Fellowship
Department of Physical Medicine and Rehabilitation
University of Pittsburgh Medical Center
Pittsburgh, Pennsylvania;
Director of Sports Medicine
California University of Pennsylvania
California, Pennsylvania

Michael A. Scarpone, DO
Medical Director
Sports Medicine Trinity Health System;
Assistant Professor
Drexel School of Medicine AGH Campus
Team Physician Pittsburgh Pirates
Steubenville, Ohio

Brian J. Shiple, DO, CAQSM, RMSK
Founder
The Center for Sports Medicine
Glenn Mills, Pennsylvania;
Assistant Clinical Professor of Family and
    Community Medicine
Temple University School of Medicine
Philadelphia, Pennsylvania

Imran James Siddiqui, MD, RMSK
Director of Clinical Care
Regenerative Orthopedics and
    Sports Medicine
Department of Physical Medicine and
    Rehabilitation
George Washington University
Washington, DC

Jay Smith, MD
Professor
Departments of Physical Medicine and
    Rehabilitation, Radiology, and Anatomy
Mayo Clinic
Rochester, Minnesota

Walter I. Sussman, DO, RMSK
Sports Medicine Physician, CAQSM
Orthopedic Care Physician Network
North Easton, Massachusetts;
Assistant Professor
Department of Physical Medicine and
    Rehabilitation
Tufts University
Boston, Massachusetts

Suad Trebinjac, MD, PhD
Associate Professor
Medical Director
Dubai Physiotherapy and Rehabilitation Center
    (DPRC);
Consultant
FIFA Medical Center of Excellence
Dubai, UAE

Andre J. van Wijnen, PhD
Professor
Department of Orthopedic Surgery
Mayo Clinic
Rochester, Minnesota

Christopher J. Visco, MD
Associate Professor
Department of Rehabilitation and Regenerative
    Medicine
Columbia University Medical Center
New York, New York

David C. Wang, DO, DABPMR
Director of Education and Training
Regenerative Orthopedics and Sports
    Medicine
Washington, DC

Christopher J. Williams, MD
Attending Physician
Regenerative Orthopedics
Centeno-Schultz Clinic
Broomfield, Colorado

Peter I-Kung Wu, MD, PhD
Resident Physician
Department of Physical Medicine and
    Rehabilitation
Spaulding Rehabilitation Hospital/Harvard
    Medical School
Charlestown, Massachusetts

Preface

The convergence of industry advancements and medical research has resulted in an exponential growth in the clinical use of regenerative medicine throughout the world. With its popularity outpacing scientific data, the need for an authoritative text on the subject has become essential. Modern-day research has tapped into a deeper and more complex understanding of cytokine- and cell-based regeneration theory that translates well into the clinical paradigm of regenerative medicine. This textbook describes the evolution of these research principles into an effective and safe clinical practice.

Today's standard treatment options in orthopedics and sports medicine, many of which are outdated and ineffective, are being replaced by regenerative medicine interventions. These ineffective and outdated treatment options include the prolonged use of anti-inflammatory medications, the use of corticosteroid injections for noninflammatory processes such as tendinopathies, the use of arthroscopic partial meniscectomy for degenerative meniscal tears, the repeated use of epidural injections with corticosteroids, and many of the spinal fusion surgeries being performed. It is clear that the current American health care system needs improvements in the delivery of care to our patients. Medical care should include a more personalized approach, as well as an overall reduction in the number of medication prescriptions and the number of surgical treatments, both of which have significant potential negative effects and significant risks.

The complexity of regenerative pathways has long been described in the medical literature. By distilling these studies, a more focused and clinically relevant paradigm for regeneration becomes apparent. The body has a remarkable natural ability to heal itself. By facilitating or accelerating this process, a practitioner can initiate and support a healing process that previously was prescribed to surgical intervention. Examples of this include meniscal and rotator cuff tears. Both common, and often resolving with a nonsurgical "watch and wait" principle, many of these injuries currently progress to surgical intervention. As meniscal and rotator cuff surgeries have high failure rates, often reaching up to 30%, they fail to provide a definitive solution in many patients. In addition, these interventions invariably alter the joint environment leading to further degenerative processes. This textbook presents nonsurgical treatment options offering a new paradigm that enhances the natural healing of these injuries and degenerative pathologies. So far, these interventions have been proven to be safe, simple, and effective, with potential economic benefits to our ailing modern health care system.

Before beginning these regenerative treatments, baseline medical knowledge is required. First, the clinician has to be able to obtain a proper medical history. Next, the clinician has to be able to perform a *comprehensive* kinetic chain-based orthopedic physical examination, which includes a full understanding of the physical exam maneuvers and the strengths and weaknesses of these maneuvers in the gathering of information. This is then followed by the ability to interpret imaging studies, including x-rays and MRIs that are directly correlated to the patient's history and examination findings. Treatment should not be driven purely by what the images show, but rather needs to be based upon the information that was gathered during the history and physical examination, as there is a plethora of information suggesting that abnormalities in images can frequently be seen in asymptomatic populations.

Clinicians interested in developing a regenerative medicine practice must be aware that the office visit with patients takes time and requires a lengthy review of the findings and *all* the treatment options available to patients. This should include the many nonsurgical and less invasive options such as diet/weight loss; vitamin supplements; orthotic, bracing, aggressive strengthening; hyaluronic injections; and the like. Some patients with biomechanical issues such as catching, locking, or joint instability may be better served with surgical treatment (perhaps enhanced with orthobiologic treatment). Clinicians need to keep up with the current scientific evidence for these treatments and provide patients with as much information as possible regarding the efficacy of these treatments that have been published in basic science, animal, and human studies. The clinician must take time with the patients to provide a *personalized* approach to their care.

Many practitioners of regenerative medicine believe in the effectiveness of these regenerative medicine methods, but often struggle to provide a holistic and evidence-based rationale for this approach. This textbook is intended as a working reference for these clinicians, offering a concise, evidence-based rationale for regenerative medicine in the world of sports medicine. Experts from a variety of renowned medical centers, including Harvard and Mayo Clinic, expound this rationale to guide the reader through this paradigm shift.

From basic science to practical pearls, the authors provide a unique insight into how modern-day regenerative medicine techniques are revolutionizing orthopedic and sports medicine treatment. Our hope is that this book will inspire a deeper awareness of the issues surrounding such a revolution: from practice management to regulatory matters. We have been fortunate to have chapter authors with great knowledge, experience, and enthusiasm in the study and clinical use of various orthobiologic treatments. We would like to thank them for their hard work and diligence in providing the most up-to-date information on their topic areas. We would also like to thank Beth Barry from Demos for first approaching us regarding this project and her assistance in getting it done.

We hope the readers of this textbook will find it a useful reference that will facilitate a thoughtful introduction to this exciting new area in orthopedic treatment, and we hope that most will consider getting involved in data collection registries or other modes of research and facilitate further advancement to improve patient outcomes. Both our individual patients and the health care system would benefit greatly.

Regenerative medicine is fundamentally a modern-day method of enhancing the human capabilities of healing. The principles of this book will provide the reader with a framework to use this understanding to fulfill the calling of all practitioners: healing the patient.

Gerard A. Malanga, MD
Victor Ibrahim, MD

CHAPTER 1

CURRENT CONCEPTS IN THE PATHOPHYSIOLOGY OF ORTHOPEDIC CONDITIONS AFFECTING TREATMENT

Christopher J. Visco and Wade Johnson

Conventional therapies for nonoperative orthopedic conditions have long been targeted to reduce inflammation with the goal of decreasing pain. It is now well known that inflammation is an important part of the healing process. Key cell signaling responsible for repair make up a component of that inflammatory milieu. Therefore, eliminating both inflammation and cell signaling with medications including nonsteroidal anti-inflammatory drugs (NSAIDs) and corticosteroids can be detrimental in the long run. As the pathophysiology of common musculoskeletal conditions has become better understood, it is increasingly possible to target specific areas of the process to improve healing.

Regenerative therapies, including platelet-rich plasma (PRP) and mesenchymal stem cells (MSCs), have been gaining popularity for orthopedic pathology in recent years; however, their use dates back decades. PRP was first developed in the 1970s, and its first documented use was for cardiac surgery in Italy in 1987 by Ferrari et al. In the 1990s, PRP began gaining popularity in maxillofacial, periodontal, and cosmetic surgery with reported significant improvements in healing. In the early 2000s, the use of PRP expanded into orthopedic conditions and the first published application of PRP for chronic tendinosis was published by Mishra and Pavelko in 2006 (1).

This chapter focuses on the science behind chronic and degenerative processes involving cartilage and tendon, as well as how these processes influence current and future management strategies. The mechanisms by which regenerative therapies exert their effects is described in detail in the later chapters.

COMMON MUSCULOSKELETAL DISORDERS IN ORTHOPEDICS

The majority of musculoskeletal disorders are managed nonoperatively in sports medicine and orthopedics. Injuries to muscle, tendon, ligament, bone, and cartilage all have nonsurgical treatment options and are potential targets for regenerative therapies including PRP and MSCs. The pathophysiology behind both acute tears and strains of muscles and ligament and chronic degenerative processes involving tendon and cartilage, including fibrocartilage and hyaline cartilage, is well documented (2–10).

TENDINOPATHY

Normal Tendon Structure

To understand the pathophysiology of tendinopathy, one must first understand the basic anatomy of a tendon. Tendons consist of bundles of collagen fibrils, which are formed from a three-polypeptide chain triple helix. The collagen fibrils are held together by proteoglycans including aggrecan and decorin, and line up in parallel and overlapping fashion forming a collagen fiber. These fibers are then bundled and enveloped in endotenon, forming a primary fiber bundle, the subfascicle, which is further bundled to form a secondary fiber bundle, known as a fascicle (Figure 1.1). Fascicles intercalate to form the tertiary structure recognizable as tendon, which is then ensheathed in the parietal layer by an epitenon.

The collagen portion of tendon is approximately 97% type I collagen, with small amounts of types II, III, IV, V, IX, and X collagen making up the various components of supportive tissues. The extracellular matrix (ECM) is made up of 65% to 80% collagen and provides strength. Elastin ensures flexibility and is present in small amounts. The remainder of ECM is known as "ground substance" and is made up primarily of water (accounting for 70% of tendon mass), with scant proteoglycans and glycoproteins. Few tendons, including the flexors and extensors of the hand and wrist, have true synovial sheaths, while others are surrounded by paratenon, with mucopolysaccharides providing lubrication between epitenon and paratenon (5). The epitenon is a fine, loose connective tissue sheath and contains the vascular, lymphatic, and nerve supply to the tendon. Paratenon is made up of type I and III collagen with the inner surface lined by synovial cells. Some tendons with a paratenon are found in close approximation to a fat pad, which includes the triceps and patellar and Achilles tendons (11,12).

The cellular component of tendons is made up of tenoblasts and tenocytes arranged in parallel rows among collagen fibers running in the long axis of the tendon. Tenoblasts are immature spindle-shaped cells with many cytoplasmic organelles reflecting their high level of metabolic activity. Tenoblasts become elongated as they age, and transform into tenocytes. Tenocytes function to synthesize collagen and the other components of the ECM, and are also very metabolically active. Together, tenoblasts and tenocytes make up 90% to 95% of the cellular component of tendons. The remaining 5% to 10% of the cellular component is made up of chondrocytes, present at the enthesis, synovial cells, located in the tendon sheath, and endothelial cells of the arterioles supplying the tendon.

There are two histologically distinct transition points in all tendons: the musculotendinous junction and the point of insertion to bone known as the "enthesis." The musculotendinous junction is rich in nerve receptors and is subject to significant mechanical stress during muscle contraction. At this junction, collagen fibers from the tendon are inserted into deep recesses within the muscle formed by myocyte processes allowing the transmission of tension created by the muscle fibers to the collagen of the tendon. This architecture reduces tensile stress exerted on the tendon, although the junction remains the weakest point of the muscle–tendon complex. The typical enthesis displays a more gradual transition from tendon to cartilage and to lamellar bone and is made up of four zones: dense tendon zone, fibrocartilage, mineralized fibrocartilage, and bone. This transition point helps to prevent collagen fiber damage and failure during stress by dispersing forces (2). Tendons also insert onto bone in the form of myo-entheses, such as the distal iliacus. Myo-entheses tend to develop degenerative pathology

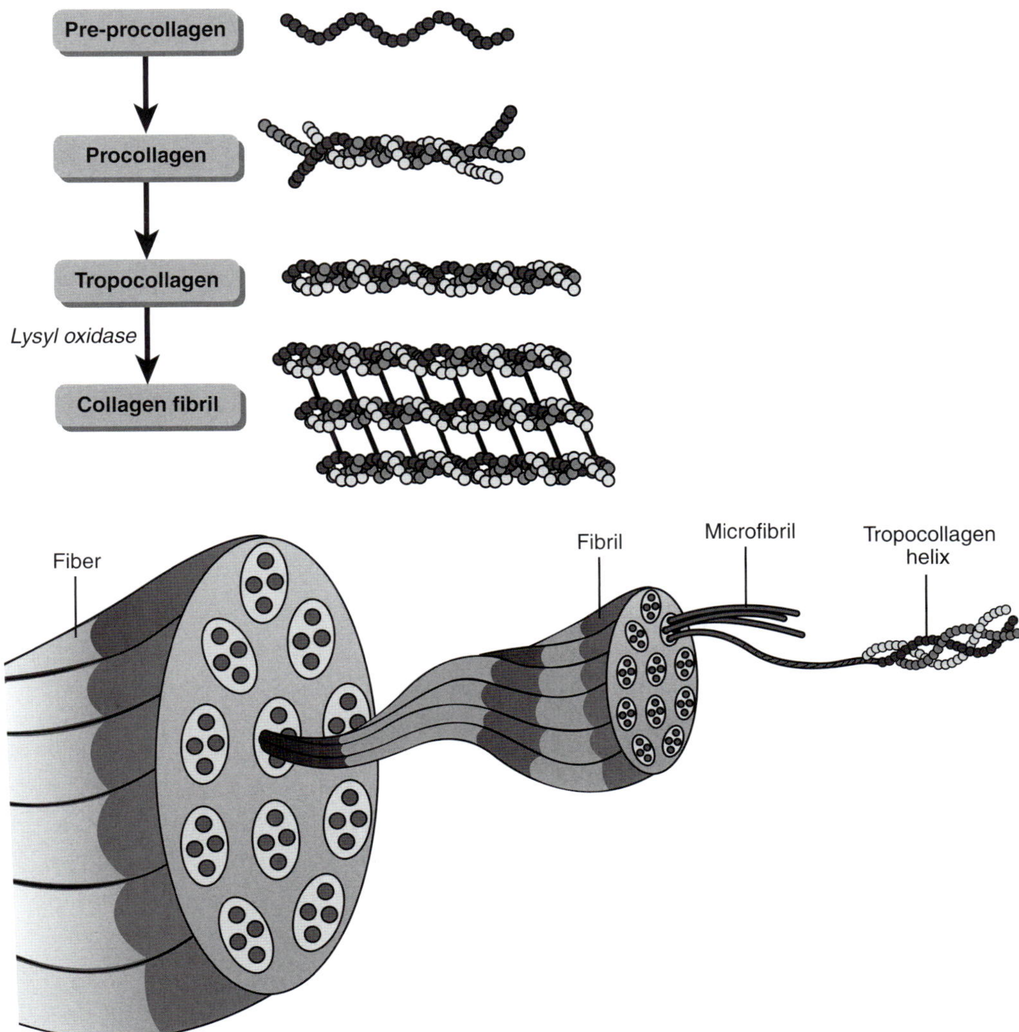

FIGURE 1.1: Tendon structure.

Source: From Ref. (13). Caldwell M, Casey E, Powell B, Shultz SJ. Sex hormones. In: Casey E, Rho M, Press J, eds. *Sex Differences in Sports Medicine.* New York, NY: Demos Medical Publishing LLC; 2016:11.

less frequently because of their superior blood supply compared to cartilaginous entheses. It is important to also note that muscle and tendon do not always insert onto bone, with muscle being able to insert directly onto ligament (e.g., vastus medialis inserting onto the medial patellofemoral ligament), and ligament inserting onto tendon (e.g., vastus lateralis onto the iliotibial band [ITB], the fibrous tract running along the lateral thigh important in stabilization of an extended, to slightly flexed, knee), and tendon onto ligament (e.g., supraspinatus onto the cuff pulley).

Tendon Blood Supply and Innervation

Intrinsic blood supply to tendon is located at the myotendinous and osteotendinous junction points; extrinsic blood supply comes from the paratenon and synovial sheath. Vessels originating in muscle supply the myotendinous junction and do not extend beyond the proximal third of the tendon, while the blood supply at the enthesis is significantly limited and located only in the insertion zone near the periosteum. Ensheathed tendons have extrinsic blood supply from major vessels forming a plexus located in the synovial sheath supplying the superficial portion of the tendon. Tendons without sheaths have extrinsic superficial vascular supply located in the paratenon. Both the extrinsic vascular supplies form communications with the intrinsic supply through penetrating branches. The musculotendinous junctions and the entheses are sites of vulnerable vascularity. Increasing age and mechanical loading may further decrease vascular supply in these areas. Entheses are also known to have significant associated fat, whether it is in the form of a fat pad, or fat at the insertional angle, or within the endotenon and epitenon. These areas are known to be richly vascularized and innervated, producing significant growth factors and proinflammatory markers in tendinopathic conditions suggesting extrinsic blood supply to the tendon (8,11).

Innervation is provided by nearby cutaneous and afferent nerves, which travel in association with arteries and arterioles (14), although some afferent nerves are found without vascular association. Small afferent nerves are located throughout the paratenon, forming plexuses with penetrating branches into the epitenon, with a distinct lack of deeper innervation. There are four types of nerve endings located within the tendons: type I Ruffini corpuscles, which are slow-adapting, low-threshold pressure sensors; type II Pacini corpuscles, which are rapidly adapting dynamic pressure sensors; type III Golgi tendon organs, which respond to tension and position; and type IV free nerve endings, which provide sensation and nociception. Golgi tendon organs are located in greatest number at the musculotendinous junction where tension is high (15).

Biomechanics

Tendons are significantly influenced by the functional demands placed on them, and as a result their structure and composition changes by location. Collagen turnover is known to be higher in tendons under greater stress such as

the supraspinatus tendon, and lower in less stressed locations such as the distal biceps tendon. Despite the differences, the metabolic rate of all tendons is limited; with oxygen consumption 7.5 times lower than the muscle, and collagen turnover time ranging from 50 to 100 days resulting in the prolongation of healing.

When a tendon is at rest, the collagen fibers are oriented in a crimped configuration, providing a buffer in which a slight elongation can occur without tension leading to fibrous damage. Collagen fibers tolerate approximately 4% elongation with the ability to return to their original configuration on release of tension. At 4% elongation, fibers begin to move longitudinally and microscopic evidence of failure of the tendon becomes evident. Once stressed to 8% elongation, macroscopic rupture occurs because of tensile failure of the fibers and interfibrillar shear failure. This effect is minimized by the presence of elastin, which can elongate up to 70% of its length without failure, and full rupture not occurring until 150% elongation. With an increasing age, tendons lose this ability to accommodate to stretch because of loss of elastic fibers and degradation of elastin by tissue elastases.

Pathophysiology of Tendinopathy

Tendinopathies are thought to develop from excessive loading and tensile strain. Repetitive loading can lead to inflammation of the tendon sheath, degeneration of the body of the tendon, or a combination of these processes. A tendon's response to repetitive loading depends on its cross-sectional area and length. Greater cross-sectional area allows a larger capacity to tolerate load before failure, and longer tendon fibers are at greater risk of elongation tendon failure. Stress on a tendon is determined by the following equation:

$$\sigma = F/A,$$

where (σ) represents stress, (F) represents the force applied on the tendon, and (A) represents the cross-sectional area of the tendon.

At most risk are the areas with poor blood supply, where microdisruption of tendon fibers, secondary to repetitive load, is not repaired efficiently. Tissue injury leads to inflammation, and the release of growth and differentiation factors (GDFs) and scleraxis (Scx) (5). Scx activates the gene encoding collagen type I within tendon fibroblasts, which promotes healing of the damaged tendon. Repetitive loading also induces noxious mechanisms, however, preventing healing. Repetitive stretch may increase substances such as prostaglandin E2, a potent inhibitor of type I collagen synthesis.

Poor blood supply predisposes damaged tendon to tissue hypoxia, which is exacerbated by elevated lactate levels in damaged tendons. Tissue hypoxia leads to an expression of vascular endothelial growth factor (VEGF). VEGF expression leads to neoangiogenesis, which is accompanied by neural ingrowth. This neural ingrowth is thought to be responsible for clinical symptoms associated with tendinopathy including pain. This is supported by evidence for increased tissue levels of glutamate, substance P, and calcitonin gene-related peptide. VEGF is also shown to upregulate matrix metalloproteinases (MMPs), which leads to degradation of ECM and further weakening of the tendon (5).

Cartilage Injury

When considering injury to cartilage, one must differentiate between two commonly injured types of cartilage: hyaline and fibrocartilage. Hyaline cartilage is found lining bony articular surfaces and is commonly affected in arthritic processes, while fibrocartilage is more commonly damaged in intervertebral discs and meniscal tissue. Both processes have significant differences in tissue composition, location, and biomechanics, and as a result, the underlying pathophysiology behind injury is unique and is discussed in the following sections.

Normal Articular Anatomy

Peripheral joints involved in osteoarthritis (OA) that are targeted with regenerative therapies are synovial joints. A synovial joint is made up of two adjacent bones surrounded by an articular capsule. This articular capsule is a fibrous connective tissue structure attached to each bone beyond the articular surface. The articular surfaces of the bones are covered with a specialized layer of hyaline cartilage allowing smooth movement between adjacent surfaces. Hyaline cartilage is made up mostly of type II collagen. The joint space is maintained with synovial fluid that is secreted from the synovial membrane lining the articular capsule. Synovial fluid also functions to provide nourishment to the poorly vascularized articular cartilage.

Hyaline cartilage lining the articular surface of bones is significantly devoid of vasculature, nerves, and lymphatics resulting in its poor ability to heal. Articular cartilage is made up of a dense ECM, consisting of approximately 80% water, with proteoglycans and collagen accounting for much of the remaining 20%. This ECM is sparsely populated with chondrocytes, responsible for the generation and repair of the articular cartilage, whose activity decreases with age (16).

Articular cartilage is divided into four zones; superficial, middle, deep, and calcified as shown in Figure 1.2.

The superficial zone is in direct contact with the synovial fluid of the joint and accounts for approximately 10% to 20% of the thickness of articular cartilage. Within the superficial zone, there is a relatively high number of flattened chondrocytes, and collagen fibers are tightly packed parallel to the articular surface allowing this zone to resist many of the tensile forces caused by joint articulation. The middle zone makes up 40% to 60% of the cartilage thickness and is composed of proteoglycans and thick collagen fibrils with very few chondrocytes present. The primary function of the middle zone is to combat compressive forces. The deep zone accounts for roughly 30% of cartilage thickness and

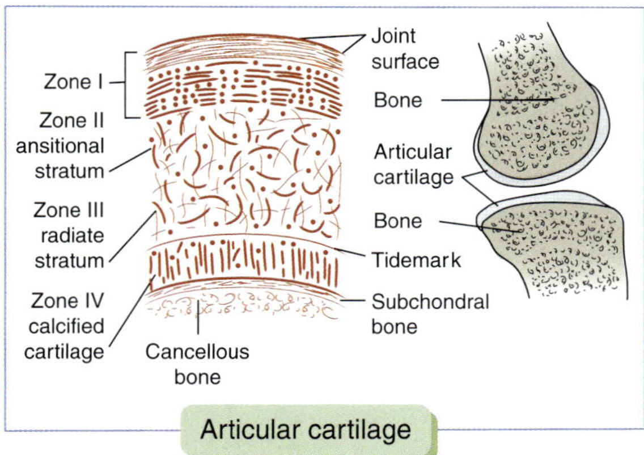

FIGURE 1.2: Cartilage zones.

Source: From Ref. (11). Caldwell M et al. Sex hormones. In: Casey E, Rho M, Press J, eds. *Sex Differences in Sports Medicine*. New York, NY: Demos Medical Publishing LLC; 2016:5.

functions primarily in combating compressive forces because of the orientation of its collagen fibrils perpendicular to the joint surface. Collagen fibrils within the deep zone have the largest diameter and highest proteoglycan content. Separating the deep zone from the calcified zone is the tidemark, which is found exclusively in joint cartilage. The calcified zone functions to anchor collagen fibrils of the deep zone to the subchondral bone and is a remnant of endochondral ossification during childhood growth.

Osteoarthritis

OA is a common orthopedic joint disorder affecting millions of individuals, with a majority of affected patients being older than 65 years. The most commonly affected joints include the hands, knees, hips, and spine. It is rarely found that OA develops from a fundamental defect in a patient's articular hyaline cartilage, as in patients with type II collagen gene defects. More commonly, the process of OA is initiated by a single trauma or repetitive microtrauma causing damage to the normal articular hyaline cartilage. Damage to the articular cartilage is one aspect of OA that is commonly targeted with regenerative therapies.

Osteoarthritis Risk Factors

One of the most significant known risk factors for the development of OA is age. As we age, there are significant changes to the components of the cartilage ECM. This is evident by the decreasing size and structural organization of proteoglycans within the ECM, as well as the buildup of advanced glycation end products, altering the biomechanical environment. As we age, chondrocytes, limited in their regenerative capability, are known to become even less active and responsive to anabolic stimuli.

Other important risk factors for the progression of OA include obesity, joint instability or malalignment, peripheral neuropathy, and presence of crystalloid joint disease. There is also evidence of genetic influence in the development of OA, including twin studies, and familial clustering patterns. Genes for the vitamin D receptor, insulin-like growth factor, fibroblast growth factor, and transforming growth factor have been identified for their involvement through association studies.

Pathophysiology

As mentioned previously, the initial insult in the process of OA is damage to the hyaline articular cartilage, often by repetitive microtrauma. This damage results in matrix fibrillation, fissure appearance, ulceration, and full-thickness loss of the joint surface. These changes are followed by an increased subchondral bone thickness, formation of new bone at joint margins (osteophytes), subchondral cyst formation, and calcification of cartilage at the junction of the hyaline cartilage and subchondral bone. It is at this junction that vascular invasion occurs contributing to an adverse biomechanical environment and further cartilage breakdown. The final stage involves synovitis with an increase in proteases and proinflammatory cytokines. MMPs, including collagenase and stromelysin, are the proteases primarily involved in ECM degradation. As the cartilage ECM breaks down, fragments are released into the synovial fluid further promoting inflammation. Proinflammatory cytokines known to be involved include interleukin-1β (IL-1β), and tumor necrosis factor-α (TNF-α), both of which are known to inhibit synthesis of ECM elements, including collagen and proteoglycans. Thus, the presence of inflammation of the synovium, highlighted by the increase in IL-1β and TNF-α, prevents the potential repair of the damaged cartilaginous matrix resulting in the progressive degeneration seen in OA.

Fibrocartilage Injury

As hyaline cartilage damage is the target for regenerative therapies in OA, fibrocartilage damage is the underlying problem and target of therapy in intervertebral disc injury, meniscal injury, and injury at the tendon–bone interface. Fibrocartilage in these locations is made up of mostly type I collagen. The commonly injured lumbar intervertebral discs are made up of a ring of fibrocartilage called the "annulus fibrosus," surrounding an inner gel-like shock-absorbing nucleus pulposus. The menisci of the knee are two C-shaped wedges with a larger, firmly fixed medial meniscus and a circular, loosely fixed lateral meniscus.

Intervertebral Disc Injury

As mentioned earlier, intervertebral discs in the lumbar spine are comprised of an outer ring of type I collagen fibrocartilage, the annulus fibrosus, encircling an inner gel of water, proteoglycans, and type II cartilage called the nucleus pulposus. The annulus fibrosus is responsible for the tensile strength of the disc, while the nucleus pulposus provides the shock-absorbing capabilities of the intervertebral disc. Intervertebral disc injury occurs through two common mechanisms: acute tearing and chronic degeneration. Injured intervertebral discs have elevated levels of inflammatory cytokines and higher activity of MMPs resulting in poor healing. Cells of the inner nucleus pulposus are especially susceptible to injury and poor healing as their nearest blood supply is approximately 8 mm away and is provided by the capillary network penetrating the subchondral plate from the adjacent vertebral bodies.

Aging, mechanical loading, lifestyle, and genetic factors play a role in disc degeneration. The concentration of cells in the annulus fibrosis decreases with age, as does the hydrophilic composition of the proteoglycans within the nucleus pulposus, which further limits the ability of the disc to influence its own healing. Calcified nucleus pulposus may herniate through the vertebral endplate forming Schmorl's nodes. This process also causes the disc to function poorly under load, resulting in an increased stress on the annulus leading to annular bulge promoting failure and tear. These changes may manifest on neuroimaging in the form of loss of disc height, and disc bulging or herniation into the spinal canal (Figure 1.3). Disc tear and herniation of intervertebral discs is associated with increased levels of IL-1, as well as osteoprotegerin and receptor activator of nuclear factor kappa-B ligand (RANKL), that are members of the TNF superfamily.

Meniscal Injury

The meniscus of the knee is composed of a large, C-shaped, fixed medial meniscus, and a smaller, round, loose lateral meniscus. Menisci are composed of three distinct zones; the peripheral component is made up mostly of type I collagen with fibroblast-like cells with modest vascularization

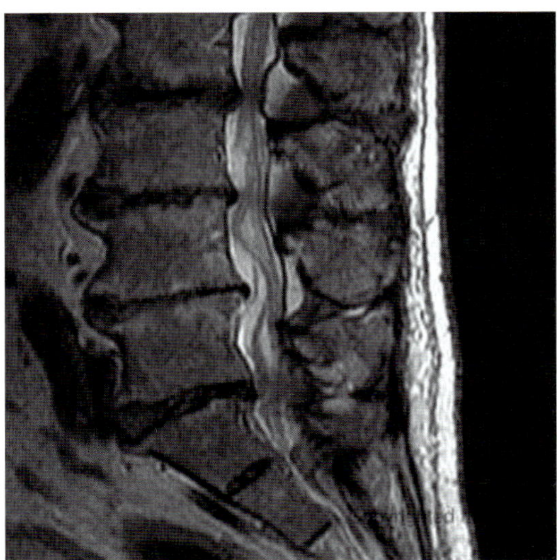

FIGURE 1.3: Loss of disc height seen in degenerative disc disease.

Source: From Ref. (17). Panagos A. *Spine*. New York, NY: Demos Medical Publishing LLC; 2009.

and is known as the "red zone," while the inner two thirds, known as the "white zone" is made up of predominantly type II collagen with chondrocyte-like cells and completely lack vascularization and neural supply. In between the red and white zones is a transition zone with characteristics of both zones and is known as the "red–white zone" (8).

At birth, menisci are highly vascularized; however, by childhood, this vascularization decreases dramatically with only 10% to 30% of the meniscus having vascular supply by the age of 10 years. In young patients, meniscal tears are commonly the result of acute sports-related injury, while older patients experience tears from more long-term degeneration. Degenerative tears tend to occur in the posterior horn and midbody of the meniscus with tears confined to the outer red zone, which is known to have more healing potential than tears involving the inner white zone owing to the difference in vascularization (8,18).

Common Treatments Currently Used

As mentioned previously, many common therapies for musculoskeletal injuries today focus on eliminating inflammation, or blocking pain, to provide symptomatic relief. These mechanisms work very well to control pain, and help patients go about their daily activities; however, they do not facilitate healing in the damaged tissue. Many of these medications are known to interfere with the inflammatory process and interrupt cell signaling, which potentially promote chronic degenerative processes.

Acetaminophen, first-line in processes such as OA, is an analgesic that works by inhibiting substance P and spinal nitric oxide. Acetaminophen has not been shown to have a direct negative effect on healing. NSAIDs also provide analgesia (through cyclooxygenase-2 [COX-2] inhibition); however, they target inflammation directly by inhibiting COX and leukotrienes to prevent the conversion of arachidonic acid to prostaglandins. This antiinflammatory action of NSAIDs may promote a cycle of chronic degradation worsening the underlying pathology that they are used to treat. Nonselective NSAIDs also block COX-1. COX-1 inhibition is known to result in reduced proteoglycan synthesis, which has been shown to have a negative effect on cartilage with long-term use in animal models (19). Chronic indomethacin use has been associated with an acceleration of joint destruction in hip OA (20). Short-term celecoxib use has been shown to result in impaired ligament healing in animal models (21). In a retrospective study of 10,000 patients, the use of nonselective NSAIDs in the first 3 months after a fracture has been associated with nonunion (22).

Steroids are commonly used in orthopedic conditions because of their potent antiinflammatory effects. Both oral steroids and locally injectable steroids are widely used to decrease inflammation, providing powerful pain relief in conditions ranging from disc herniation to tendonitis. Corticosteroids have been widely shown to interfere with the healing of tissues throughout the body. With regard to cartilage repair, systemic corticosteroids reduce circulating insulin-like growth factor 1 (IGF-1) levels and induce IGF-1 resistance leading to decreased chondrocyte production and matrix synthesis

(23). Glucocorticoids are known to impair collagen synthesis, and locally injectable corticosteroids have been shown to reduce synthesis of proteoglycans, and protein in cartilage (24).

In addition to the direct effects on inflammation and signaling, it is also important to note the systemic effects of glucocorticoids, especially in long-term use. Adrenal suppression via inhibition of the hypothalamic–pituitary–adrenal (HPA) axis can be seen with high dose, long-term oral corticosteroid administration. This occurs as exogenous glucocorticoids inhibit the hypothalamic production of corticotropin-releasing hormone (CRH), thus decreasing adrenocorticotropic hormone (ACTH) stimulation of adrenal activity. The result is a decreased cortisol and endogenous sex hormone production manifested by malaise, weakness, fatigue, myalgias, and arthralgias, as well as many other symptoms. Mineralocorticoid production by the adrenals, including aldosterone, is less affected as the renin–angiotensin system remains intact (25). In addition, the production and release of growth hormone inhibited with suppression of the HPA axis is an important catabolic hormone promoting protein synthesis.

NSAIDs, steroids, and other systemically absorbed antiinflammatory medications are to be avoided when considering PRP and MSC injection owing to their interference with inflammation and the cell signaling involved. This also includes inhaled corticosteroid medications for breathing disorders that have systemic absorption from the lung. One study has shown no effect on the delivery of growth factors following a PRP injection in patients on aspirin and clopidogrel (26).

Surgical Management

In degenerative disease involving tendon and cartilage, including meniscus, articular cartilage, and intervertebral disc disease, surgical intervention is generally reserved for cases recalcitrant to conservative care. Considering the overall incidence of tendinosis, surgical intervention is rarely indicated and has varying degrees of efficacy with certain procedures known to have significantly higher rates of positive outcomes than others.

Surgical correction of tendinopathy is typically reserved for cases without improvement even after 6 months of conservative management (27). Surgical correction classically involves incising the paratenon, removing adhesions, and debriding degenerative tissue (28). This is often, although not always, accompanied by introducing longitudinal incisions in the tendon to promote a healing response. The efficacy of surgical management for tendinopathy has been drawn into question as a systematic review of 26 studies investigating surgical correction of patellar tendinopathy has revealed that studies with more positive results correlate with poorer study quality (27). Adverse effects may also be more prevalent in certain conditions, particularly in excision of calcific tendons, which has a subsequent higher rate of rupture compared to nonoperative care (29).

Degenerative disorders of articular cartilage have many surgical options for management, with the most common surgically corrected joints being the hip and knee. Arthroscopic debridement of knee OA with or without associated meniscal tear is a common practice that is not supported by randomized trials (30). These options should be approached with caution in light of significant potential for complications with surgical intervention and limited benefits, particularly in individuals older than 60 years who demonstrate worse outcome (31). Total joint arthroplasty is the most common definitive treatment currently used for OA at the hip and knee. Total hip and knee arthroplasty for end-stage OA is associated with significant pain relief and improved function at 12 months compared to classic conservative therapies including physical therapy, oral NSAIDs, steroid injection, and viscosupplementation alone (32). However, there are significant adverse events associated with total joint arthroplasty including, but not limited to, surgical site infection, periprosthetic fracture, venous thromboembolism requiring prophylactic anticoagulation, and, very rarely, death (30,32).

Surgical intervention in acute meniscal tears is commonly performed when symptoms are refractory to conservative care, and become frequent and interfere with daily function. Often this is done to prevent further damage to articular cartilage predisposing a patient to the development of OA. Surgical correction of chronic degenerative meniscal tears in the absence of significant arthritis, however, has not been shown to be beneficial when compared to physical therapy alone when evaluating for pain or function (30,33). Furthermore, studies comparing surgical management of acute tears to degenerative tears in patients older than 50 years old have revealed significantly positive results for acute tears versus little benefit for degenerative tears at 6-year follow up (30,33).

Surgical intervention is also commonly used for degenerative disease of intervertebral discs. Nonspecific low back pain without radicular symptoms is commonly attributed to degenerative disease of the intervertebral discs and rates of spinal fusions for this type of pain is on the rise. Lumbar fusion, including resection of the degenerate disc, with or without instrumentation has not been shown to have any improved outcomes when compared with nonsurgical management in regards to pain or function (34). Spinal fusion is also known to predispose spinal segments adjacent to the fusion to long-term degenerative changes, often leading to revision and extension of previous spinal fusions (34).

OTHER CONCEPTS AFFECTING THERAPY

Smoking

Cigarette smoking is known to influence a prothrombotic state but increasing platelet activity, elevating fibrinogen concentration in the blood, and inhibiting tissue plasminogen activator release from the endothelium. Smoking also delays healing in tissues by up to 60%, and several studies have revealed different ways in which this delay occurs. One component of cigarette smoking, nicotine, has been shown to interfere with stem cell differentiation into chondrocytes. Smokers have also been demonstrated to have up to 50% fewer circulating stem cells than nonsmokers.

Alcohol

The negative effects of heavy alcohol use on MSCs are well documented. Heavy alcohol use has been shown to decrease activity and number of MSCs, as well as limit their multipotent potential. More moderate alcohol use and its effect on MSCs is less well known. Dose-dependent inhibition of platelet aggregation is also a well-known phenomenon secondary to alcohol consumption. As a result of these known effects, it is commonly recommended to avoid alcohol after PRP and stem cell injection.

Exercise

It is widely accepted that a quality rehabilitation program after injection helps to maximize the effects of regenerative therapy. Early after injection, usually in the first 3 to 5 days after injection, it is common to have a therapy program focusing on joint protection and gentle range of motion. Exercise then progresses to initial strengthening and neuromuscular control, through 2 weeks postinjection, and finally to dynamic motion and sport-specific movements after 2 weeks postinjection.

Sleep and Metabolic Derangements

Sleep is known to play a major role in the healing process. During sleep, anabolic properties in the body are highest, evident by low levels of cortisol and catecholamines. Catecholamines interfere with cell division that is integral to the healing process. Growth hormone is also secreted in significant amounts during deep sleep, which aids in the mobilization of free fatty acids for energy and increases protein synthesis. Deprivation of sleep has been shown to lead to a loss of total body nitrogen and, as a result, protein (35). Studies involving mice have shown that sleep deprivation inhibits migration and homing of implanted multipotent stem cells.

Diet and other metabolic disturbances can play a major role in the differentiation potential and effectiveness of MSC injections. In studies on mice, obesity was shown to have a negative effect on adipogenic, osteogenic, and chondrogenic potential of harvested MSCs (36). In contrast to obesity, malnutrition also has a detrimental effect on tissue healing. Protein malnutrition is known to interfere with collagen formation. Adequate glucose is required to provide the energy required for new tissue deposition and angiogenesis; however, hyperglycemia has been associated with poor tendon healing in rat models (37).

CONCLUSION

As demonstrated throughout this chapter, conservative therapies for degenerative orthopedic disorders have classically targeted reducing inflammation to relieve pain to improve function. Although therapies reducing inflammation are successful at transiently improving symptoms, which may allow improved function in the short-term, the potential long-term detrimental effects are well documented. The varying response to surgical interventions for degenerative disease, as well as their potential risks, has also been well established. The importance of the inflammatory milieu in the healing process continues to be better understood, leading to advancements in conservative therapies. The promotion of the body's healing capabilities by utilizing the inflammatory cascade is the target of recent advancements in regenerative therapy. These concepts are further discussed in the subsequent chapters.

REFERENCES

1. Mishra A, Pavelko T. Treatment of chronic elbow tendinosis with buffered platelet-rich plasma. *Am J Sports Med*. 2006;34(11):1774–1778.
2. Sharma P, Maffulli N. Biology of tendon injury: healing, modeling and remodeling. *J Musculoskelet Neuronal Interact*. 2006;6(2):181–190.
3. Johnson WE, Roberts S. Human intervertebral disc cell morphology and cytoskeletal composition: a preliminary study of regional variations in health and disease. *J Anat*. 2003;203(6):605–612.
4. Raj PP. Intervertebral disc: anatomy-physiology-pathophysiology-treatment. *Pain Pract*. 2008; 8(1):18–44.
5. Abate M, Silbernagel KG, Siljeholm K, et al. Pathogenesis of tendinopathies: inflammation or degeneration? *Arthritis Res Ther*. 2009;11(235). http://arthritis-research.biomedcentral.com/articles/10.1186/ar2723
6. Martel-Pelletier J. Pathophysiology of osteoarthritis. *Osteoarthritis Cartilage*. 2004;12:S31–S33.
7. Goldring SR, Goldring MB. Clinical aspects, pathology and pathophysiology of osteoarthritis. *J Musculoskelet Neuronal Interact*. 2006;6(4): 376–378.
8. Makris EA, Hadidi P, Athanasiou KA. The knee meniscus: structure-function, pathophysiology, current repair techniques, and prospects for regeneration. *Biomaterials*. 2011;32(30): 7411–7431.
9. Page P. Pathophysiology of acute exercise-induced muscular injury: clinical implications. *J Athl Train*. 1995;30(1):29–34.
10. Cereatti A, Rippani FR, Margheritini F. Pathophysiology of ligament injuries. In: F Margheritini & R Rossi (Eds.) *Orthopedic Sports Medicine*. Milan, Italy: Springer; 2011:41–47.
11. Benjamin M, Redman S, Milz S, et al. Adipose tissue at entheses: the rheumatological implications of its distribution. A potential site of pain and stress dissipation? *Ann Rheum Dis*. 2004;63(12):1549–1555.
12. Shaw HM, Santer RM, Watson AH, et al. Adipose tissue at entheses: the innervation and cell composition of the retromalleolar fat pad associated with the rat Achilles tendon. *J Anat*. 2007;211(4):436–443.
13. Caldwell M, Casey E, Powell B, Shultz SJ. Sex hormones. In: Casey E, Rho M, Press J, eds. *Sex*

Differences in Sports Medicine. New York, NY: Demos Medical Publishing LLC; 2016:11.

14. Danielson P. Innervation patterns and locally produced signal substances in the human patellar tendon. https://www.diva-portal.org/smash/get/diva2:140418/FULLTEXT01.pdf

15. Benjamin M, Kaiser E, Milz S. Structure-function relationships in tendons: a review. *J Anat.* 2008;212(3):211–228.

16. Loeser RF. Aging and osteoarthritis: the role of chondrocyte senescence and aging changes in the cartilage matrix. *Osteoarthritis Cartilage.* 2009;17(8):971–979.

17. Panagos A. *Spine.* New York, NY: Demos Medical Publishing LLC; 2009.

18. Fox AJ, Bedi A, Rodeo SA. The basic science of human knee menisci. *Sports Health.* 2012; 4(4):340–351.

19. Mastbergen S, Jansen N, Bijlsma J, et al. Differential direct effects of cyclo-oxygenase-1/ 2 inhibition on proteoglycan turnover of human osteoarthritic cartilage: an in vitro study. *Arthritis Res Ther.* 2005;8(R2). http://arthritis-research .biomedcentral.com/articles/10.1186/ar1846

20. Huskisson EC, Berry H, Gishen P, et al. Effects of antiinflammatory drugs on the progression of osteoarthritis of the knee. LINK Study Group. Longitudinal Investigation of Nonsteroidal Antiinflammatory Drugs in Knee Osteoarthritis. *J Rheumatol.* 1995;22(10):1941–1946.

21. Elder CL, Dahners LE, Weinhold PS. A cyclooxygenase-2 inhibitor impairs ligament healing in the rat. *Am J Sports Med.* 2001;29(6): 801–805.

22. Bhattacharyya T, Levin R, Vrahas MS, et al. Nonsteroidal antiinflammatory drugs and nonunion of humeral shaft fractures. *Arthritis Rheum.* 2005;53(3):364–367.

23. Olney RC. Mechanisms of impaired growth: effect of steroids on bone and cartilage. *Horm Res.* 2009;72(Suppl 1):30–35.

24. Behrens F, Shepard N, Mitchell N. Alterations of rabbit articular cartilage by intra-articular injections of glucocorticoids. *J Bone Joint Surg Am.* 1975;57(1):70–76.

25. Raff H, Sharma S, Niemann L. Physiological basis for the etiology, diagnosis, and treatment of adrenal disorders: Cushing's syndrome, adrenal insufficiency, and congenital adrenal hyperplasia. http://www.ncbi.nlm.nih.gov/pmc/articles/ PMC4215264

26. Smith CW, Binford RS, Holt DW, et al. Quality assessment of platelet rich plasma during antiplatelet therapy. *Perfusion.* 2007;22(1):41–50.

27. Coleman BD, Khan KM, Maffulli N, et al. Studies of surgical outcome after patellar tendinopathy: clinical significance of methodological deficiencies and guidelines for future studies. Victorian Institute of Sport Tendon Study Group. *Scand J Med Sci Sports.* 2000;10(1):2–11.

28. Nelen G, Martens M, Burssens A. Surgical treatment of chronic Achilles tendinitis. *Am J Sports Med.* 1989;17(6):754–759.

29. Gohr CM, Fahey M, Rosenthal AK. Calcific tendonitis: a model. *Connect Tissue Res.* 2007; 48(6):286–291.

30. Herrlin S, Hållander M, Wange P, et al. Arthroscopic or conservative treatment of degenerative medial meniscal tears: a prospective randomised trial. *Knee Surg Sports Traumatol Arthrosc.* 2007;15(4):393–401.

31. Redmond JM, Gupta A, Cregar WM, et al. Arthroscopic treatment of labral tears in patients aged 60 years or older. *Arthroscopy.* 2015;31(10): 1921–1927.

32. Skou ST, Roos EM, Laursen MB, et al. A randomized, controlled trial of total knee replacement. *N Engl J Med.* 2015;373(17):1597–1606.

33. Moseley JB, O'Malley K, Petersen NJ, et al. A controlled trial of arthroscopic surgery for osteoarthritis of the knee. *N Engl J Med.* 2002;347(2):81–88.

34. Mirza SK, Deyo RA. Systematic review of randomized trials comparing lumbar fusion surgery to nonoperative care for treatment of chronic back pain. *Spine.* 2007;32(7):816–823.

35. Adam K, Oswald I. Sleep helps healing. *Br Med J (Clin Res Ed).* 1984;289(6456):1400–1401.

36. Wu CL, Diekman BO, Jain D, et al. Diet-induced obesity alters the differentiation potential of stem cells isolated from bone marrow, adipose tissue and infrapatellar fat pad: the effects of free fatty acids. *Int J Obes (Lond).* 2013;37(8):1079–1087.

37. Egemen O, Ozkaya O, Ozturk MB, et al. The biomechanical and histological effects of diabetes on tendon healing: experimental study in rats. *J Hand Microsurg.* 2012;4(2):60–64.

CHAPTER 2

UNDERSTANDING REGENERATIVE MEDICINE TERMINOLOGY

Jay Smith and Andre J. van Wijnen

The field of regenerative medicine is relatively new but expanding rapidly. Multiple journals dedicated entirely to stem cell research and articles pertaining to regenerative medicine are becoming commonplace in major academic journals. Many clinicians who have had no previous education in regenerative medicine are challenged by the unfamiliar and at times seemingly intentionally obscure terminology encountered as they try to extract clinically relevant information from the scientific literature. The primary purpose of this chapter is to introduce the reader to common terminology used in the literature and during lectures and discussions pertaining to regenerative medicine. Readers understanding the terminology and related concepts discussed herein should feel confident that they have acquired a solid foundation to digest the scientific literature and engage in conversations pertaining to clinical regenerative medicine. Although written to read in a form conducive to reading in its entirety, the chapter can be used for reference as the terms are listed in alphabetical order. In addition, by necessity the chapter is representative and not comprehensive.

COMMON REGENERATIVE MEDICINE TERMINOLOGY

21st Century Cures Act—Refers to a law passed in late 2016 that includes sections relevant to regenerative medicine (Sections 3033–3036). These sections of the Act in many ways reflect some of the language that had been previously proposed in the REGROW ACT, which was introduced in early 2016 but has not been passed as of the time of this writing. With respect to regenerative medicine, the purpose of the 21st Century Cures Act is essentially threefold: (a) accelerate approval of Regenerative Advanced Therapies, (b) mandate the development of guidelines with respect to the regulatory treatment of medical devices used to manufacture biologic agents, and (c) mandate the development of standards and consensus definitions for regenerative agents. The Act defines a "Regenerative Advanced Therapy" as a non-361-regulated regenerative medicine therapy that is used to treat a "serious or life threatening condition," and which has preliminary clinical evidence suggesting the potential to meet an unmet clinical need for that condition. On submitting an IND

(Investigational New Drug application) for the biologic to the Food and Drug Administration (FDA), the manufacturer can request that the product be considered a Regenerative Advanced Therapy. The FDA then assesses the evidence and determines the designation. If designated as a Regenerative Advanced Therapy, the drug qualifies for expedited approval and the FDA is required to develop an appropriate approval pathway for the drug, which may not, in contradistinction to past situations, necessarily include a requirement for prospective, randomized controlled trials. The law mandates that the FDA must develop an approval pathway in conjunction with the manufacturer, and that approval may in some situations be granted based on registry data, collective clinical experience, and similar forms of documentation short of prospective, randomized, controlled trials. This constitutes the primary mechanism by which the 21st Century Cures Act has the potential to accelerate approval of selective biologic agents.

21 CFR Part 1271—Refers to title 21 of the code of federal regulations (CFR), which outlines regulatory pathway for human cells, tissues, and cellular and tissue-based products (HCT/Ps). All entities using HCT/Ps must comply with Food and Drug Administration (FDA) regulatory requirements concerning the manufacturing and delivery of HCT/Ps. 21 CFR 1271.10 identifies the criteria for regulation of HCT/Ps solely under section 361 of the Public Health Service (PHS) Act and 21 CFR Part 1271. To qualify as a "361" regulated HCT/P, a HCT/P must be (a) minimally manipulated, (b) intended for homologous use, (c) manufactured without combining the HCT/P with substances other than water, crystalloids, or a sterilizing, preserving or storage agent, *and* (d) either does not have a systemic effect and is not dependent on living cells for its primary function, or is autologous, allogeneic from a first- or second-degree relative, or is for reproductive use. HCT/Ps meeting all of these criteria are considered "361" regulated and do not require premarket approval (PMA) by the FDA. Any HCT/Ps failing the "361 test" and not qualifying for the "Same Day Surgical Exemption"

(21 CFR 1271.15) are regulated under section 351 of the PHS Act and are considered to be "drugs." HCT/Ps regulated under 351 must undergo the same process as commercially manufactured drugs, including submission of a biologic license application (BLA) to the FDA for PMA before manufacture and delivery. From a practical standpoint, a HCT/P is generally regulated as either a "361" or "351." For example, based on the contemporary interpretation of FDA guidelines, bone marrow aspirate concentrate (BMAC) produced by aspirating and centrifuging bone marrow for autologous injection into a joint may be regulated as a "361." The manufacturer (who may be a physician or a health care provider in the office setting), is not required to obtain PMA from the FDA but is required to register with the FDA and follow appropriate standard operating procedures when manufacturing the HCT/P. However, if the bone marrow mesenchymal stem cells (MSCs) contained in the BMAC are isolated and culture expanded, the final product (i.e., culture-expanded bone marrow MSCs) used for similar purposes would render the product a "351" because the HCT/P is now "more than minimally manipulated" because of culture expansion. This product could not be used to treat patients without FDA approval.

Adipose-Derived Stem Cells (ADSCs**)**—Also referred to as "Adipose-Derived Mesenchymal Stem Cells (AMSCs)," these are MSCs isolated from the stromal vascular fraction (SVF) of homogenized adipose tissue (Figure 2.1). ADSCs are located in the capillary and perivascular adventitia of large blood vessels within adipose tissues and are thought to derive from pericytes. ADSCs share common characteristics with bone marrow–derived MSCs (BMSCs) with respect to the expression of common cell surface markers, gene expression profiles, and differentiation potential (Figure 2.2). Compared to BMSCs, ADSCs are present in higher numbers per unit volume of tissue, more rapidly proliferate in culture, and are less susceptible to senescence secondary to culture expansion. These benefits have resulted in an increased interest in the use of ADSCs for regenerative medicine to be delivered

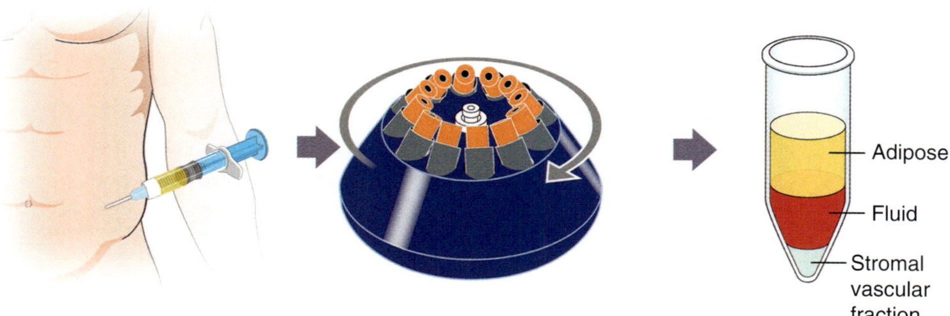

FIGURE 2.1: Adipose tissue may be aspirated from the abdominal wall or other region (i.e., lipoaspiration) and processed via enzymatic digestion and centrifugation to produce SVF. Following centrifugation, the SVF pellet can be removed from the bottom of the separation tube and directly used for regenerative purposes, or be further processed to isolate the relatively large number of ADSCs it contains. The SVF pellet contains not only a large number of ADSCs but also many other progenitor cells, which may also have therapeutic benefits.

ADSCs, adipose-derived mesenchymal stem cells; SVF, stromal vascular fraction.

Source: Mayo Clinic, Rochester, Minnesota. © Mayo Clinic. Used with permission.

in the form of SVF or culture-expanded ADSCs. However, clinical trials directly comparing ADSCs and BMSCs for musculoskeletal applications are currently lacking in the peer-reviewed literature.

Adipose Tissue—The fatty tissue located throughout the body is known as "adipose tissue." It contains adipose/fat cells surrounded by stromal tissue consisting of connective tissue and a rich vascular network. With respect to regenerative medicine, adipose tissue has gained increased attention in recent years owing to the relatively large number of MSCs per unit volume of adipose tissue compared to bone marrow. Most of these MSCs are associated with the blood vessel walls. Adipose tissue may be processed to produce smaller portions of otherwise intact adipose tissue for the purposes of performing a fat graft or lipotransfer. This is a common procedure in plastic surgery and has also been used in regenerative medicine. It may even be additionally processed via enzymatic or nonenzymatic means to remove the adipose cells, blood cells, and oils, resulting in stromal vascular fraction (SVF) (Figure 2.1). SVF contains a relatively high concentration of adipose-derived stem cells (ADSCs), as well as a variety of additional progenitor cells and stromal elements. SVF can be further processed to extract the ADSCs for culture expansion. Currently, the

manufacturing of SVF and culture-expanded ADSCs is considered "more than minimally manipulated" in the context of FDA guidelines and is, therefore, regulated as "351 HCT/Ps."

Adult Stem Cells (ASCs)—Multipotent stem cells that are capable of differentiating into multiple cell types. Examples include MSCs (Figure 2.3), fetal stem cells obtained from umbilical cord blood (UCB, not to be confused with embryonic stem cells), amniotic stem cells, and hematopoietic stem cells (HSCs). ASCs can be isolated from their respective tissues and used for regenerative purposes. Although ASCs share many characteristics, potentially clinically significant differences exist among ASCs obtained from different sources. Compared to embryonic stem cells that are pluripotent and can produce all cells in the body, multipotent ASCs can produce only some cell types based on their origin and niche. Their multipotent nature also renders them less susceptible to malignant transformation.

Allogeneic—Refers to a situation in which a biologic agent is obtained from one individual and subsequently delivered to a different individual. Allogeneic biologic treatments are susceptible to immune responses (e.g., rejection), which may endanger the recipient and/or reduce the

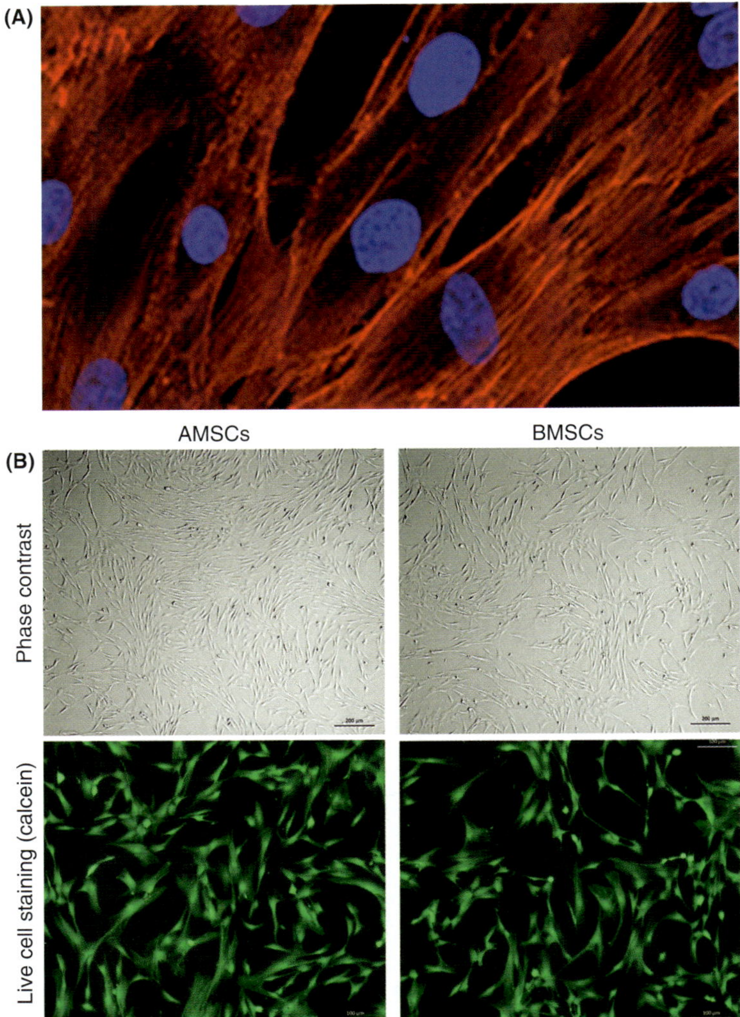

FIGURE 2.2: (A) Culture-expanded ADSCs with special staining to highlight the fibroblastic appearance of the cells, as well as their large nuclei. The fibroblastic appearance is characteristic of mesenchymal stem cells. (B) Upper two panels represent phase contrast microscopy of adipose-derived mesenchymal stem cells (ADSCs, or here AMSCs) and BMSCs, whereas the two lower panels represent correlative stained images. Note the similar morphologic, fibroblastic features of the ADSCs/AMSCs and BMSCs. MSCs from different sources throughout the body share many morphological, immunophyenotypic, and functional features.

ADSCs, adipose-derived mesenchymal stem cells; AMSCs, adipose-derived mesenchymal stem cells; BMSCs, bone marrow–derived mesenchymal stem cells; MSCs, mesenchymal stem cells.

Source: Mayo Clinic, Rochester, Minnesota. © Mayo Clinic. Used with permission.

efficacy of treatment. MSCs are characteristically immunoprivileged because of their low expression of major histocompatibility complex 1 (MHC1), and lack of expression of major histocompatibility complex 2 (MHC2). The low immunogenicity of MSCs provides the opportunity to develop allogeneic MSC-based treatments without the need for immunosuppression.

It is important to note that the characteristic of being immunoprivileged applies only to purified MSCs; unpurified cell-based products like bone marrow aspirate (BMA), BMAC, and SVF contain additional cells and proteins that render the product immunoreactive and preclude allogeneic use. An additional advantage of allogeneic MSC-based treatments is the ability to acquire

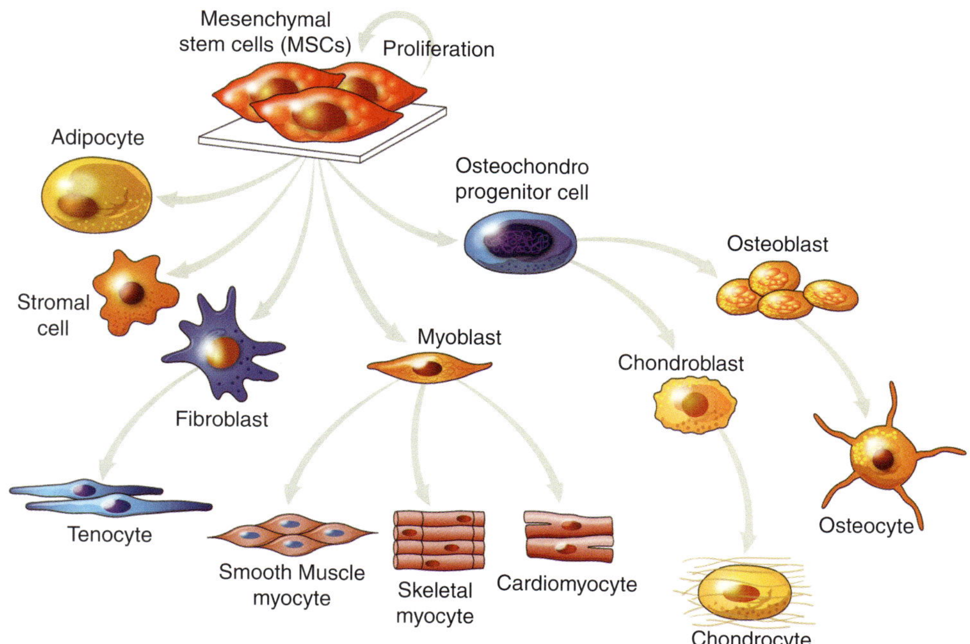

FIGURE 2.3: MSCs, also called "mesenchymal stromal cells," are ASCs that can self-replicate (proliferation), as well as differentiate into cells of various tissue types (multipotency), including major musculoskeletal tissues.

ASCs, adult stem cells; MSCs, mesenchymal stem cells.

Source: Mayo Clinic, Rochester, Minnesota. © Mayo Clinic. Used with permission.

MSCs from younger, healthy individuals, and stockpile them for more timely delivery. Several commercial products based on allogeneic MSCs are currently in various phases of development.

Amniotic Stem Cells—See **Adult Stem Cells**

Apoptosis—Programmed cell death. Apoptosis refers to cells that are dying. In the context of regenerative medicine, apoptotic cells can be considered to be cells that are so "sick" or old that they are starting to die. It is obviously undesirable as it renders the cell incapable of fulfilling its anticipated therapeutic functions. Apoptotic cells are commonly detected by Annexin V staining and flow cytometry. Cells that stain positive for Annexin V are apoptotic. Of note, MSCs have antiapoptotic properties and may be able to "heal" cells that are apoptotic.

Autologous—According to 21 CFR 1271.3(a), autologous means "the implantation, transplantation,

infusion, or transfer of human cells or tissue back into the individual from whom the cells or tissues were recovered." In other words, autologous refers to a situation in which a biologic agent is obtained from the same individual to whom it is subsequently delivered. Compared with allogeneic, in which the biologic agent is obtained from a donor of the same species, and xenogenic, in which the agent is obtained from a donor of a different species. Manufacturing culture-expanded BMSCs from patient A and delivering them to patient A would be autologous, whereas manufacturing BMSCs from patient A and delivering them to patient B would be allogeneic. Manufacturing BMSCs from patient A and delivering them to a rabbit as part of a preclinical trial would be xenogenic. Of note, "autologous use" is one of the requirements for a biologic agent to be regulated as a 361 product by the FDA (see 21 CFR 1271).

Biologic License Application (BLA)—A BLA is a request to the FDA for permission to introduce a biologic agent considered by the FDA to be a drug (i.e., "351" product, see 21 CFR 1271) into clinical practice. Although the foundation of the BLA lies with the regulations for interstate commerce, from a practical standpoint, any biologic agent that is determined by FDA guidelines to be regulated under section 351 of the PHS act must submit a BLA to the FDA before clinical implementation. This is the same pathway that pharmaceutical companies must follow to bring new drugs to market.

Bone Marrow Aspirate Concentrate (BMAC)— It is also known as "bone marrow concentrate" (BMC). It is a concentrated form of BMA-containing MSCs (Figure 2.3), HSCs, endothelial progenitor cells, plasma, and a variety of soluble bioactive substances. Adult bone marrow consists of plasma and blood cells at various stages of differentiation. The cellular component of bone marrow can be divided into nucleated and nonnucleated cells, with white blood cells and their precursors accounting for the overwhelming majority of the nucleated cell fraction (nucleated red blood cells and megakaryocytes are also present but make up only a small portion of the nucleated cell fraction). Bone marrow MSCs (BMSCs) and HSCs also reside in the nucleated cell fraction, but BMSCs account for only 1/10,000 to 1/50,000 nucleated cells, with the density of BMSCs being reduced by age, disease, certain medications, and other patient-specific factors. Nonetheless, "nucleated cell counts," "total nucleated cell (TNC) counts," and more specifically "mononuclear cell counts" are commonly used as a surrogate measure of the number of BMSCs contained in a BMAC preparation. BMAC is most commonly obtained by aspirating bone marrow from the pelvic bone, and processing it through density gradient centrifugation to reduce the unwanted fluid and cellular fractions. BMAC can then be injected as a same day procedure. Based on the presumption that BMSCs are the primary mediators of the therapeutic effects of BMAC, several techniques have been proposed to increase the yield of BMSCs in BMAC, including using an aspiration technique consisting of multiple low volume, high pressure aspirations.

BMSCs can also be isolated from BMAC and culture expanded to produce large numbers of BMSCs for therapeutic use. With respect to FDA guidelines, culture expansion of BMSCs is considered "more than minimally manipulated," resulting in the BMSCs being regulated as a "351" product (i.e., a drug, see 21 CFR 2171).

Bone Marrow Mesenchymal Stem Cells (BMSCs)—In addition of being referred to as "bone marrow–derived mesenchymal stem cells," BMSCs are MSCs isolated from BMA or BMAC. BMSCs are closely adherent to the bony trabeculae of the marrow cavities, an analogous location to the "stroma" in which ADSCs and pericytes are located. BMSCs share common characteristics with ADSCs including their presumed pericyte origin, expression of common cell surface markers, gene expression profiles, and differentiation potential (Figure 2.2). Compared to ADSCs, BMSCs are present in lower numbers per unit volume of tissue, proliferate more slowly in culture, and may be more susceptible to the effects of aging. BMSCs are produced by aspirating bone marrow (see Bone Marrow Aspirate Concentrate) and isolating the BMSCs for culture expansion. Clinical trials directly comparing ADSCs and BMSCs for musculoskeletal applications are currently lacking in the peer-reviewed literature.

CD Markers—See **Cluster of Differentiation Markers**.

Cell Therapy/Cell-Based Therapy—It is the introduction of new cells into the body for therapeutic benefit. One of the earliest cellular therapies was the use of blood transfusions. With respect to regenerative medicine, platelet-rich plasma (PRP), BMAC, SVF, and culture-expanded MSCs are all categorized as cell-based therapeutic agents (although technically platelets are not cells—see Platelets).

Center for Biologics Evaluation and Research (CBER)—CBER is the section within the FDA that oversees human cells, tissues, and cell and tissue products (HCT/Ps).

Cluster of Differentiation Markers (CD Markers)—CD stands for "cluster of differentiation," and is a protocol for characterizing cells based on the molecules that appear on their surface. Using immunophenotyping techniques such as flow cytometry, the phenotypic identity of a cell can be identified. For example, according to the International Society for Cellular Therapy (ISCT), MSCs are characterized by the expression of markers CD73, CD90, and CD105, and absence of hematopoietic markers such as CD14, CD34, and CD45.

Colony-Forming Units (CFUs)—From the perspective of regenerative medicine, the CFU number provides a measure of the number of stem cells in a given patient sample (e.g., BMAC, SVF) relative to the total number of cells in the specimen. The abbreviation CFU is frequently followed by a letter (e.g., colony-forming units-fibroblast [CFU-F]), indicating what types of cells are forming the colonies. The types of cells that grow in CFUs depend on the biological source sample and the mix of growth factors in the cell culture medium. CFU assays are performed by seeding cells on plastic culture dishes at very low density. The cultures are allowed to grow for several days after which the plate is stained with a dye (e.g., Crystal Violet, which colors cells purple). The dye allows easy visualization of any cells that grew by light microscopy. Only those cells capable of dividing often enough to form clusters of cells (colonies) are detected by this method. Hence, the method deselects for senescent ("aged") or quiescent ("dormant") cells, or cells only capable of very slowly dividing. The number of colonies that are formed is considered a direct reflection of the number of stem cells that was present in the original cell suspension.

Culture Expansion—The process by which isolated MSCs are stimulated to proliferate in order to increase the number of MSCs available for therapeutic use. As the number of MSCs that may be obtained through bone marrow aspiration or fat grafting/lipotransfer is relatively small (roughly thousands to hundreds of thousands), researchers have used culture expansion to manufacture large doses of MSCs for clinical research or therapeutic benefit (roughly millions to hundreds of millions). Culture expansion is most commonly performed by isolating MSCs from bone marrow or adipose tissue, transferring them to a plastic culture flask with appropriate growth media, and allowing them to proliferate to cover the plastic flask surface. Once the MSCs become confluent (i.e., completing covering the plastic flask surface) they are removed and reseeded into additional flasks with culture media. A single cycle of cell collection, seeding, and feeding is referred to as a "passage." Culture-expanded MSCs are typically used following passages 3 to 5 because MSCs may become senescent and/or exhibit an increased risk of genetic alterations following excessive expansion (greater than passage 7–10). In many cases, MSCs are culture expanded to passage 3 to 5, and then cryopreserved for later use.

Embryonic Stem Cells (ESCs)—These are pluripotent stem cells derived from the blastocyst following egg fertilization. ESCs can differentiate into any cell located in the human body, in contradistinction to ASCs, which are multipotent, and therefore possess a more restricted range of differentiation potential. The pluripotency of ESCs makes them potentially powerful vehicles for cell-based therapy. However, the use of ESCs remains ethically controversial and they have been associated with an increased risk of malignant transformation.

Exosome—It is a cell-derived vesicle with a diameter of approximately 30 to 150 nanometers. In the context of regenerative medicine, MSCs produce and secrete exosomes containing a variety of bioactive molecules, as well as genetic material in the form of microRNA (miRNA). Exosome contents can be modified by MSCs based on environmental cues and are a major vehicle by which MSCs powerfully influence cells in their local environment—referred to as "paracrine effects." Stimulating MSCs to produce condition-specific exosomes for therapeutic benefit represents an active area of research in regenerative medicine.

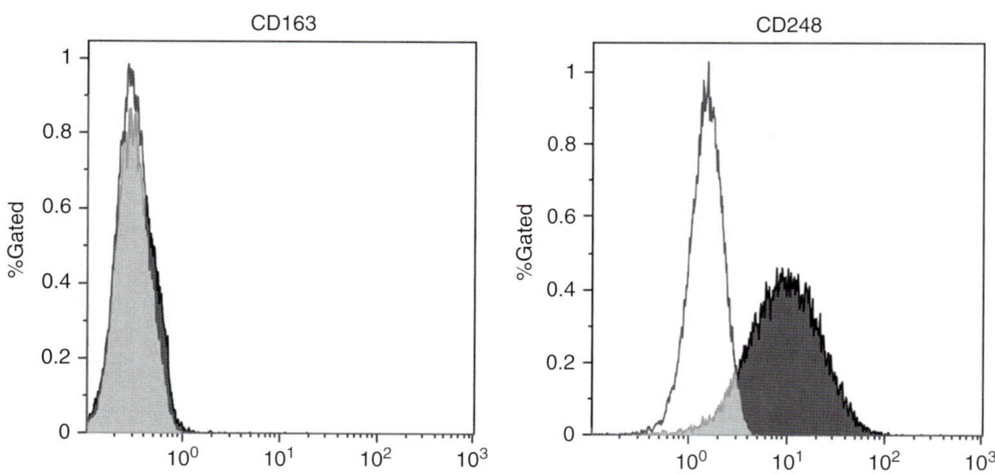

FIGURE 2.4: Flow cytometry/FACS results from adipose-derived mesenchymal stem cells obtained from stromal vascular fraction, demonstrating the absence of cell surface marker CD163 (a macrophage marker) and the presence of marker CD248 (a pericyte marker). The peak on the left represents a negative control. Thus, all the cells in the sample are negative for CD163, as indicated by the overlap of the sample peak and the negative control peak. On the contrary, the cells in the sample are generally positive for CD248.

FACS, flow-assisted cell sorting.

Source: Mayo Clinic, Rochester, Minnesota. © Mayo Clinic. Used with permission.

Fat Graft—It is the transfer of autologous adipose tissue/fat from one portion of the body to another. Fat grafts can vary in size and shape but by definition maintain the native microstructure of the donor tissue consisting of adipose cells, ADSCs, and other cells embedded in their stromal "niche." Fat grafting has also been referred to as "lipotransfer," although the latter term is more commonly used to refer to the transfer of relatively small volumes of smaller fat grafts.

Flow Cytometry/Fluorescence-Activated Cell Sorting (FACS)—Flow cytometry or FACS is a sophisticated technique to characterize the homogeneity and properties of cell populations (cytometry), as well as to select or deselect specific subpopulations (sorting) (Figure 2.4). In regenerative medicine, FACS sorting is used for quality control of stem cell populations to ensure that the cells selected for culture expansion and subsequent treatment have specific cell surface markers that are characteristic for desired stem cells (see Cluster of Differentiation Markers). The basic principle underlying FACS is that laser light is beamed at a liquid stream of a cell suspension (in a "flow cell") and the interaction of the light with the cell is recorded by a detector that reports the events (i.e., presence of a desired characteristic), and can also send a signal to sort the cell from other cells. Cells are sorted by an electromagnetic signal (electrostatic deflection) that changes the direction of the stream, resulting in the collection of cells in a separate vessel. They can be characterized for a range of attributes, including size and shape (through forward and side scatter of light), DNA content (by staining with fluorescent dyes that intercalate into DNA), intracellular proteins (in permeabilized fixed cells), or cell surface markers (using antibodies against more than 300 different known cell surface antigens—see Cluster of Differentiation Markers). Cell surface antigens are particularly useful in applications using live stem cells in which specific subpopulations need to be sorted for subsequent growth in cell culture. For example, using FACS, ADSCs can be identified and sorted from SVF by identifying MSC surface markers such as CD73, CD90, and CD105.

Food and Drug Administration (FDA**)**—The governmental body charged with the oversight and regulation of biologic products, including HCT/Ps. The FDA enforces laws enacted by Congress that regulate food, drugs, medical devices, blood, biological products, and cosmetics.

Good Manufacturing Practice (GMP)—It is also referred to as "current Good Manufacturing Practice" (cGMP). cGMP is a set of regulations that ensure the proper design, monitoring, and control of manufacturing processes for biologic products. cGMP ensures the identity, purity, potency/strength, and safety of the manufactured products. Its facilities are necessary to isolate and culture expand MSCs.

Hematopoietic Stem Cells (HSCs)—ASCs located primarily in the bone marrow and blood, and which are responsible for the continued renewal of blood and immune cells. Similar to other ASCs, HSCs are multipotent and can be identified through immunophenotyping to identify a characteristic set of cell surface molecules, such as CD14, CD34, and CD45 (see Cluster of Differentiation Markers). Transplantation of HSCs has been performed for many years to restore the bone marrow and blood in cancer patients following ablative chemotherapy (i.e., "stem cell transplant" or "bone marrow transplant"). From a regenerative medicine perspective, HSCs are prevalent in BMAC and may be responsible for some of the therapeutic effects of BMAC. HSCs can also be found in peripheral blood and umbilical cord blood, where they can be isolated and used for therapeutic purposes.

Homing—It is the migration of MSCs to target areas within the body. As discussed earlier, MSCs reside in all tissues throughout the body in association with the regional vasculature. The perivascular location of MSCs allows them to respond to vascular signals transmitted from distant sites in the body. In response to such signals, MSCs may become activated, detach from the perivascular tissue, and travel to distant regions to exert their influence on the injured tissues and

cells, including tissue resident stem cells. This process is referred to as "homing" and is controlled by a variety of chemical-signaling pathways, most notably the stromal-derived factor-1 (SDF-1)-chemokine receptor type 4 (CXCR4) pathway. Although homing provides a mechanism by which intravascular injection/infusion can be used to deliver MSCs to remote regions, many injected/infused MSCs are trapped in the lungs, liver, and spleen. It can also occur regionally, in which MSCs can specifically relocate to an injured or inflamed region within an organ or space (e.g., joint).

Homologous—This term means "the same" or "substantially the same." With respect to FDA regulations for HCT/Ps, homologous is defined in 21 CFR Part 1271.3(c) as the "replacement or supplementation of a recipient's cells or tissue with an HTC/P that performs the same basic function in the recipient as in the donor." Whether an HCT/P is used in a homologous or nonhomologous manner is one criterion that determines regulation of the HCT/P under section 361 versus 351 of the PHS act (see 21 CFR Part 1271). Of note, as the definition of homologous is currently based on function, the cells or tissues do not have to be delivered to the same site or a homologous location.

Human Cells, Tissues, and Cell and HCT/Ps—The FDA is charged with the oversight and regulation of HCT/Ps and defines HCT/Ps under 21 CFR 1271.3(d) as "articles containing or consisting of human cells or tissues that are intended for implantation, transplantation, infusion or transfer to a human recipient," with some few exceptions such as vascularized human organs for transplantation and minimally manipulated bone marrow intended for homologous use. The FDA is charged with the oversight and regulation of HCT/Ps, including the determination of whether HCT/Ps are regulated under section 361 or 351 of the PHS act (see 21 CFR Part 1271).

Induced Pluripotent Stem Cells (iPSCs**)**—These are reprogrammed, autologous, adult MSCs that exhibit embryonic stem cell–like properties. Owing to their expanded therapeutic potential compared to adult multipotent stem cells, iPSCs are being actively researched for multiple clinical applications.

Lipoaspiration—It is the process by which adipose tissue is removed from the body. Lipoaspiration typically involves infiltration of the subcutaneous fat with a tumescent solution consisting of sterile normal saline, lidocaine, and epinephrine. The tumescent solution provides local anesthesia and transitions the adipose tissue into a more liquid phase, facilitating removal via a small cannula and a manual or mechanical suction. Lipoaspiration may also be used to refer to liposuction, although the former term may imply the use of manual suction (e.g., syringe) to remove relatively small volumes of adipose tissue and the latter term may imply the use of mechanical suction to remove larger amounts of tissue. The removed tissue is referred to as "lipoaspirate." The lipoaspirate may be discarded or, with respect to regenerative medicine, can be used to perform fat grafting/lipotransfer (see Fat Graft) or to manufacture SVF or ADSCs (Figure 2.1).

Liposuction—See **Lipoaspiration**.

Lipotransfer—See **Fat Graft**.

Mesenchymal Stem Cells (MSCs**)**—They are also called "mesenchymal stromal cells." MSCs are ASCs that are multipotent and located throughout the body. They are particularly numerous in adipose and bone marrow, where they can be harvested and culture expanded for research or therapeutic purposes, in the form of ADSCs and BMSCs, respectively. MSCs are characterized by their fibroblastic morphology (thin and elongated) (Figures 2.2 and 2.3); plastic adherence; low immunogenicity; antiinflammatory, antiapoptotic, antifibrotic, and immunomodulatory effects; ability to self-replicate; propensity to differentiate into multiple cell types of mesenchymal origin (e.g., chondrocytes, osteocytes, and adipocytes); ability to migrate or "home"

to sites of injury or inflammation; extensive, adaptive, paracrine activity; and expression of surface molecules (see Cluster of Differentiation Markers, although there is no single, MSC-specific surface marker). The primary purpose of MSCs is to replace lost or damaged cells and tissues within their local environment. Given the significant interaction between MSCs and their resident niche, the phenotypic profile of MSCs from different tissues and different regions of the body is not identical. However, for the most part the clinical significance of these phenotypic differences remains unknown. As previously discussed, MSCs share many characteristics with pericytes, including their localization to the perivascular tissues and expression of pericyte markers such as CD248. Consequently, current evidence suggests that all MSCs are derived from pericytes.

microRNA (miRNA**)**—It is a small noncoding RNA molecule containing 15 to 30 nucleotides that regulates gene expression. MSCs secrete miRNA within exosomes (see Exosome). Following uptake of the MSC-generated exosomes and their contained miRNA by regional cells, the miRNA can exert profound and powerful effects on cellular function. This form of paracrine signalling is thought to represent a major mechanism by which MSCs influence the local environment.

Minimally Manipulated—With respect to FDA guidelines for HCT/Ps as defined in 21 CFR Part 1271.3(f) minimal manipulation is defined "for structural tissue, processing that does not alter the original relevant characteristics of the tissue related to the tissue's utility for reconstruction, repair, or replacement; and for cells and nonstructural tissues, processing that does not alter the relevant biological characteristics of cells or tissues." Examples of minimal manipulation include density gradient separation, centrifugation, and cell sorting or selection, whereas generation of SVF from adipose tissue via enzymatic digestion or culture expansion of MSCs represents more than minimal manipulation.

Whether a HCT/P is minimally manipulated or more than minimally manipulated is one criterion that determines regulation of the HCT/P under section 361 versus 351 of the PHS Act (see 21 CFR Part 1271).

Niche—It is a place or position. With respect to regenerative medicine, "niche" commonly refers to the environment in which the stem cell resides or functions. There are significant interactions between the stem cell and the niche in which it resides. By nature, stem cells are responsive to their niche, which explains phenotypical differences among stem cells residing in different parts of the body and also the ability of stem cells to relocate or home to a new environment, interpret environmental signals, and execute an adaptive response for therapeutic or regenerative purposes.

Off-Label—In the context of regenerative medicine, it is used to describe a non-FDA-approved therapeutic use of a biologic agent. For example, the injection of BMAC into the knee to treat knee osteoarthritis is not approved by the FDA and therefore considered "off label." Although the manufacturing of many currently available 361-compliant (see 21 CFR Part 1271) HCT/Ps can be performed using FDA 510K–cleared devices and kits, the delivery of these HCT/Ps to patients represents "off label" use. "Off-label" is not equivalent to "illegal," as off-label use of commercially available medications is common and considered to constitute the practice of medicine. From a practical perspective, the use of an off-label therapy should be disclosed to the patient during the informed consent process, and many third-party payers do not reimburse for off-label treatments.

Orthobiologics—The term is commonly used to describe the spectrum of regenerative agents used to treat orthopedic/musculoskeletal disorders, including but not limited to PRP, BMAC, platelet lysate (PL), fat grafts, and MSCs.

Paracrine—Paracrine signaling is a form of cell-to-cell communication by which a cell produces a signal to induce changes in nearby cells. Paracrine signally can occur through direct cell-to-cell contact or the release of bioactive factors that subsequently travel to and interact with nearby cells. Current evidence suggests that MSCs exert the majority of their therapeutic and regenerative effects through paracrine signaling rather than differentiation into new cell types. Through paracrine signaling, MSCs exert immunomodulatory, antiapoptotic, antifibrotic/anti-scarring, and trophic effects (proliferation and differentiation) on resident cells. Many of these paracrine effects are mediated via exosomes.

Passage—In a technical sense, it is the act of transferring a population of cells from one culture plate to another. This is typically done when cells in the original culture have grown to a density where they begin to inhibit each other's growth (i.e., they have become confluent). At this point, cells are dislodged from the first plate, placed into suspension, and counted. Equal cell numbers are then replated on new cell culture dishes. In regenerative medicine, passage number is a proxy for the number of cell divisions that a population has undergone. Typically, the lower the passage number the better, because the cells are more pristine. However, the cells that have not undergone cell culture at all (primary cells) may contain contaminants because cell culture purifies cell populations by selection of the fittest (only cells that are favored to grow will grow). The number of doublings (embodied in "passage") is very important, because stem cells derived from patients are not immortal and have only a restricted number of cell doublings. The latter is known as "Hayflick's limit": Cells can divide about 30 times before they become terminally aged (senescent) or perish. The molecular reason is that cells gradually lose telomeres from chromosome ends (i.e., protective repetitive sequences at the end of the DNA that function as protective caps). This loss creates chromosomal damage. Typically, stem cells from patients can undergo about 9 to 10 passages before they become senescent. In keeping with Hayflick's limit (30 cell divisions), this means that cells typically undergo about three rounds of cell division per culturing period ("passage"). As ASCs divide about once every 24 to 30 hours, a typical culturing period takes about 4 days, during which the original cell number has been expanded by about 10-fold. From a practical perspective, MSCs are often culture expanded to passage 3 to 5, then cryopreserved for later use.

Pericyte—These are ubiquitous perivascular cells adherent to blood vessels. Recent research suggests that MSCs are derived from pericytes and are similarly located in the perivascular tissues. The perivascular position of MSCs allows them to monitor local, regional, and distant environmental conditions and rapidly respond to injury or inflammation.

Platelet—Although commonly referred to as a type of "blood cell," platelets are small non-nucleated bodies derived from bone marrow megakaryocytes and released into the blood stream, where they circulate for 5 to 9 days before being replaced. Owing to their ubiquitous nature within the blood stream, platelets represent the "first responders" to injury or inflammation. Platelets contain hundreds of bioactive factors such as growth factors, cytokines, and chemokines located within their alpha- and dense-granules. In response to an injury or inflammation, platelets mobilize and manufacture, and release appropriate bioactive factors to promote hemostasis, initiate and modulate the inflammatory response, activate resident MSCs, recruit MSCs from distant regions (see Homing), and promote tissue healing. The multiple beneficial properties of platelets led to the development of PRP as a regenerative agent to modulate inflammation and promote healing.

Platelet Lysate (PL)—It is also known as human platelet lystate (HPL). A derivative of platelet concentrate whereby platelets are concentrated and lysed to concentrate growth factors, cytokines, plasma protein nutrients, and other platelet products into a cell-free liquid. HPL is typically produced by lysing platelets via multiple freeze-thaw cycles, inducing a fibrin clot production by adding calcium chloride, and centrifuging to precipitate cell and tissue debris. The supernatant layer represents the HPL that further represents the cell- and tissue-free products of the platelets. Autologous HPL may be used as an alternative or adjunct to PRP or other biologic agents, whereas pooled allogeneic HPL is now the most commonly used culture media for the expansion of MSCs.

Platelet-Rich Plasma (PRP)—It is a solution containing a greater than normal concentration of platelets. PRP injections are commonly used to deliver supraphysiologic doses of platelet-derived bioactive factors capable of modulating inflammation and promoting tissue healing. PRP is currently produced by density gradient centrifugation, during which whole blood is separated into different cell-plasma fractions, including a platelet-rich layer. A variety of commercially available, FDA 510K approved centrifuge–PRP kit combinations exist, among which there are significant differences in the amount of whole blood required for processing, processing time, and ability to concentrate platelets, remove red blood cells, and remove white blood cells (WBC) or WBC-polymorphonuclear cell sub-types. Although there is no universally agreed on or scientifically validated definition of PRP, some authors have proposed that PRP should contain at least 1 million platelets per microliter (normal is 150,000–350,000 platelets/mL) with a concomitant increase in growth factors and cytokines. However, other authors have emphasized that the total dose of platelets in PRP may be more important than the actual concentration. In the laboratory, PRP can stimulate the proliferation and differentiation of MSCs, either increase or decrease inflammation, and promote tissue healing. Clinically, PRP has been injected into a variety of tendons, ligaments, and joints to improve pain and function, with variable clinical results. Some of these differences may be clinically significant, such as the goal of minimizing the number of red blood cells in PRP used for intra-articular injection. There are currently no FDA-approved indications for PRP to treat musculoskeletal disorders (i.e., regenerative PRP injections are considered "off label").

Potency—In the context of stem cells, it is used to describe the potential for the stem cell to differentiate into various cell types. Pluripotent stem cells are located in the blastocyst during embryonic development and are capable of differentiating into any cell in the human body. ESCs are an example of pluripotent stem cells. Multipotent cells are more differentiated than pluripotent cells but are still capable of differentiating into multiple tissue types. ASCs are multipotent stem cells and include MSCs, fetal stem cells obtained from UCB (not to be confused with embryonic stem cells), amniotic stem cells, and HSCs. As stem cell potency is reduced, the ability of the stem cell to differentiate into various tissue types is also reduced. However, in some cases appropriate stimuli may alter the potency of stem cells, such as the case in iPSCs (see Induced Pluripotent Stem Cells).

Prolotherapy—It is also called "proliferative therapy." Prolotherapy is performed by injecting irritant solutions that stimulate a low-grade inflammatory reaction to promote tissue proliferation and healing. Perhaps the most common prolotherapy injectate is hyperosmolar dextrose, although a multitude of proliferants have been used (e.g., sodium morrhuate).

Senescence—"Aging," often used in the context of proliferating MSCs to describe the aging effects of repeated division and replication during culture expansion. Senescent MSCs can be identified through laboratory testing (e.g., shortening of telomeres), and cell senescence implies suboptimal therapeutic potential. In addition, in some situations cell senescence may be associated with an increased risk of malignant transformation. Consequently, there is a limit to which MSCs can be expanded in culture (i.e., the number of passages) and following culture expansion, they should be tested for purity and to detect the senescent phenotype (see Good Manufacturing Practice).

Stroma—In regenerative medicine, it generally refers to the part of a tissue or organ that serves a structural role. For example, adipose tissue consists of adipose cells surrounded by stroma, which consists of a connective tissue framework providing cell support, as well as the vasculature supplying blood and nutrients to the cells. As MSCs are currently considered to arise from pericytes and localize to the stroma tissues throughout the body, some authors/researchers advocate use of the term "mesenchymal stromal cells" rather than "MSCs." From a practical standpoint, these terms can be used interchangeably.

Stromal Vascular Fraction (SVF)—It is a component of lipoaspirate containing a high concentration of ADSCs in addition to multiple progenitor cells and cell components. SVF is most commonly produced from lipoaspirate through enzymatic (i.e., collagenase) digestion, lysis of red blood cells, filtering, and centrifugation to free the ADSCs from the stroma, and precipitate the ADSCs and other cells into a small pellet (Figure 2.1). This SVF pellet is then used for therapeutic or research purposes to deliver a high dose of ADSCs and other progenitor cells to an injured or inflamed region. Although SVF can deliver a significantly higher dose of MSCs than BMAC or fat grafts/lipoaspirates, SVF is currently regulated as a 351 HCT/P (i.e., a "drug") by the FDA because of the use of "more than minimal manipulation" of the adipose tissue during manufacturing of the SVF. Nonenzymatic methods of obtaining SVF have been developed, but require further analysis with respect to equivalency and regulatory pathway.

Telomere—These are caps at the end of each strand of DNA in cell chromosomes. Telomeres protect the chromosomes and shorten over time with accumulated cell division cycles. Consequently, telomere shortening reflects the age of the cell and is used to assess cell senescence.

Viability—It is a term used to denote whether a cell is alive or dead. In comparison, apoptosis refers to cells that are "sick" or "aging" to the point that they are in the process of dying (see Apoptosis section). Although apoptotic cells may be saved by the actions of MSCs in certain circumstances, cells that are no longer viable cannot be revived—only replaced. Common methods to assess cell viability include Trypan blue staining and DAPI (4′, 6-diamidino-2-phenylindole) staining.

Xenogenic—It refers to a biologic agent that is obtained from an animal of one species and delivered to an animal of a second species. Xenogenic treatments are currently limited exclusively to research settings. A common example would be the treatment of rabbits with human MSCs (hMSCs) to study the effect of hMSCs in knee osteoarthritis. Xenogenic treatments allow researchers to examine and document the effect of human HCT/Ps in animal models.

ACKNOWLEDGMENTS

We thank our colleagues, as well as present and former members of our laboratories, including Wenchun Qu, Holly Ryan, Tao Wu, Hai Nie, Min Su, Rebekah Samsonraj, Janet Denbeigh, and Amel Dudakovic, for stimulating discussions. This work was supported by the Mayo Clinic Center of Regenerative Medicine and generous philanthropic gifts of William and Karen Eby.

CHAPTER 3

REGULATORY ISSUES REGARDING THE CLINICAL USE OF REGENERATIVE TREATMENTS

Karl M. Nobert

THE LAW AS IT RELATES TO REGENERATIVE MEDICINE IN THE UNITED STATES

Historical Basis for Federal Regulation and Oversight

The Food and Drug Administration (FDA) conducted an extensive evidence-based risk analysis before implementing criteria for the regulation of human cells, tissues, and cellular and tissue-based products (HCT/Ps), which can be found in the Code of Federal Regulations (CFR) at 21 CFR Part 1271. These criteria, if met, allow certain HCT/Ps to be regulated solely under Section 361 of the Public Health and Safety (PHS) Act and Part 1271 for the prevention of communicable disease transmission rather than pursuant to the premarketing requirements under the Federal Food, Drug and Cosmetic Act (FDCA) for drug, biological, or medical device products. In the relevant part, Section 1271.10(a) sets forth the criteria as follows:

(a) An HCT/P is regulated solely under Section 361 of the PHS Act and the regulations in this part if it meets all of the following criteria:

(1) The HCT/P is minimally manipulated.

(2) The HCT/P is intended for homologous use only, as reflected by the labeling, advertising, or other indications of the manufacturer's objective intent.

(3) The manufacture of the HCT/P does not involve the combination of the cells or tissues with another article, except for water; crystalloids; or a sterilizing, preserving, or storage agent, provided that the addition of water; crystalloids; or the sterilizing, preserving, or storage agent does not raise new clinical safety concerns with respect to the HCT/P.

(4) Either:

(i) The HCT/P does not have a systemic effect and is not dependent on the metabolic activity of living cells for its primary function; or

(ii) The HCT/P has a systemic effect or is dependent on the metabolic activity of living cells for its primary function, and:

(1) Is for autologous use

(2) Is for allogeneic use in a first- or second-degree blood relative or

(3) Is for reproductive use.

Before finalizing these criteria and the regulations of Part 1271, the FDA gathered extensive data and information from the industry and other stakeholders to identify the types of HCT/Ps that could be regulated solely for communicable disease transmission and without any premarket review.[1] First, FDA acknowledged the long-time use and available information about certain cell- and tissue-based products. In its 1997 "Proposed Approach to the Regulation of Cellular and Tissue-Based Products" for human use, the FDA stated:

> Tissues have long been transplanted in medicine for widespread uses—such as skin replacement after severe burns, tendons and ligaments to repair injuries, heart valves to replace defective ones, corneas to restore eyesight, and the use of human semen and implantation of eggs to help infertile couples start a family. . . .

The Proposed Approach further stated that:

> . . . Except for a small number of tissues previously regulated as devices since 1993, FDA's regulation of the *conventional tissues* used for replacement purposes has focused on preventing the transmission of communicable disease, as authorized by the Public Health Service Act (PHS Act)."[2] . . .

Again, emphasizing that conventional tissue products are of lower risk, and not new biotechnology products, the FDA stated:

> . . . In recent years, scientists have developed new techniques, many derived from biotechnology that enhance and expand the use of human cells and tissues as therapeutic products. These new techniques hold the promise of some day providing therapies for cancer, AIDS, Parkinson's Disease, hemophilia, anemia, diabetes, and other serious conditions. . . . *[Only the] most conventional and reproductive tissues would not be subject to premarket approval requirements.*[3] . . . [Emphasis added]

For example, the FDA stated, "many structural tissue-based products are conventional tissues having a *long and established history of safe use in the medical community*," and therefore, would not need safety data and premarket authorization.[4] The use of bone to treat orthopedic conditions is an example of such a conventional tissue.

In the Proposed Approach, the FDA also addressed stem cell products and acknowledged the lack of information available to design any streamlined oversight. The FDA stated that data would be required before certain stem cell products could be regulated in the future by product-class-specific processing controls and product standards.[5] The FDA has yet to propose such special controls. Instead, by choosing homologous use as one criterion for the "down-regulation" of certain HCT/Ps, the FDA concluded there was a sufficient basis on which to predict a product's behavior; and, therefore, a basis to conclude such a product could be considered lower risk thus supporting exemption from premarket notification and approval requirements.[6]

The Meaning and Proposed Application of FDA's "Minimal Manipulation" Standard for Analyzing Product Safety and Risk

As noted earlier, Section 1271.10(a) of the regulations sets forth the criteria that the FDA relies on for evaluating the safety and potential risks of an HCT/P. Given the current uncertainty of the meaning and scope of some of the included criteria, it may be helpful to examine more clearly the practical application of the terms and difficulties the FDA itself has faced in applying the criteria to specific HCT/P products.

Minimal Manipulation

Under 21 Section 1271.3(f)(2), "minimal manipulation [of HCT/Ps] means: . . . [f]or cells or non-structural tissues, processing that does not alter the relevant biological characteristics of cells or tissues."[7]

In practice, this definition has been anything but clear. The HCT/P regulatory scheme was fully implemented before 2005, and since then the FDA has received many questions from individual manufacturers about the classification of their products. In September 2006, the FDA published and implemented *Guidance for Industry and FDA Staff—Minimal Manipulation of Structural Tissue (Jurisdictional Update),* in which the FDA stated:

> FDA has received several RFD's [Requests for Designation] requesting a determination of whether or not certain HCT/Ps will be regulated solely under section 361 of the PHS Act based on the manipulation the product undergoes during processing. . . . For purposes of determining whether a structural tissue product is minimally manipulated, a tissue characteristic is "original" if it is present in the tissue in the donor. A tissue characteristic is "relevant" if it could have a meaningful bearing on how the tissue performs when utilized for reconstruction, repair, or replacement. A characteristic of structural tissue would be relevant when it could *potentially increase or decrease the utility* of the original tissue for reconstruction, repair or replacement.
>
> Accordingly, FDA's determination of whether structural tissue is eligible for regulation solely under section 361 of the PHS Act has encompassed a consideration of all the potential effects, both *positive and negative,* of the alteration of a particular characteristic on the utility of the tissue for reconstruction, repair, or replacement, that is, changing the characteristic could improve or diminish the tissue's utility.[8] [Emphasis added]

An improvement to the utility of a HCT/P, such as decellularization to preclude an immune response, being considered minimal manipulation was a concept never before articulated by the FDA. A narrow interpretation of what would increase the utility or result in a positive change to a relevant characteristic could lead to the regulation of conventional HCT/Ps as drug, biological, or medical device products.

Not surprisingly, the FDA continued to receive the questions. The Tissue Reference Group (TRG) was and continues to be responsible for responding to such questions. The TRG publishes summaries of its responses, which provide its recommendations as to the regulatory status of a specific product. Since 2006, the FDA has issued 22 such recommendations specific to minimal manipulation alone, which are posted on the TRG webpage.[9] Examples include:

FY 2014:
Ground adipose tissue that is defatted and decellularized is more than minimally manipulated and, therefore, is not a 361 HCT/P because the processing alters the original relevant characteristics of the adipose tissue's utility for reconstruction, repair, or replacement.

FY 2013:
An allogeneic, decellularized adipose tissue matrix product is more than minimally manipulated and therefore not a 361 HCT/P because the processing alters the original, relevant characteristics of the adipose tissue's utility for reconstruction, repair, or replacement.

Bone marrow–derived mesenchymal stem cells expanded in culture are more than minimally manipulated and therefore not a 361 HCT/P.

FY 2012:
A cell selection process that results in activation of the T-cell receptor (TCR) does not meet the definition of minimal manipulation, as defined in 21 CFR 1271.3(f), because TCR activation alters the relevant biological characteristics of the selected cell population.

FY 2008:
Allogeneic demineralized bone matrix combined with human collagen derived from the same donor is a medical device. Processing of the carrier alters the original relevant characteristics of the demineralized bone matrix and this constitutes more than minimal manipulation.

FY 2006:

Umbilical cord stem cells treated with enzyme to increase engraftment are considered biological products and are subject to Investigational New Drug Applications (INDs) and Biologic License Applications (BLAs) because this processing constitutes more than minimal manipulation.

The FDA acknowledged that the Jurisdictional Update did not adequately clarify the meaning of minimal manipulation when it issued, on December 23, 2014, a Draft Guidance on minimal manipulation of HCT/Ps (HCT/P Draft Guidance) to try again to clarify the meaning of minimal manipulation.[10] Among other things, the HCT/P Draft Guidance states that "extraction or separation of cells from structural tissue in which the remaining structural tissue's relevant characteristics relating to reconstruction, repair, or replacement are changed generally would [not] be considered minimal manipulation."[11] For example, the FDA found that "[b]one marrow-derived mesenchymal stem cells expanded in culture are more than minimally manipulated and therefore not a 361 HCT/P."[12]

The HCT/P Draft Guidance, however, warns that determining minimal manipulation is not so easy. The FDA states that, "[w]hile some structural tissue may undergo processing that alters the cellular or extracellular matrix components without altering the original relevant characteristics of the tissue, the same processing may alter the original relevant characteristics of a different tissue." There is little more in the HCT/P Draft Guidance to understand under what circumstances a process would be more-than-minimal manipulation when it is considered minimal manipulation in another context.

Homologous Use

The term "homologous use" is defined for HCT/Ps under 21 Section §1271.3(c), which states:

Homologous use means the repair, reconstruction, replacement, or supplementation of a recipient's cells or tissues with an HCT/P that performs the same basic function or functions in the recipient as in the donor.

As an example of the definition's application, the TRG concluded in 2008 that "[a]utologous adipose tissue enzyme digested and processed for urinary incontinence and treatment of impotence . . . . is a non-homologous use."[13]

Homologous use also suggests effectiveness of the cell-based product to function the same way when reimplanted. For example, autologous adipose-derived adult stem cells are being used to treat traumatic and degenerative diseases, including bowed tendons, ligament injuries, osteoarthritis, and osteochondral defects. Such products are currently being marketed without any preapproval from the FDA. Although it is certain that the FDA would not agree, as stem cells have the potential to differentiate into different cells, one could argue that these uses, in fact any use, would be homologous.

For obvious reasons, additional information and interpretation is needed from the FDA to fully understand the meaning and scope of "homologous use."

SUPPORTING CASE LAW: *UNITED STATES V. REGENERATIVE SCIENCES, LLC*[14]

In a February 2014 decision, the DC Court of Appeals affirmed that the FDA has regulatory jurisdiction over cell-based products exceeding its "more-than-minimally manipulated" standard, thus subjecting them to premarket review and approval. The case is important because of its potential to directly impact physicians and medical researchers practicing in this field.

The case involved two physicians using cultured stem cells to treat patients for various orthopedic conditions and diseases. They argued that they were offering a "procedure" allowed within the practice of medicine and not a product falling within the FDA regulatory jurisdiction. The performed procedure involved the extraction of bone marrow from a patient and the isolation of mesenchymal stem cells (MSCs) for culturing in a solution, in which other substances are added to encourage growth and differentiation. On achieving a sufficient numbers of cells for reinjection, the antibiotic doxycycline was added to prevent bacterial contamination. The resulting mixture was then injected into the same patient at the site of the damaged tissue.

The Court found that, although derived from and returned to the same patient, the cultured cells exceeded the earlier standard rendering them an unapproved drug product and their use a violation of federal law. This was because (a) the culturing of MSCs "is designed to determine the growth and biological characteristics of the resulting cell population," and (b) the substances added to the cultured stem cells "affect the differentiation of bone marrow cells."

Citing concerns about the possible use of unsafe, contaminated, or harmful products to treat patients, the Court found in favor of the FDA ceding it a regulatory oversight. It did this by relying on the existing federal statute that gives authority to the FDA for the establishment of regulatory requirements to prevent the introduction, transmission, and spread of communicable diseases. This has the effect of resulting in a review process in which manufacturers (here, the physicians themselves) are subject to inspection, and are required to show that their cell-based products are manufactured in a manner to assure their purity and potency.

By contrast, cell- and tissue-based products that are truly minimally manipulated and, thus, fall beneath the adopted standard are exempt from the FDA's rigorous drug approval process. The Court rejected every argument made by the two physicians in this case. They had argued that the FDA does not have the legal authority to implement regulations covering such autologous therapies because the "procedure" involves simply the patient's own stem cells being returned to the very same patient. They argued that the performed procedure was within the practice of medicine and, therefore, not an FDA-regulated product.

Key takeaways from the case include:

- Practicing physicians and medical researchers may be subject to FDA regulatory oversight if deemed to be using cell-based procedures that exceed the "more-than-minimal manipulation" standard.
- The FDA has regulatory jurisdiction over the use of cell-based products and therapies in the United States.
- The argument that such procedures are within the practicing of medicine and outside of the FDA's purview were rejected by the Court.

Federal regulation trumps that of any laws, rules, or guidelines adopted by the individual states or state medical boards.

Those who "manufacture" cell-based products or offer cell-based procedures, including physicians within their own clinics, exceeding the adopted standard, are subject to facility inspection and must comply with the FDA's regulatory requirements.

FDA'S CURRENT SHOWING OF ENFORCEMENT DISCRETION AND ITS SCOPE

Although the offering of several forms of regenerative medicine today is technically in violation of the law as articulated in both the regulations and the Regenerative Sciences case, it appears that the FDA is currently showing some certain level of "enforcement discretion" with respect to autologous cell-based therapies that do not pose a significant and immediate danger to the patients. This is most likely because of the current absence of an FDA cell-based drug product in the market. However, this likely will change as human and veterinary products begin to come in the market. For the time being, the FDA seems to be taking enforcement action opposing only the most egregious patient therapies that attract attention because of exaggerated disease or treatment-marketing claims, poor facility inspections, and patient injury.

Enforcement discretion at its basic level is a decision by a government authority not to take authorized enforcement action in specific cases. The FDA's "decision not to prosecute or enforce [the FDCA in all cases], whether through civil or criminal process, is a decision generally committed to an agency's absolute discretion."[15] Such agency action is reviewable by a court only when there is a "meaningful standard against which to judge the agency's exercise of discretion."[16] The FDCA provides such a standard and thus limits the discretion the FDA may exercise.

FDA REGULATORY ENFORCEMENT AND THE POTENTIAL RISK FOR PHYSICIANS

On December 30, 2015, the FDA issued warning letters to three physician-owned and operated stem cell treatment centers in California, Florida, and New York asserting that they had unlawfully recovered and processed adipose tissue to perform stem cell therapy on patients. These incidents are significant because they signal a departure from the FDA's former practice of exercising little to no regulatory oversight (often referred to as "enforcement discretion") of the physicians/clinicians offering these therapies to patients, replacing it with a more active approach to compliance and potential enforcement.

The centers were harvesting and using autologous stromal vascular fraction (SVF) for intravenous (IV) and intrathecal injections, and nasal or oral nebulization. These procedures were offered for a variety of serious conditions including, but not limited to, autism, Parkinson's disease, pulmonary fibrosis, chronic obstructive pulmonary disease, multiple sclerosis, cerebral palsy, and amyotrophic lateral sclerosis. Their use as treatments rendered them as drugs for which FDA review and approval is required.[17]

For regulatory purposes the products were also considered drugs because of the manner in which they were manufactured. This was because the company's processing altered the original relevant characteristics of the adipose tissue relating to the tissue's utility for reconstruction, repair, or replacement.

The FDA also found that the centers were failing to follow Agency's requirements covering the processing and manufacturing of adipose tissue for stem cell treatments.[18]

The centers were warned that failure to promptly correct these violations could result in regulatory action without further notice including action such as product and equipment seizure, injunction or criminal prosection in the most serious cases of failure to comply. In the near term, it seems clear that the FDA intends to increase its regulatory oversight and enforcement activities in this area, thus exposing clinicians who fail to comply to considerable risk.

NOTES

1. *See* 1997 Proposed Approach to Cellular and Tissue-Based Products. Retrieved from http://www.fda.gov/downloads/biologicsbloodvaccines/guidancecomplianceregulatoryinformation/guidances/tissue/ucm062601.pdf
2. *Id.,*p. 8. Examples of conventional tissues include skin as a wound covering and bone for orthopedic conditions.
3. *Id.,* pp. 5–6.
4. *Id.,* p. 20. *See* Transcript "Open Public Meeting: Manipulation and homologous use in spine and other orthopedic Reconstruction and Repair," August 2, 2000, p. 40.
5. *Id.,* p. 11.
6. *Id.,* p. 19.
7. *See* Draft Guidance for Industry and FDA Staff: Minimal Manipulation of Human Cells, Tissues, and Cellular and Tissue-Based Products (HCT/P Draft Guidance), December 23, 2014, p. 8. Retrieved from http://www.fda.gov/biologicsbloodvaccines/guidancecomplianceregulatoryinformation/guidances/cellularandgenetherapy/ucm427692.htm. Interestingly, the HCT/P regulation, unlike the proposed Draft Guidance, provides another definition of minimal manipulation for structural tissue. Minimal manipulation "[f]or structural tissue, [means] processing that does not alter the original relevant characteristics of the tissue relating to the tissue's utility for reconstruction, repair, or replacement." Although cells generally would be considered nonstructural, the FDA has proposed in the HCT/P Draft Guidance for the minimal manipulation of HCT/Ps that "if you isolate cells from

structural tissue, you should apply the definition of minimal manipulation for structural tissue."

8. Guidance for Industry and FDA Staff—Minimal Manipulation of Structural Tissue (Jurisdictional Update) (September 2006). Retrieved from http://www.fda.gov/regulatoryinformation/guidances/ucm126197.htm

9. The TRG does not publish its responses to protect the confidentiality of persons who ask the TRG for a recommendation as to the classification of its products. Instead, the TRG publishes brief summaries of its recommendations. For a summary of all of the TRG's recommendations, including those listed here, *see* TRG Update. Retrieved from http://www.fda.gov/BiologicsBloodVaccines/TissueTissueProducts/RegulationofTissues/ucm152857.htm

10. *See* Draft Guidance for Industry and FDA Staff: Minimal Manipulation of Human Cells, Tissues, and Cellular and Tissue-Based Products, December 23, 2014. Retrieved from http://www.fda.gov/biologicsbloodvaccines/guidancecomplianceregulatoryinformation/guidances/cellularandgenetherapy/ucm427692.htm. This HCT/P Draft Guidance would replace the Jurisdictional Update if finalized.

11. *Id.*, p. 5.

12. *See* TRG Update at http://www.fda.gov/BiologicsBloodVaccines/TissueTissueProducts/RegulationofTissues/ucm152857.htm

13. *Id.*

14. U.S. *v.* Regenerative Scis., LLC, 741 F.3D 1314 (D.C. Cir. 2014). In its decision, the court also affirmed the lower court's decision ruling that the U.S. District Court did not err in permanently enjoining the company for violating federal drug regulations.

15. 5 U.S.C. § 701(a).

16. Heckler *v.* Chaney, 470 U.S. 821, 828 (1985).

17. Section 201(g) of the FD&C Act [21 U.S.C. 321(g)] and a biological product as defined in Section 351(i) of the PHS Act [42 U.S.C. 262(i)].

18. Included in the regulations, these requirements are referred to as current Good Manufacturing Practice (cGMPs) and current Good Tissue Practice (cGTPs).

CHAPTER 4

CLINICAL AND ADMINISTRATIVE CONSIDERATIONS IN PERFORMING REGENERATIVE PROCEDURES

Leah M. Kujawski, Michael A. Scarpone, and David C. Wang

Beyond the usual medical office equipment, regenerative medicine clinics require a more unique staff and distinctive equipment. Basic regenerative medicine requirements include laboratory fume hoods, refrigerators, blood draw stations, and related supplies. Patient rooms should be designed to support the main objective of efficient patient care and compliance with federal and state guidelines.

LABORATORY

Laboratories have to be separate from patient care spaces with a secure door that can be fully closed and locked (Figure 4.1). Appropriate storage cabinets that can be locked are necessary to store various medications, chemicals, and phlebotomy supplies (syringes, needles, local anesthetics, other injectable solutions, and medications used for regenerative medicine). A separately designated space for a phlebotomy station, with a comfortable blood draw chair and all appropriate supplies directly accessible, will improve the efficiency and comfort of the blood-drawing process. Similarly, the centrifuge, hood, cell counter, sink, and other devices for tissue preparation should be positioned in a space-efficient layout requiring minimal movement between preparation steps, which optimizes time efficiency and minimizes the chances for contamination.

The Occupational Safety and Health Administration (OSHA) has developed several requirements that medical clinics with laboratories must meet. OSHA policies and standard operating procedures (SOPs) for clinical staff should be posted in each laboratory and must be updated annually to maintain compliance.[1] Laboratories used for stem cell procedure preparation should meet Centers for Disease Control and Prevention (CDC) requirements in order to maintain compliance as a biosafety level-2 laboratory.[2] A nonporous work space must be used

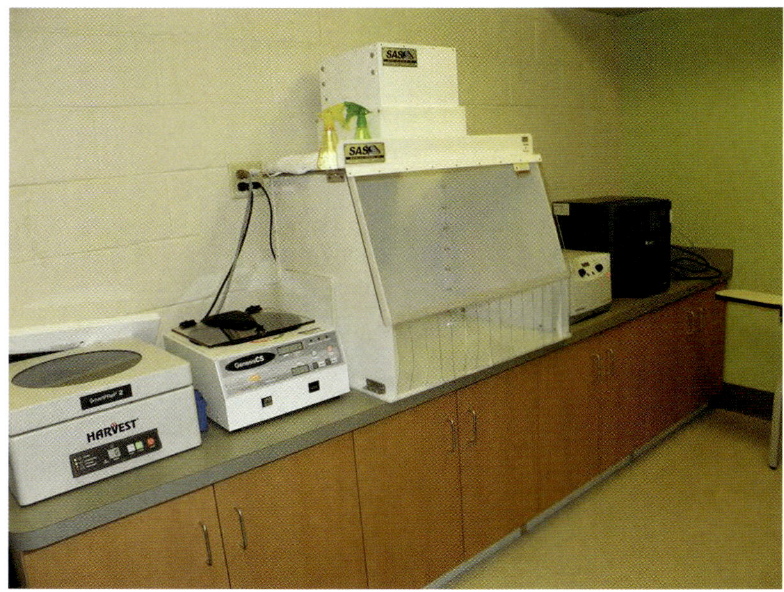

FIGURE 4.1: Blood draw and processing room: equipped for blood draw and tissue preparation, including centrifuge, sterile hood, and coulter cell counter.

to prepare injections and is recommended to be at a comfortable standing height.[3] Additionally, sharp containers as well as biohazard boxes are traditionally kept in the laboratory, along with personal protective equipment (PPE), including masks, eyeshields or goggles, gloves, and gowns. A sink with an eye-flushing station should be in close proximity to the laboratory, as these are required for hand hygiene and eye flushing in the event of an eye splash injury. If glass containers are present, dedicated cleaning equipment for shattered glass, such as a small broom and dust pan, must be kept in the laboratory and must be labeled "for glass use only."

An autoclave may be necessary for larger, high-volume practices. In the early start-up phase of a regenerative practice, disposable equipment/tools may be more cost-effective because maintenance and routine cleaning are an ongoing expense. Another option for cost control may be the use of an outside autoclave facility (hospital, surgical center, etc.) that charges a simple fee per use. Each practice should perform a cost analysis to determine what is best for its situation. A high-quality refrigerator dedicated for storage of biological samples is necessary for certain procedures, including stem cell allografts and certain platelet lysate preparations. A −80°C freezer may be required if storing tissues such as amniotic stem cells. As per OSHA, "food and drink shall not be kept in refrigerators, freezers, shelves, cabinets or on countertops or benchtops where blood or other potentially infectious materials are present".[4] OSHA-compliant biohazard labeling is required to maintain safety standards.

EXAM ROOMS

Each room should have adequate space (approximately 10 ft × 12 ft or larger) to allow for maneuvering of the diagnostic ultrasound machine (Figure 4.2). Smaller, less-expensive portable ultrasound units are advised in the early stages of a regenerative practice to provide maximum versatility for minimal cost. A full discussion of diagnostic ultrasound units is beyond the scope of this text, but there are numerous resources available to assist in the decision of obtaining this valuable equipment. A moderate-sized (30–42 in.) high-definition flat screen TV of at least 1080p resolution can be positioned at the eye level, at approximately a 90° offset from the ultrasound unit (generally placing it across the treatment table from the clinician) to allow for

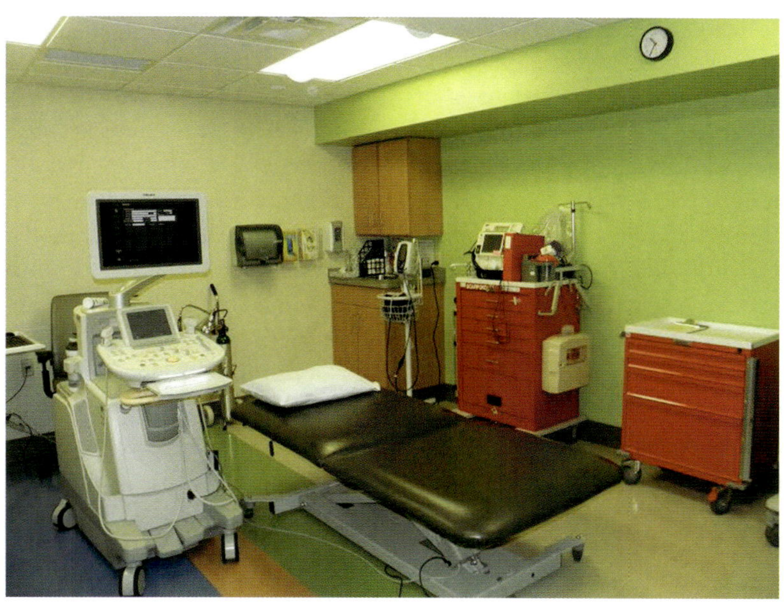

FIGURE 4.2: Procedure room: equipped with MSK ultrasound and conscious sedation capabilities if necessary. MSK, musculoskeletal.

improved ergonomics during ultrasound-guided procedures. Other recommended room equipment and supplies include the usual, such as an electric high-low exam table, pneumatic wheeled stool, sink, patient gowns, disposable paper shorts, towels, table paper, disposable chucks, body pads, and bolsters. Recommendations for a larger, more well-equipped procedure room include dimensions of at least 14 × 14 ft to 15 × 15 ft, with a more powerful cart-based ultrasound, fluoroscopy equipment, and appropriate fluoroscopy procedure table. It should have an advanced cardiac life support (ACLS)-recommended mobile emergency resuscitation station ("crash cart"), pulse oximeter, supplemental oxygen, and supplies and equipment to perform intravenous catheter placement and potentially conscious sedation for more advanced procedures. Each room should have sterile procedure supplies, including drapes, probe covers, gowns, and gloves.

LOCATION AND ANCILLARY SERVICES

Because of the novel nature of a regenerative medicine practice, the office should ideally be located in a highly accessible, relatively populated region with proximity to high-traffic areas, public transportation, airports, and other medical facilities, which can increase access to referring physicians. Accessibility to advanced imaging (x-ray, CT, and MRI) is important for timely diagnostic confirmation when needed. Close proximity to respected physical therapy, massage therapy, chiropractic, nutritional counseling, integrative medicine, and athletic and personal training facilities can provide opportunities for developing important cross-referral networks.

STAFFING

As with any other medical practice, having well-trained and motivated staff will ease patient care and optimize practice efficiency. For all staff involved in patient communication, implementing standardized scripted answers for frequently asked questions can maintain clear and cohesive communication within the practice. Given the novel and as-of-yet not well-recognized nature of regenerative medicine among the general public, specific staff education on communicating with patients about what regenerative medicine is; the basics of the relevant science and research; what to expect before, during, and after treatment; and cost considerations is of particular importance. Staffing considerations can be categorized into two divisions—clinical and administrative.

Clinical staff, in particular certified medical assistants (CMAs), can help a practice flourish by performing systematic patient intake documentation, preparing and maintaining supplies and equipment for regenerative and nonregenerative procedures, assisting in postprocedural care, addressing patient questions and concerns, and enhancing the overall patient experience with empathic and supportive care. Because the unique physiologic effects of regenerative procedures will often result in temporary increased pain and stiffness postprocedure, it is important that clinical staff are knowledgeable in how to counsel and comfort patients when they experience these reactions, and how to differentiate them from true adverse effects such as infection or tissue injury. Due to the stringent nature of properly preparing cellular samples for regenerative therapies, a high level of quality control in protocols and techniques is critical. Therefore, designating a practice-wide clinical manager who can ensure consistency in CMA performance can be very valuable. Practices that provide conscious sedation will need an anesthesiologist or certified registered nurse anesthetist (CRNA) and RNs with training in conscious sedation management on site.

Administrative staff, including front-desk and telephone reception, billing/coding, legal and compliance, and marketing, must be experienced in handling the many atypical aspects of regenerative medicine services. At the time of this writing, regenerative therapies are generally not covered by insurance providers, whereas other concomitant services, including medical evaluation and management, diagnostic ultrasound examination, and nonregenerative procedures, typically are covered. As such, administrative staff will need to confidently guide patients through the insurance implications and financial considerations of their course of treatment. Billing specialists who are intimately familiar with the differences between standard covered services and noncovered regenerative procedures, as well as the latest updates in ever-changing local coverage determinations, can be critical to maintaining the financial and medicolegal stability of a regenerative practice. Having a staff member assume official responsibility as the compliance officer is also recommended, because of the complexity of federal guidelines and importance of maintaining compliance on a consistent basis (see the following section).

ADMINISTRATIVE CONSIDERATIONS

Informed Consent

Despite the potential positive impact of regenerative medicine on musculoskeletal health, it is still not considered standard of care. Therefore, obtaining informed consent from patients before any regenerative procedure is of particular importance. Although informed consent is generally the standard practice for any medical procedure, consent for regenerative therapies must address specific issues that are characteristic to these procedures. As with other procedures, written informed consent to treat should define the specific procedure(s) planned, discuss risks/complications, benefits, and alternative treatments, and be signed by the patient and a witness such as the CMA or treating clinician after any patient questions are answered. Regarding potential complications, those typically cited with any needle-based percutaneous procedure include posttreatment pain/soreness/stiffness/swelling, vasovagal reactions, worsening of symptoms, infection, bruising, bleeding, blood vessel injury, nerve injury, organ injury/puncture, dural injury/puncture, and spinal headache with spinal injections, allergic/anaphylactic reaction, and death. Complications specific to regenerative procedures include more significant posttreatment pain/soreness/stiffness/swelling due to activation of the patient's inflammatory healing response, transient elevated blood sugar in diabetics with dextrose prolotherapy (although this has not been demonstrated in the medical literature), vasovagal reactions specifically during phlebotomy for platelet-rich plasma (PRP), increased local pain at stem cell harvesting sites, and bony injury and fracture at bone marrow aspiration sites. The consent form should address all therapies that could potentially be performed during the duration of the patient's treatment, or alternatively, separate forms can be utilized for each individual therapy. Ideally, the form(s) are signed and updated each time a patient undergoes a procedure.

In addition to an informed consent to treat, patients should also sign a financial consent form (e.g., an Advanced Beneficiary Notice) with their new patient intake paperwork. This form should clearly state that regenerative therapies are generally not covered services, nor reimbursable by health insurance providers, and that the patient is responsible for providing payment for any such noncovered services. The form should outline what the potential cost of therapies could be, as well as the expectation of when payment is due. Any changes in the financial obligations for a patient should be presented in writing and should be signed prior to the patient receiving any type of regenerative therapies.

Occupational Safety and Health Administration

Because regenerative medicine is not generally considered standard of care as previously mentioned, it is especially prudent to consistently maintain proper compliance with all federal standards. Each state jurisdiction may also have separate regulations in addition to federal requirements. A regenerative medicine office must have an OSHA binder containing policy requirements as well as an Emergency Action Plan (EAP), Exposure Control Plan (ECP), Bloodborne Pathogens Program (BBP), Hazard Communication Program (HCP), Lockout/

Tag-out Program, Sharps Injury Log, and Respiratory Program.[5] Complete requirements and guidelines may be researched at OSHA.org. OSHA is regulated by the Department of Labor (DOL) and updated regulations are frequent—be advised to follow these updates and implement all new requirements. An annual OSHA meeting must be held for all employees including physicians, and attendance records for those meetings must be kept on file. Implementation of OSHA policies is required and must be documented in order to remain compliant. Offices may have a single consultation visit from an OSHA reviewer, without official repercussions, to evaluate their level of compliance.

Centers for Disease Control and Prevention

Although OSHA regulations are federal law, the CDC and other agencies implement public health laws passed by Congress through federal regulations.[6] The CDC publishes both regulations and recommendations. Regulations are rules for which medical practices can be held accountable, and are federally mandated. Recommendations are best medical practice guidelines, but are not federally required. Understanding the difference between regulations and recommendations can be important when establishing practice policies. The Federal Register has a searchable list of all regulations that are active or that may be under review or revision.[7]

Health Insurance Portability and Accountability Act

To improve the efficiency and effectiveness of the health care system, the Health Insurance Portability and Accountability Act of 1996 (HIPAA), Public Law 104–191, included Administrative Simplification provisions that required Department of Health and Human Services (HHS) to adopt national standards for electronic health care transactions and code sets, unique health identifiers, and security.[8] HIPAA is regulated by the HHS. Having a HIPAA compliant electronic medical record (EMR), policies in place to protect protected health information (PHI), and educated staff dedicated to adhering to HIPAA policies are required to maintain HIPAA compliance. Within the medical office, HIPAA policies must be updated annually, and staff educated on all changes to existing policies. Patients must be informed of office adherence to HIPAA policies. For a medical office to legally be able to release patients' medical records to entities other than themselves, the patients must each sign a HIPAA release form identifying which individuals are authorized to receive PHI. HIPAA releases updates quarterly and offices must be vigilant to keep their policies and physical implementations updated. There are three primary HIPAA compliance measures that medical practices must address: there must be policies written for employees to understand and implement, all electronic devices and platforms used by office staff for patient care must be tested and found secure according to HIPAA standards, and there must be regularly documented physical implementation of written policies.

Clinical Laboratory Improvement Amendments

Clinical Laboratory Improvement Amendments (CLIA) regulate laboratory testing and require that clinical laboratories obtain a certificate before accepting materials derived from the human body for the purpose of providing information for the diagnosis, prevention, or treatment of any disease or the impairment of, or assessment of the health of human beings.[9] CLIA require clinical laboratories to be certified by their state as well as the Center for Medicare and Medicaid Services (CMS) before they can accept human samples for diagnostic testing. Laboratories can obtain multiple types of CLIA

certificates, based on the kinds of diagnostic tests they conduct.[10] Three federal agencies are responsible for regulating CLIA: The Food and Drug Administration (FDA), CMS, and CDC. Each federal agency has a part in ensuring laboratory testing, but CMS-regulated policies are likely the most relevant for medical office operations. Issuing laboratory certificates, conducting inspections, enforcing compliance, and publishing CLIA rules and regulations are some of CMS's main responsibilities.

The specific type of biologic material handled in the office laboratory, and whether the specimens will be used to diagnose, prevent, or treat specific diseases, dictates whether the laboratory needs to pursue CLIA certification. At the time of this writing, regenerative medicine practices do not require a CLIA-certified laboratory. However, if the office tests specimens for the purpose of diagnosis, then a CLIA certification would need to be obtained.

Joint Commission Standards

Joint Commission (formerly Joint Commission on Accreditation of Health Care Organizations [JCAHO]) accreditation is federally mandated only when an office accepts Medicare and/or Medicaid. Joint Commission accreditation can be earned by many types of health care organizations, including hospitals, doctors' offices, nursing homes, office-based surgery centers, behavioral health treatment facilities, and providers of home care services.[11] Health care organizations that achieve accreditation through Joint Commission–deemed status surveys are determined to meet or exceed Medicare and Medicaid requirements.[12] There are voluntary accreditation options for multiple types of clinics, such as ambulatory surgical centers, home health agencies, and hospice agencies. At the time of this writing, regenerative medicine private practice offices do not require Joint Commission accreditation.

NOTES

1. 29 CFR 1910.1030(d)(1).
2. Page 43, OSHA Laboratory Safety Guidelines.
3. Laboratory Safety—Ergonomics for the prevention of musculoskeletal disorders in laboratories fact sheet.
4. 29 CFR 1910.1030.
5. https://www.osha.gov/as/opa/worker/employer-responsibility.html
6. http://www.hhs.gov/hipaa/for-professionals/index.html
7. http://www.cdc.gov/regulations/index.html
8. https://www.federalregister.gov/documents/search?conditions%5Bagency_ids%5D%5B%5D=44&conditions%5Btype%5D%5B%5D=RULE&conditions%5Btype%5D%5B%5D=PRORULE&order=oldest
9. Administrative Procedures for CLIA Categorization—Guidance for industry and food and drug administration staff (introduction referencing 42 CFR Part 493).
10. http://www.fda.gov/MedicalDevices/DeviceRegulationandGuidance/IVDRegulatoryAssistance/ucm124105.htm
11. https://www.jointcommission.org/achievethegoldseal.aspx
12. https://www.jointcommission.org/facts_about_federal_deemed_status_and_state_recognition

CHAPTER 5

REGENERATIVE MEDICINE IN THE CANINE: A TRANSLATIONAL MODEL

Sherman O. Canapp, Jr. and Brittany Jean Carr

THE USE OF BIOLOGICS IN THE CANINE

A number of animal models have been used to explore the various potential applications of regenerative medicine procedures. One of the most seemingly applicable and robust models is that of dog. Many of the principles explored in this model have direct human applications and are explored in detail throughout this chapter. The use of biologics for canine sports medicine has continued to increase significantly over the past 5 to 10 years. It appears that the same benefits noted from biologics in equine and human sports medicine have now been recognized and adopted in canines. In particular, regenerative medicine therapies such as platelet-rich plasma (PRP) and adipose and bone marrow–derived stem cell (BMSC) therapies have grown in popularity, with literature supporting their use for osteoarthritis (OA) and soft tissue injuries. Hyaluronic acid (HA) has also increased in use over the past 5 to 10 years in the canine, specifically as treatment for OA and postsurgical synovial fluid replacement.

PLATELET-RICH PLASMA

PRP is an autogenous fluid concentrate composed primarily of platelets and growth factors. PRP has been shown to support healing by supplying growth factors, cytokines, chemokines, and other bioactive compounds (1–7). Although PRP's first clinical applications were limited to dentistry to improve bone healing, PRP now has much broader clinical applications, extending to orthopedic surgery and sports medicine. Recent studies have shown PRP to be efficacious in managing both OA and soft tissue injuries (3,4,7–31).

Platelets play roles in both hemostasis and wound healing by releasing growth factors to stimulate other cells of the body to migrate to the area of trauma and facilitate tissue healing. These growth factors include platelet-derived growth factor (PDGF), transforming growth factor-β1 (TGF-β1), TGF-β2, vascular endothelial growth factor (VEGF), basic fibroblastic growth factor (bFGF), and epidermal growth factor (EGF) (1–4,6). These growth factors have been shown to act either individually or synergistically to enhance cellular migration and proliferation, angiogenesis, and matrix deposition to promote tendon and wound healing, aid in bone healing, and counteract the cartilage breakdown that is associated with OA (2–8,10–13,19–22,26,29,31). Thus, PRP has been used to manage a number of orthopedic conditions. The application PRP for soft tissue healing has been studied (10,11,19,20,21,24–27,30). A recent double-blinded, randomized, controlled trial showed that patients with patellar tendinopathy treated with PRP had greater function and less pain than patients in the control group (11). Multiple studies in animal models as well as in human patients have documented the use of PRP for OA (7,8,12–18,22,23). One recent prospective, blinded, randomized trial showed a single dose of PRP to be more effective than a placebo for improving function in humans with knee OA (22). Furthermore, recent studies have also shown that platelets recruit, stimulate, and provide a scaffold for stem cells, supporting PRP's use in combination with stem cells to aid in cartilage, bone, and soft tissue healing (27,31–39).

The Optimal PRP Product

Previous studies have reported that PRP should have anywhere from a four- to sevenfold increase in platelets (2–4,6). However, inclusion or exclusion of mononuclear cells, neutrophils, and red blood cells (RBCs) have been found to also affect the inflammatory responses after PRP injection and hence, alter the efficacy of the product for various applications (2,5,10,19–22,40–44).

RBC concentration in the PRP product is of particular importance (40). A recent study found a higher RBC concentration in PRP increases the concentrations of unwanted inflammatory mediators, specifically interleukin-1 (IL-1) and TGF-α. This study also showed that synoviocytes treated with RBC concentrate had significantly more synoviocyte death when compared with leukocyte-rich PRP (LR-PRP), leukocyte-poor PRP (LP-PRP), and phosphate-buffered saline (PBS) (40).

The effect of leukocyte concentration in PRP products has also been of recent interest. Recent studies have shown LR-PRP is associated with increased pro-inflammatory mediators, including IL-1β, IL-6, IL-8 interferon gamma (IFN-γ), and tumor necrosis factor alpha (TNF-α) (1,2,5,10,40,41). An increase in leukocyte concentration in PRP is also associated with increased metalloproteinase (MMP-3 and MMP-13) gene expression and less cartilage oligomeric matrix protein (COMP) and decorin gene expression (10,36,45,46). This is thought to be attributed largely to the presence of neutrophils. Furthermore, an increased concentration of neutrophils in PRP has also been shown to be positively correlated with an increased MMP-9 concentration, which degrades collagen and other extracellular matrix (ECM) molecules (20,36,41,45). Another recent study found that LR-PRP causes significantly more synoviocyte death when compared with LP-PRP and PBS (40). Thus, LP-PRP has been thought to be more beneficial than LR-PRP in counteracting inflammation associated with OA (10,19,20,40,45). However, much debate remains over the ideal neutrophil concentration.

The effect of monocyte and lymphocyte concentration in a PRP product also remains largely unknown. Platelets activate peripheral blood mononuclear cells (lymphocytes, monocytes, and macrophages) to help stimulate collagen production, which is believed to be mediated by an increase in IL-6 expression (47,48). Thus, monocytes increase cellular metabolism and collagen production in fibroblasts and a decrease in release of anti-angiogenic cytokines interferon-γ and IL-12 (47,48). However, the role of monocytes and lymphocytes in PRP therapy remains unclear.

Multiple commercial PRP separation systems have been developed for both human and equine use. Different commercially available PRP separation systems have been found to yield different concentrations of platelets, white blood cell (WBC), and growth factors (6,43). Additionally, there is limited research supporting the validation of human and equine PRP systems for canine use. Recent studies have found that human and equine PRP systems do not yield similar or reliable results in the canine (44,49,50). In one study, key parameters of the PRP product from five of the most commonly used commercial canine PRP systems in healthy, adult canines were compared. PRP concentration results varied among systems. The systems with the highest platelet yield were SmartPReP®2 ACP+ and CRT Pure PRP. However, although SmartPReP®2 ACP+ yielded a 219% mean increase in platelets and 85% decrease in RBC from baseline, this system failed to reduce neutrophil concentrations. CRT Pure PRP yields a 550% mean increase in platelets while removing greater than 95% of the RBC and 85% of neutrophils. However, no claims regarding the efficacy of PRP therapy in canines or the efficacy of the PRP formulations evaluated can be deduced from these studies. Further study is also indicated to assess the concentrations of growth factors and cytokines in the commercial canine PRP products and determine the concentration of platelets and growth factors required for therapeutic effect.

Platelet-Rich Plasma in the Canine

Recently more studies have been published to support the use of PRP in dogs for both soft tissue injury and OA. The use of PRP for anterior cruciate ligament (ACL) injury in dogs has been investigated. One study showed that dogs treated with one single intra-articular injection of leukoreduced PRP had less pain, lameness, effusion, and synovial inflammatory and degradative biomarkers at 8 weeks posttreatment when compared to dogs treated with rest and nonsteroidal anti-inflammatory drugs (NSAIDs) (51). Another study found that dogs who underwent a partial ACL transection and meniscal release in one knee and received five weekly leukoreduced PRP injections had significantly improved orthopedic examination findings, less synovitis and evidence of ACL repair arthroscopically, and less severe changes histopathology 6 months posttreatment compared to dogs who were

treated with saline (52). Other similar studies have found that the use of PRP enhances autograft revascularization and reinnervation in dogs who underwent ACL reconstruction (53,54). The use of PRP for supraspinatus tendinopathy (ST) in dogs has also been documented. One recent study showed that in dogs with ST treated with a single PRP ultrasound-guided injection had subjective (owner-assessed) improvement in lameness and function in 40% of dogs with improved tendon heterogeneity and in 60% of dogs with improved tendon echogenicity 6 weeks following treatment (55). Limited literature regarding the use of PRP for OA and cartilage lesions in dogs is available. One study showed that in dogs with experimentally induced full thickness cartilage defects treated with either leukocyte and platelet-rich plasma (L-PRP) or leukocyte and platelet-rich fibrin (L-PRF) had significantly better mean macroscopic and microscopic scores compared to controls at 4 and 16 weeks posttreatment (56). Although the results of these studies are encouraging, more studies are needed to evaluate the efficacy of PRP therapy and further define its clinical applications in canines.

Administration of PRP

PRP therapy is a minimally invasive procedure that typically can be performed on an outpatient basis. It is often performed as a series of one to three injections, with 2 weeks between each injection. If PRP is being used to manage moderate to severe OA, in my experience about 50% of dogs require more than one injection for significant improvement.

Typically in dogs, most commercial systems require anywhere from 9 to 60 mL of blood to be collected from the jugular vein using an 18-gauge needle or butterfly needle, processed, and prepared for injection. Once the PRP is processed, the area to be treated is clipped and aseptically prepared. Sedation or general anesthesia may be required for injection, depending on the location of the injection.

For OA, PRP joint injections are usually performed without sedation; however, some joints, such as the hip, require sedation and may also require advanced imaging (fluoroscopy) for guidance. If one is not familiar with joint injections, it is wise to sedate patients until comfort with the procedure is obtained.

PRP has been used for tendon and ligament injuries, and is most commonly used for low-grade strains or sprains. For soft tissue injuries, ultrasonography guidance is used to ensure accuracy of the injection because PRP is most effective when administered directly into the lesion. Sedation is also required because the PRP injections are ultrasound guided and the patient must remain still.

The most common side effect is discomfort associated with the injection, which can be managed with pain medications, if needed, and typically resolves within 12 to 24 hours of the injection. NSAIDs and steroids need to be avoided 2 weeks before and after PRP therapy as NSAIDs have been shown to alter platelet function (57). Finally, a dedicated rehabilitation therapy program is often recommended in conjunction with PRP therapy to achieve and maintain the fullest musculoskeletal potential and performance level. Because the effects of certain modalities on PRP have not been well documented, therapeutic ultrasound, electrostimulation, and hydrotherapy are not recommended for the first 4 weeks following PRP therapy.

STEM CELL THERAPY

Almost all veterinary research has focused on adult stem cells, specifically mesenchymal stem cells (MSCs), derived from bone marrow (BM-MSCs) or adipose tissue. Recent studies have demonstrated the efficacy of stem cell therapy for canine OA (58–66). The use of stem cell therapy for elbow OA in dogs has been investigated (58–60). One study in dogs with elbow OA caused by spontaneous fragmented coronoid process demonstrated that those that underwent arthroscopic fragment removal and a proximal ulnar ostectomy and received stromal vascular fraction (SVF) or allogeneic stem cells had a

more favorable outcome than those treated with surgery alone (58). Other studies performed in dogs with chronic OA found significant improvement in dogs treated with adipose-derived MSCs (59,60). Studies have also evaluated the use of MSC for hip OA. In one recent study, dogs with hip OA that received a single intra-articular injection of adipose-derived cultured stem cells had a better outcome than control patients and those that received plasma rich in growth factors (PRGF) (61). A randomized, double-blinded, multicenter, controlled trial showed that dogs with chronic hip OA treated with adipose-derived stem cell therapy had significantly improved lameness scored and compiled scores for lameness, pain, and range of motion compared with control dogs (62). Two recent studies found that dogs with hip OA that were treated with a single intra-articular injection of adipose-derived cultured stem cells had significantly reduced lameness quantified by force plate at day 180 following treatment (63,64). The use of stem cell therapy for knee OA has also been evaluated (65,66). One study showed that in dogs with ACL transections, dogs that were treated with adipose-derived MSCs and PRP therapy had significantly more ECM synthesis and chondrocyte proliferation histiologically (65). Another study showed that dogs with chronic stifle OA that were treated with porcine adipose-derived stem cells had reduced lameness quantified by force plate at 12 weeks following treatment (66).

Recent studies have also evaluated the use of stem cell therapy for soft tissue injury. One case study in a dog with a gastrocnemius strain treated with BM-MSC therapy concluded that stem cell therapy with a custom, progressive, dynamic orthosis may be a viable, minimally invasive treatment option (67). Stem cell therapy has also been evaluated for the use of ST in dogs. In a recent study, 55 dogs with ST were treated with adipose-derived progenitor cells (ADPCs) and PRP (68). At 90 days following ultrasound-guided injection of ADPCs-PRP, a significant increase in total pressure index percentage (TPI%) was noted in the injured (treated) forelimb and shoulder diagnostic musculoskeletal ultrasound revealed a significant reduction in tendon size (area cm squared) and significant improvement in fiber pattern of the affected supraspinatus tendon (68). Stem cell therapy has also been used in dogs with partial ACL ruptures (69).

The most common places from which to harvest adult-derived MSCs are the patient's bone marrows or adipose tissue. To date, no evidence supports superiority of one over the other in terms of viability or efficacy of the derived stem cells. However, adipose tissue may be a preferred source in dogs for several reasons, including ease of access, low morbidity and pain associated with collection, and high-yielding MSC count (especially falciform). Once the sample is obtained, it is processed and prepared for injection. Both BMSCs and adipose-derived stem cells can be processed onsite or shipped to a university or private company for processing, culturing, and banking for future use (70).

As with other forms of regenerative medicine, stem cell therapy is a minimally invasive procedure that typically can be performed on an outpatient basis with or without sedation, depending on the location of the injection. In addition, because recent studies have shown that PRP recruits and stimulates stem cells, PRP is often combined with stem cells before injection to both activate and act as a scaffold for the stem cells (71–77).

Both SVF and ADPC are used in the dog. To date, no studies show superiority of adipose-derived SVF versus culture-expanded adipose-derived MSCs for treatment of canine orthopedic conditions. Both SVF and ADPC can be injected directly into the injured tissue or joint or can be administered by the intravenous (IV) route. However, recent studies have shown that stem cells given by IV do not actually reach joints or injured tissues (78). Thus, the authors currently do not recommend giving stem cells by IV for orthopedic applications.

BM-MSCs are most commonly used in equine regenerative medicine but can also be used in dogs. The two primary techniques for canine BM-MSC therapy are bone marrow aspirate concentrate (BMAC) and cultured-expanded. Only 2% to 4% of the mononuclear cell population of bone marrow is considered an MSC. The BMAC technique evolved such that the nucleated cellular portion of tissue aspirates obtained from bone marrow was concentrated and then applied to the injured tissue. This therapy is appealing for several reasons. BMAC can be processed quickly for faster therapeutic application. Processing takes only 1 to 2 hours if it can be performed in-house by using a commercially available kit, which allows the practitioner to initiate therapy 3 to 4 weeks earlier than can be done with culture-expanded cells. These cells are not manipulated in culture to the extent that culture-expanded cells are, meaning that they do not undergo adherence, expansion, or trypsinization through multiple passages, which can alter cellular phenotype. Alternatively, BM-MSCs can be isolated, cultured, and expanded. This yields a more homogenous population with a larger quantity of cells for injection. To date, no studies show superiority of BMAC over culture-expanded BM-MSCs in the treatment of canine orthopedic conditions. Also, there have been no studies documenting the superiority of BMSCs over adipose derived stem cells, nor has there been a study documenting the number of stem cells needed for treating soft tissue injuries or OA.

Stem Cell and PRP Combination Therapy

MSCs have potent anti-inflammatory, anti-fibrosis, pro-angiogenic properties, and can integrate into tissues and contribute to healing (79). MSCs require growth factor supplementation for growth in vitro, and the tendinopathy environment may not allow for optimal MSC cell growth and integration (80). Moreover, MSCs prefer to connect into a three-dimensional fibrous environment (81). PRP can provide both growth factors to promote MSC engraftment, as well as a fibrin scaffold for MSCs to attach to on injection and platelet activation. PRP has been shown to release its growth factors 5 days after activation, while MSCs have been demonstrated to survive at the injection site at least 30 days after injection, thus giving both an early and sustained stimulus for healing (82). Synergy between stem cells and PRP has been reported (83–86). Certain growth factors and cytokines released from platelets bind to receptors on the surface of stem cells and initiate a cascade involving signal transduction, gene expression and stem cell proliferation, migration, and differentiation. In addition, PRP provides a delivery vehicle and three-dimensional scaffold to support cell survival and proper differentiation (36). For these reasons, PRP combination therapy together with MSCs is commonly used.

Administration of Stem Cell Therapy

Injection of stem cells and PRP is a minimally invasive procedure that typically can be performed on an outpatient basis. Sedation or general anesthesia may be required, depending on the location of the injection. Joint injections are usually performed without sedation; however, some joints, such as the hip, require sedation and may also require advanced imaging (fluoroscopy) for guidance. If one is not familiar with joint injections, it is wise to sedate patients until comfort with the procedure is obtained. For soft tissue injuries, sedation is often required and ultrasonography guidance ensures accuracy of the injection because both PRP and stem cells are most effective when administered directly into the site of injury. The most common side effect is mild discomfort associated with the injection, which typically resolves within 12 to 24 hours.

Rehabilitation Therapy Following Stem Cell Therapy

A dedicated rehabilitation therapy program guided by trained and certified individuals in canine rehabilitation is often recommended for 12 weeks after regenerative medicine therapy, depending on the diagnosed condition. Rehabilitation therapy should be performed weekly in conjunction with an at-home exercise program. Rehabilitation therapy helps to speed healing by decreasing inflammation and swelling, building muscle mass, increasing range of motion, and improving overall comfort. These therapy sessions often include manual therapies, standard isometric exercises, and class IIIb laser therapy. Class IIIb low-level laser therapy is recommended because recent studies have shown it can stimulate stem cell differentiation, proliferation, and viability (87). Certain therapies are contraindicated within the first 8 weeks of regenerative medicine therapy because their effects on stem cells and PRP have not been fully studied; these therapies include Class IV low-level laser therapy, underwater treadmill therapy, therapeutic ultrasound, shockwave therapy, neuromuscular electrical stimulation/transcutaneous electrical neurostimulation, and NSAIDs. Once the tissue has healed, as confirmed via orthopedic examination, gait analysis, and diagnostic ultrasonography and/or needle arthroscopy, the rehabilitation program focuses on strengthening and conditioning. After appropriate muscle mass has been attained, dogs are cleared for retraining and return to sport. On average, patients treated with regenerative medicine therapy typically return to competition or normal activity within 4 to 6 months of treatment.

HYALURONIC ACID

Viscosupplementation with HA for the treatment of OA is commonly used in dogs and based on improving the rheologic properties within the joint. HA has been thought to slow the progression of OA and decrease inflammation within the joint (88–95). Specifically, it increases the joint fluid viscosity, increases cartilage (glycosaminoglycan [GAG]) formation, and decreases degradative enzymes and cytokines (88,89,92–95). Several clinical studies in humans have demonstrated relief of joint pain associated with OA following intra-articular injections of HA (96–99). Limited information regarding the effects of intra-articular HA on naturally occurring OA in dogs is available; however, several experimental studies using intra-articular HA in dogs have been reported (88–91,100,101). Results from these studies have also demonstrated decreases in pain, lameness, osteophytosis, synovial hyperemia and hypertrophy, GAG, and cartilage degradation (88–91,100,101). However, the mechanism by which HA produces beneficial effects remains controversial (90,97,100,101).

Hyaluronic Acid in the Canine

Studies evaluating the effects of intra-articular HA in dogs have used doses ranging from 10 mg to 20 mg and treatment periods ranging from 3 to 16 weekly injections (91,100,101). The injections must be given under sterile conditions with the dogs under heavy sedation or general anesthesia. Complications from these injections may include temporary increased pain and lameness and septic arthritis. Reportedly, more than 70% of dogs respond well to HA and improvement can be noted for more than 6 months following administration (91).

Administration of Hyaluronic Acid

Intra-articular injection of HA is a minimally invasive procedure that typically can be performed on an outpatient basis. The authors perform a series of three weekly injections. Sedation or general anesthesia may be required, depending on the location of the injection. Joint injections are usually performed without sedation; however, some joints, such as the hip, require sedation and may also require advanced imaging (fluoroscopy) for guidance. If one is not familiar with joint injections, it is wise to sedate patients until comfort with the procedure is obtained. The most common side effect is mild discomfort associated with the injection, which typically resolves within 12 to 24 hours.

BIOLOGICS FOR OA

OA is an extremely common condition in canines affecting one out of five adult canines (102,103). Similar to humans, there is no cure for OA but rather a multimodal approach to management long term. Management in canines includes various exercise programs; weight management; rehabilitation therapy including manual therapy, modalities and hydrotherapy; oral joint modifying agents; nonsteroidal anti-inflammatory medications; surgical treatment; and most recently intra-articular injections.

A rapidly growing component to the multimodal approach of managing OA is the use of intra-articular biologics. Injections are performed under aseptic technique (shaved and prepped). Injections may be performed awake for the shoulder, elbow, carpus, and stifle; however, the hip and hock typically require sedation or anesthesia, as they are more challenging to perform. Injections may be performed blind under landmark-guided palpation techniques, fluoroscopic, radiographic, or ultrasound guidance.

Some of the earliest reports of such products in the canine were with HA. Early studies on the effects of HA utilized the canine as a model for OA. These reports revealed a significant decrease in pain, lameness, inflammation, and gross and microscopic degradation of cartilage lesions (88–91,100,101). The HA treatment protocol for canine OA is similar to that in humans and equine in that it is commonly performed as a series, typically weekly for 3 weeks. The Dalton size of the HA molecule is smaller (approximately 700,000–900,000) than in humans and horses; therefore the replacement molecular size is also usually equivalent or larger in dose. The typical dose for the average size canine is 1 mL or 10 mg intra-articular (IA).

The use of PRP for the treatment of OA has also grown substantially over the past 3 to 5 years. In the author's experience, patients with mild to moderate OA will have improved comfort and function following a single injection of PRP for 4 to 6 months. If a patient has no objective clinical improvement following a single injection of PRP within 2 weeks, another PRP injection is usually recommended. If a patient shows no objective improvement following three injections of PRP, stem cell therapy is usually recommended.

Adipose-derived progenitor stem cells (ADSC) and BMSCs are also gaining in popularity for the treatment of OA in the canine. The first reported use of IA ADSC was by Black et al. for the treatments of hip and elbow OA (62). Since that time, numerous other reports have demonstrated the efficacy of these biologics for OA treatment (51–56,58–69).

In veterinary medicine, ADSC may include both SVF and culture-expanded mesenchymal cells. To date, there is no report in the canine literature that shows superiority of one technology over the other for the treatment of OA in the canine. Unlike in humans, where the adipose tissue is collected via liposuction, in the canine it is typically collected via a surgical approach obtaining the falciform ligament or various subcutaneous tissue locations. The adipose tissue may then be processed immediately "patient-side" mechanically and enzymatically (SVF), or processed through culture expansion over a 2-week period in a laboratory.

For BMSC both BMAC and culture expansion are commonly used. The bone marrow is typically collected from the femur or humerus as the ilium gives less volume and is challenging to target in canines. The bone marrow may then be processed immediately "patient-side" mechanically through centrifuge separation (BMAC), or processed through culture expansion over a 3-week period of time in a laboratory. To date, there is no report in the canine literature that shows superiority of one technology over the other for the treatment of OA in the canine.

Regardless of the technology being used, ADPC versus BDSC or "patient-side" versus culture expansion for the treatment of OA in the canine, it is simply that: a treatment. It is another "tool in our toolbox" toward the multimodal approach to treating OA. It is important for clients/owners of canine patients to realize that the use of stem cells in the canine will not be cured, but rather improved. The stem cells are not capable of "regenerating the joint," but rather decreasing the inflammatory mediators and pain associated with the OA cascade. Clinically, it appears that a single injection of stem cells can improve patients for 6 to 12 months at which time a booster stem cell injection will be required. Combining PRP with the stem cells does seem to achieve a stronger and longer lasting effect. In addition, repeating the stem cell/PRP combination injection with serial PRP injections does seem to subjectively also achieve a stronger and longer lasting effect.

BIOLOGICS FOR SOFT TISSUE INJURY

It is reported that tendon and ligament injuries account for nearly 45% of all musculoskeletal injuries in humans yearly in the United States (103). Similarly, soft tissue injuries are common conditions afflicting sporting, performance, and active dogs due to the repetitive forces placed on tendons and ligaments during activities (104,105). A previous survey with agility dogs found that 32% of the population had some degree of orthopedic lameness during training, and that 53% of those evaluated by a veterinarian were due to muscle or tendon injury (104). Tendons and ligaments are susceptible to major stress during sports, and if injured through repetitive microtrauma, heal slowly due to poor vascularity compared with other connective tissues. Although tendon ruptures or avulsions are typically treated through primary surgical repair, this is not typically an option for intratendinous lesions. Intratendonous lesions typically heal by secondary intention or fibrosis rather than regeneration (73,74). Because of the loss of organized matrix, these tissues have lost their elasticity and are predisposed to reinjury. Many of these injuries are treated conservatively with regenerative medicine therapy. The use of biologics gives new hope for extending the careers and improving the quality of life of the canine athlete.

For tendon injections sedation or general anesthesia is usually required. The injections are always performed under ultrasound guidance unless they are performed during open surgery to augment the repair location. The fenestration technique is typically utilized in canine tendon injections. Intra-articular tendons such as the subscapualris tendon are most commonly treated through an intra-aricular injection. For collateral ligaments, injections are also most commonly performed under ultrasound guidance unless during open surgery to augment the repair location. Intra-articular ligaments such as the cranial cruciate ligament (CCL) are most commonly treated through an intra-articular injection.

Stem Cell Therapy for Soft Tissue Injury

To date there does not appear to be any evidence in the canine literature showing superiority of adipose versus bone marrow for the source of stem cells. There also appears to be no conclusive evidence in the canine literature of superiority of culture-expanded versus patient-side bench top processing. It is well documented in the literature that there are significantly more adult mesenchymal cells present in a culture-expanded sample versus patient-side SFV or BMAC processing. Our research shows the typical dose for a culture-expanded fat or bone marrow sample is approximately 5 million cells/mL (106). In contrast, the dose of stem cells following SVF preparation is approximately 344,000 MSC/mL while BMAC showed roughly 4,800 MSC/mL (106). Despite this huge difference in the amount of cells, our positive clinical outcomes and objective outcome measures in our studies show the same positive healing pattern for tendon and ligament injuries with cultured cells as we see with SVF and BMAC. Therefore, it may be possible that it is not the cell type (bone marrow vs. adipose), or the quantity of cells present in the sample but simply that the cells are viable, and targeted to the appropriate lesion under ultrasound guidance.

Although we have not identified a significant difference in positive patient outcomes with cultured versus patient-side processing (SVF and BMAC), we do see substantial practical benefits to patient-side techniques over culture expansion. The major advantages to the use of culture expansion include: it provides a homogeneous population of cells; yields a large cell volume of 5 to 10 million cells/mL; there are safety and controlled processing standards; and there is opportunity to bank cells for future use. The disadvantages of culture expansion, however, include: longer turn-around time (2–3 weeks), which means the clients/patients must return for treatment at a later date (in many situations then requiring two anesthesia events); shipping issues (where cells can become damaged or lost in transport); more expensive (as there are additional laboratory and transport fees); some believe cultured cells have less "regenerative capabilities" compared to fresh cells. The final disadvantage of cultured cells is the concern by the FDA regarding cell manipulation as well as transporting cells across state lines.

Based on the pros and cons outlined previously, it may be clear that in-house patient-side processing may have practical clinical advantages over culture expansion. There are also pros and cons when comparing the patient-side techniques (SVF vs. BMAC). The advantages of SVF are that it is a fairly easy surgical procedure to collect the adipose tissue and SVF contains a larger volume of mesenchymal cells compared to BMAC. The disadvantages include: higher collection morbidity; collection must be performed in the operating room (higher procedural costs); longer collection procedure; longer processing time (1.5–3 hr); no established controlled processing; kits and enzymes are more expensive; cells are manipulated by using enzymes and may be considered a "drug" by the FDA in the future. Alternatively, the advantages of BMAC include: ease of collection from femur or humerus; less collection morbidity; can be performed in treatment room versus operating room (less operational costs); quick collection time; quick processing time (15 minutes); self contained system.

Stem Cell and PRP Combination Therapy for Soft Tissue Injury

Stem cell and PRP combination therapy is often chosen for soft tissue injuries. Since there is no documented superior ratio, the authors use PRP and stem cells in a 1:1 ratio. Combination therapy provides the stem cells for regeneration, growth factors needed for upregulation, and scaffold to maintain the cells in the injected location and allow for soft tissue engraftment.

COMMONLY TREATED SOFT TISSUE INJURIES IN THE CANINE

Active canines experience many of the same soft tissue injuries to which humans are susceptible. Rotator cuff (supraspinatus, subscapularis, and biceps), iliopsoas, and Achilles are the most common tendon injuries in the canine that are treated with biologics. CCL (similar to ACL) partial tears and carpal (wrist) and tarsal (ankle) collateral ligament grade II sprains are the most commonly treated ligaments in the canine.

Rotator Cuff Injury in the Canine

Rotator cuff injury is a common cause of forelimb lameness in dogs. The etiology is thought to be repeated strain activity and overuse from chronic repetitive activity, with a failure of adequate remodeling (107–110). Like in humans, it can be challenging to treat and recurrence is not uncommon. Although inflammation may play a role in the initiation of ST, it generally is not involved in the propagation and progression of the disease process. Histology of pathologic supraspinatus tendons shows absent to minimal inflammation with hypocellularity, a loss of tightly bundled collagen appearance, an increased proteoglycan content, and a lack of neovascularization in response to injury (110–119). Tendons damaged from repeated strain demonstrate discontinuous, disorganized tendon fibers with little to no inflammation, occasional mineralization within the tendon, and bony remodeling at its insertion site in chronic cases (111–118). In chronic cases, calcification at the site of insertion has been well documented in both humans and dogs (114,119–122).

Diagnostic musculoskeletal ultrasonography is a relatively new technique that has been used and validated for the diagnosis of rotator cuff injury in both humans and dogs (107,123–130). Musculoskeletal ultrasound provides a noninvasive definitive diagnosis of rotator cuff injury, and allows for facile and cost-effective sequential exams to assess response to treatment. Changes in size, shape, and echogenicity of the tendon found on diagnostic ultrasound all may indicate rotator cuff injury (131). Based on these findings, recommendations for treatment are made.

Previous reports on the treatment of ST in dogs have included surgical management, in which recurrence was not uncommon. Regarding conservative medical management, a retrospective study on 327 ST cases in dogs revealed 75% failed to respond to rest and NSAIDs and 40% failed to respond to a dedicated rehabilitation therapy program (132). This may suggest that conservative management is often insufficient to treat ST. Recent studies have suggested the potential efficacy of biologic regenerative therapies in humans (133,134). Meta-analysis of MSC effects on tendon healing suggests that stem cells increase collagen fiber density, enhance tissue architecture, restore a nearly normal tendon–bone interface, and improve biomechanical strength (135). In addition to the effects of MSCs on tendons, there is evidence demonstrating that MSCs survive when extracted and placed into the tendon environment and that cells can be stored for later use. Although the evidence for use of stem cells in tendons remains limited due to low clinical trial data, dozens of preclinical studies in humans strongly support its potential role in tendon healing. One recent study in which a single PRP injection for ST was performed in 10 dogs showed a subjective (owner-assessed) improvement in lameness and function in 40% of dogs with improved tendon heterogenicity and in 60% of dogs with improved echogenicity (136).

One recent retrospective study in dogs described the effects of ADPCs and PRP combination therapy for the treatment of ST in dogs (68). Following ultrasound-guided injection of ADPC-PRP, objective gait analysis was available on 25 of the 55 dogs at 90 days post–ADPC-PRP therapy. Following treatment, a significant increase in TPI% was noted in the injured (treated) forelimb at 90 days posttreatment. At 90 days following treatment, 88% of cases had no significant difference in TPI% of the injured limb to the contralateral limb. The remaining 12% of cases had significantly improved. Bilateral shoulder diagnostic musculoskeletal ultrasound revealed a significant reduction in tendon size (area cm squared) in the treated tendon at 90 days following treatment when compared to the initial area cm squared. All cases showed significant improvement in fiber pattern of the affected supraspinatus tendon by the ultrasound shoulder pathology rating scale. Based on the objective gait analysis and diagnostic ultrasound results, ADPC-PRP therapy appears to be promising for dogs with ST, especially those that have failed to respond to conservative management and rehabilitation therapy.

Typically, grade II to III strains and/or those that have failed previous conservative management with rest, medication, and rehabilitation therapy, regenerative medicine will be recommended. Injection of stem cells and PRP is a minimally invasive procedure that typically can be performed on an outpatient basis. Sedation is often required and ultrasonography guidance ensures accuracy of the injection because both PRP and stem cells are most effective when administered directly into the site of injury. The most common side effect is mild discomfort associated with the injection, which typically resolves within 12 to 24 hours.

A dedicated rehabilitation therapy program guided by trained and certified individuals in canine rehabilitation is often recommended for 12 weeks after regenerative medicine therapy. Rehabilitation therapy should be performed weekly in conjunction with an at-home exercise program. Rehabilitation therapy helps to speed healing by decreasing inflammation and swelling, building muscle mass, increasing range of motion, and improving overall comfort. These therapy sessions often include manual therapies, standard isometric exercises, and class IIIb laser therapy. Class IIIb low-level laser therapy is recommended because recent studies have shown it can stimulate stem cell differentiation, proliferation, and viability (87). Once the tissue has healed, as confirmed via orthopedic examination, gait analysis, and diagnostic ultrasonography, the rehabilitation program focuses on strengthening and conditioning. After appropriate muscle mass has been attained, dogs are cleared for retraining and return to sport. On average, patients diagnosed with an iliopsoas tendinopathy that are treated with regenerative medicine therapy typically return to competition or normal activity within 4 to 6 months of treatment.

Iliopsoas Tendinopathy

Thirty-two percent of hind limb muscle strains in dogs involve the iliopsoas muscle group (137). The muscle is prone to acute strain injuries from excessive stretch while engaged in eccentric contraction, wherein the external forces being driven across the muscle overload the contractile force of the muscle itself (138–142). The fibers of the muscle may then become disrupted and lose continuity, with additional disruption of the vascular supply leading to interstitial hemorrhage and swelling (141). Acute and chronic injury to the iliopsoas muscle groups has been a topic of interest in recent years with an increasing volume of literature pertaining to diagnosis and treatment of this condition.

Clinical presentation with iliopsoas discomfort can include gait abnormalities and lameness with decreased coxofemoral extension. Grade I strains have intact architecture with myositis and bruising. Such strains are generally the result of repeated muscle contractions resulting in mild muscle cell damage at the sarcomere. These injuries are rarely noted or diagnosed asides from athletic or performance animals, and generally resolve with appropriate rest in less than 1 week. Grade II strains have myositis with some fascial tearing. Grade III strains involve fascial tearing, muscle fiber disruption, and hematoma formation (143).

Descriptions of imaging modalities for iliopsoas pathologies have been reported (144–154). In particular, ultrasound evaluation using an 18 mHz probe has become a valuable and practical tool in assessing the iliopsoas and surrounding musculature and has been shown to be an accurate diagnostic tool in the assessment of acute and chronic iliopsoas strain, correlating well with historical and physical examination findings (147,150). Diagnostic ultrasound can be utilized to confirm a diagnosis, grade the pathology present, establish an appropriate treatment strategy, and monitor the patient's progress during recovery.

Achilles Tendinopathy

Achilles tendinopathy is commonly seen in the performance dog. In dogs, the injury can be acute or chronic and involve either part of the tendon or the entire tendon (155–157). Most Achilles tendon injuries are reported to occur in medium- to large-breed dogs, either during normal activity or as a result of trauma (155–157). Overuse due to chronic repetitive activity is believed to be an important factor in Achilles tendinopathy in the performance dog (155). Activities such as quick turns, landing from jumps, and jump-turn combinations often place soft tissue structures under extreme stress and can result in a strain injury (155–157). Strain injuries reduce the tensile strength of tendons, predisposing them to further injury. Repeated strain leads to disruption of the tendon fibers, causing pain and inflammation. Partial rupture, with one or more tendon components intact, has been most commonly reported in dogs (155). Regardless, rupture of one or more of the structures can be a debilitating injury.

Recently, regenerative medicine therapy has been used to help treat Achilles tendon injuries in both human and veterinary medicine. Recent studies using PRP to treat Achilles tendinopathy in rats have shown that rats treated with PRP have greater maturation of tendon callus, stronger mechanical resistance, enhanced neovascularization, and improved histiologic appearance (158–161). One study in dogs with Achilles tendinopathy treated with PRP showed that dogs treated with PRP had histiologically improved tendon healing and returned dogs to function sooner than control dogs (162). PRP has also been used to treat humans with Achilles tendinopathy. One recent case series of 27 patients diagnosed with recalcitrant Achilles tendinopathy showed that PRP injections produced good overall results for the treatment of chronic recalcitrant Achilles tendinopathy with a stable outcome up to a medium-term follow-up (163). A recent review also supported a strong positive effect of PRP for Achilles tendon rupture and showed that PRP treatments increased proliferation, DNA levels, and GAG levels (164).

Stem cell therapy has also shown great promise for treatment of Achilles tendon injuries. Studies have been performed in rats with Achilles tendinopathy treated with stem cell and PRP therapy and have shown stem cell and PRP therapy encourage earlier mechanical strength and functional restoration (165–167). Both BMAC and ADPCs have been evaluated in rabbits with Achilles tendinopathy. In one recent study where ADPCs were used to augment surgical repair, rabbits that were also treated with ADPCs had significantly increased neovascularization, decreased inflammation, and increased structural organization of the surgical repair compared to rabbits treated with surgery alone (168). One case report in a dog with an acute gastrocnemius tendon strain treated with autologous MSCs and a custom orthosis reported improvement on force plate gait analysis and serial diagnostic ultrasound evaluations and return to full function (169). Treatment of Achilles tendinopathy with stem cell therapy has also been reported in humans. Excellent outcomes and a mean return to sport at 5.9+/−1.8 months was reported in one retrospective study where BMAC was used to augment surgical repair of 27 patients with Achilles tendon ruptures (170). Although the application of regenerative medicine appears promising, future randomized, blinded, and controlled studies are still needed to fully elucidate the indications, effects, and applications of biologics for Achilles tendon injuries.

Treatment for Achilles tendon injury in the dog is based on the degree of injury as indicated on musculoskeletal ultrasound. For grade I strains, rest, nonsteroidal anti-inflammatory medications, and rehabilitation therapy with low-level laser therapy with or without a support wrap is indicated. Grade II strains often require the aforementioned therapies and regenerative medicine therapy (often PRP with or without stem cell therapy). For grade III strains (full tears or avulsion), surgical reconstruction with adjunct regenerative medicine therapy (PRP with or without stem cell therapy) is recommended. Multiple surgical repair techniques have been described. Surgery performed is often dependent on the degree of injury and structures injured seen on diagnostic ultrasound and intraoperatively. Regenerative medicine therapy is performed either intraoperatively or immediately following surgery using ultrasound guidance to inject PRP and/or stem cells directly into the site of surgical repair. Following surgery and regenerative medicine, healing time is approximately 16 weeks. During this time, patients are placed in a splinted bandage for the first 6 weeks and then transitioned to a custom hinged brace that can be dynamized over the recovery period to gradually allow for more range of motion at the tarsus and engagement of the Achilles tendon mechanism. During recovery patients are also entered into a rehabilitation therapy program. Therapy sessions often include manual therapy, standard isometric exercises, gentle passive range of motion (PROM), and class III-b laser therapy. Rehabilitation therapy should be performed weekly in conjunction with an at-home exercise program.

Once the tissue has healed, as confirmed via diagnostic ultrasound, the rehabilitation program focuses on strengthening and conditioning.

Once a normal fiber pattern and appropriate muscle mass have been attained, dogs are then cleared for retraining and return to sport. On average, patients treated with surgery and/or regenerative medicine therapy typically return to competition within 6 months of treatment completion.

Cranial Cruciate Ligament Injuries

The CCL rupture is one of the most common causes of hind limb lameness and the most common stifle joint injury in dogs (171–173). Surgical intervention has been established as the gold standard to correct the instability, restore the stifle to function, and delay the onset of OA (174–179). The progression of OA has been documented as a known long-term complication of surgery (176,180–189). Although surgical stabilization is commonly chosen for an unstable stifle, or a complete tear, much debate remains as to how to proceed with an early partial tear where a functional, stable stifle remains. While a partial tear is likely to progress to a complete tear if left untreated due to the degenerative cascade of effects that occurs, surgically "stabilizing" a stable stifle could be deemed overkill. Thus, treatment of an early partial CCL tear with regenerative medicine has been explored as several studies report that MSCs are an optimal source for ligament regeneration due to their high proliferation and collagen production potential and ability to quickly differentiate into ligament fibroblasts (190,191).

Numerous animal studies have been conducted to evaluate the regeneration potential of MSCs, which have revealed that MSCs result in cell engraftment in the CCL, meniscus, and cartilage when injected intra-articularly (192,193). Another study found that intra-articularly injected MSCs can accelerate the healing of partial ACL tears in rats when evaluated biomechanically and histologically (194). Similar results were found following an intra-articular injection of either fresh bone marrow cells or cultured MSCs in rats, where labeled cells were later located within the ACL, both histologically normal and with more mature spindle cells (195). Human clinical studies show similar potential, where patients have shown improvement in objective measures of ACL integrity and subjective outcomes after bone marrow MSC injection of grade I through III ACL tears (196). Safety for clinical use has been verified with no neoplastic complications (197).

PRP provides growth factors to enhance and promote MSC engraftment, providing a synergistic effect. Growth factors improve cell proliferation, promote an anabolic phase of cells, and stimulate MSC differentiation into fibroblasts (198–201). Additionally, PRP provides a three-dimensional scaffold for MSCs to facilitate differentiation and cell survival during delivery (202). A recent study showed that several intra-articular injections of PRP alone indicated evidence of CCL repair and remodeling in dogs (203). These findings promote the use of PRP in combination with MSCs to aid in ligament healing.

Furthermore, a recent retrospective study was performed in dogs to evaluate the use of autologous BMAC or ADPCs with PRP combination for the treatment of early partial CCL tears (69). Gait analysis data revealed that 90 days post-treatment dogs placed equal pressure on both hind limbs, which was a significant difference from baseline where the affected limb was placing significantly less pressure (69). Second-look stifle arthroscopy revealed a fully regenerated CCL in 69% of dogs, significant improvement in 8%, while 23% failed. Additionally, it was found that after a mean time of 1.8 years, 17% of dogs had a Helsinki Chronic Pain Index (HCPI) greater than or equal to 12 indicating chronic pain, while 83% had an HCPI less than 12 indicating normal locomotion and comfort (69). All owners believed their dog to have an excellent or very good quality of life, and that their dog had an excellent or good outcome posttreatment (69). Although these studies provide promise to the use of regenerative medicine as an alternative treatment option to traditional surgical intervention of early partial CCL tears in dogs, the results raise additional questions. Further studies are needed to determine if these are reproducible in a well-populated randomized, blinded, and controlled trial.

In all patients with a suspected early partial tear, stifle arthroscopy is recommended to confirm the partial tear and rule out other concurrent stifle pathology such as a meniscal tear. During arthroscopy, the torn portion (percent) of the CCL is measured using the standardized L probe. If less than or equal to 50% of the cranio-medial band of the CCL is determined to be damaged, typically stem cell and PRP combination therapy is recommended. However, if a greater than 50% tear is observed, surgical stabilization is often recommended. Following arthroscopy, if the patient is deemed to be a good candidate for regenerative medicine, fat or bone marrow and blood can be collected for stem cell and PRP processing. Injection of stem cells and PRP is a minimally invasive procedure that can be performed either the same day as arthroscopy if in-house processing is available, or, if same day treatment is not available or elected, stem cell and PRP collection, processing, and injection typically can be performed on an outpatient basis. In the majority of cases, stem cells and PRP are aseptically injected into the stifle joint; however, they can also be injected directly into the CCL with arthroscopic guidance. The most common side effect is mild discomfort associated with the injection, which typically resolves within 12 to 24 hours.

Following regenerative medicine therapy, a dedicated rehabilitation therapy program guided by trained and certified individuals in canine rehabilitation is often recommended for 12 weeks. During this time, patients are often placed in a custom, controlled-range-of-motion-hinged stifle brace to further protect the stifle during healing. Rehabilitation therapy should be performed weekly in conjunction with an at-home exercise program. Rehabilitation therapy helps to speed healing by decreasing inflammation and swelling, building muscle mass, increasing range of motion, and improving overall comfort. These therapy sessions often include manual therapies, standard isometric exercises, and class IIIb laser therapy. Class IIIb low-level laser therapy is recommended because recent studies have shown it can stimulate stem cell differentiation, proliferation, and viability (87). Once the CCL has healed, as confirmed via orthopedic examination, gait analysis, and second-look arthroscopy, the rehabilitation program focuses on strengthening and conditioning. After appropriate muscle mass has been attained, the dogs are cleared for retraining and return to sport. On average, patients diagnosed with an early partial CCL injury that are treated with regenerative medicine therapy typically return to competition or normal activity within 4 to 6 months of treatment.

Stifle Collateral Ligament Injuries

Collateral ligament injuries of the knee are commonly seen in humans, particularly athletes (204–206). Injury of the collateral ligaments of the stifle is less common in the dog. However, just as in the human, collateral ligament injuries are usually secondary to trauma which places excessive varus or valgus stress on the joint. Diagnosis is usually suspected with physical examination findings consistent with medial or lateral instability and confirmed on diagnostic ultrasound. Surgical repair is typically recommended for complete ruptures or avulsions. However, regenerative medicine is typically recommended for lower grade sprains (grade I and II).

To date there are no published studies regarding the use of biologics in dogs with medial or lateral collateral ligament injuries. However, there are studies in other animal models and humans. In one recent case report, a football (soccer) player with a high grade MCL injury that was treated with multiple PRP injections achieved full range of motion, complete function, and returned to sport at 25 days following treatment (207). Studies in rats with MCL injury treated with MSC have shown that MSC could accelerate the functional healing of the ligament (208–210). Further randomized, controlled,

blinded studies in dogs and humans are indicated to define the role and efficacy of biologics in collateral ligament injury.

Treatment for collateral ligament injury in the dog is based on the degree of injury as indicated on musculoskeletal ultrasound. For grade I sprains, rest, nonsteroidal anti-inflammatory medications, and rehabilitation therapy with low-level laser therapy is indicated. For grade II sprains often require the aforementioned therapies and regenerative medicine therapy (often PRP with or without stem cell therapy). For grade III strains (full tears or avulsion), surgical reconstruction with adjunct regenerative medicine therapy (PRP with or without stem cell therapy) is recommended. Regenerative medicine therapy is performed either intraoperatively or immediately following surgery using ultrasound guidance to inject PRP and/or stem cells directly into the site of surgical repair. Following surgery and regenerative medicine, healing time is approximately 16 weeks. During recovery patients are entered into a rehabilitation therapy program. Therapy sessions often include manual therapy, standard isometric exercises, gentle PROM, and class III-b laser therapy. Rehabilitation therapy should be performed weekly in conjunction with an at-home exercise program. Once the tissue has healed, as confirmed via diagnostic ultrasound, the rehabilitation program focuses on strengthening and conditioning. Once a normal fiber pattern and appropriate muscle mass have been attained, dogs are then cleared for retraining and return to sport. On average, patients treated with surgery and/or regenerative medicine therapy typically return to competition within 6 months of treatment completion.

CONCLUSION

The use of biologics for canine sports medicine has continued to increase significantly and the results of research studies and clinical reports are encouraging. Regenerative medicine therapy has been used in adjunct to surgical repair and/or rehabilitation therapy with promising outcomes. Future directions should include randomized, blinded, placebo-controlled studies to further define the indications, applications, mechanisms of action, and efficacy of biologics for OA and soft tissue injury in the performance canine.

REFERENCES

1. Boswell SG, Cole BJ, Sundman EA, et al. Platelet-rich plasma: a milieu of bioactive factors. *Arthroscopy*. 2012;28(3):429–439.
2. Dohan Ehrenfest DM, Doglioli P, de Peppo GM, et al. Choukroun's platelet-rich fibrin (PRF) stimulates *in vitro* proliferation and differentiation of human oral bone mesenchymal stem cell in a dose-dependent way. *Arch Oral Biol*. 2010;55(3):185–194.
3. Filardo G, Kon E, Roffi A, et al. Platelet rich plasma: why intra-articular? A systematic review of preclinical studies and clinical evidence on PRP for joint degeneration. *Knee Surg Sports Traumatol Arthrosc*. 2013;23:2459. doi:10.1007/s00167-013-2743-1
4. Hsu WK, Mishra A, Rodeo SR, et al. Platelet-rich plasma in orthopaedic applications: evidence-based recommendations for treatment. *J Am Acad Orthop Surg*. 2013;21(12):739–748.
5. McLellan J, Plevin S. Does it matter which platelet-rich plasma we use? *Equine Vet Educ*. 2011;23(2):101–104.
6. Pelletier MH, Malhotra A, Brighton T, et al. Platelet function and constituents of platelet rich plasma. *Int J Sports Med*. 2013;34(1):74–80.
7. Sundman EA, Cole BJ, Karas V, et al. The anti-inflammatory and matrix restorative mechanisms of platelet-rich plasma in osteoarthritis. *Am J Sports Med*. 2014;42(1):35–41.
8. Abrams GD, Frank RM, Fortier LA, et al. Platelet-rich plasma for articular cartilage repair. *Sports Med Arthrosc*. 2013;21(4):213–219.
9. Cho K, Kim JM, Kim MH, et al. Scintigraphic evaluation of osseointegrative response around calcium phosphate-coated titanium implants in tibia bone: effect of platelet-rich plasma on bone healing in dogs. *Eur Surg Res*. 2013;51(3–4):138–145.
10. Dragoo JL, Braun HJ, Durham JL, et al. Comparison of the acute inflammatory response of two commercial platelet-rich plasma systems in healthy rabbit tendons. *Am J Sports Med*. 2012;40(6):1274–1281.
11. Dragoo JL, Wasterlain AS, Braun HJ, et al. Platelet-rich plasma as a treatment for patellar tendinopathy: a double-blind, randomized controlled trial. *Am J Sports Med*. 2014;42(3):610–618.
12. Filardo G, Kon E, Di Martino A, et al. Platelet-rich plasma vs hyaluronic acid to treat knee degenerative pathology: study design and preliminary results of a randomized controlled trial. *BMC Musculoskelet Disord*. 2012;13:229. doi:10.1186/1471-2474-13-229
13. Filardo G, Kon E, Buda R, et al. Platelet-rich plasma intra-articular knee injections for the treatment of degenerative cartilage lesions and osteoarthritis. *Knee Surg Sports Traumatol Arthrosc*. 2011;19(4):528–535.
14. Franklin SP, Cook JL. Prospective trial of autologous conditioned plasma versus hyaluronan plus corticosteroid for elbow osteoarthritis in dogs. *Can Vet J*. 2013;54(9):881–884.
15. Jang SJ, Kim JD, Cha SS. Platelet-rich plasma (PRP) injections as an effective treatment for early osteoarthritis. *Eur J Orthop Surg Traumatol*. 2013;23(5):573–580.
16. Khoshbin A, Leroux T, Wasserstein D, et al. The efficacy of platelet-rich plasma in the treatment of symptomatic knee osteoarthritis: a systematic review with quantitative synthesis. *Arthroscopy*. 2013;29(12):2037–2048.
17. Kon E, Buda R, Filardo G, et al. Platelet-rich plasma: intra-articular knee injections produced favorable results on degenerative cartilage lesions. *Knee Surg Sports Traumatol Arthrosc*. 2010;18(4):472–479.
18. Kon E, Mandelbaum B, Buda R, et al. Platelet-rich plasma intra-articular injection versus hyaluronic acid viscosupplementation as treatments for cartilage pathology: from early degeneration to osteoarthritis. *Arthroscopy*. 2011;27(11):1490–1501.
19. McCarrel T, Fortier L. Temporal growth factor release from platelet-rich plasma, trehalose lyophilized platelets, and bone marrow aspirate and their effect on tendon and ligament gene expression. *J Orthop Res*. 2009;27(8):1033–1042.
20. McCarrel TM, Minas T, Fortier LA. Optimization of leukocyte concentration in platelet-rich plasma for the treatment of tendinopathy. *J Bone Joint Surg Am*. 2012;94(19):e143–e148.

21. Mishra A, Pavelko T. Treatment of chronic elbow tendinosis with buffered platelet-rich plasma. *Am J Sports Med.* 2006;34(11):1774–1778.

22. Patel S, Dhillon MS, Aggarwal S, et al. Treatment with platelet-rich plasma is more effective than placebo for knee osteoarthritis: a prospective, double-blind, randomized trial. *Am J Sports Med.* 2013;41(2):356–364.

23. Raeissadat SA, Rayegani SM, Babaee M, et al. The effect of platelet-rich plasma on pain, function, and quality of life of patients with knee osteoarthritis. *Pain Res Treat.* 2013;1:1–7.

24. Randelli P, Arrigoni P, Ragone V, et al. Platelet rich plasma in arthroscopic rotator cuff repair: a prospective RCT study, 2-year follow-up. *J Shoulder Elbow Surg.* 2011;20(4):518–528.

25. Sampson S, Gerhardt M, Mandelbaum B. Platelet rich plasma injection grafts for musculoskeletal injuries: a review. *Curr Rev Musculoskelet Med.* 2008;1(3–4):165–174.

26. Silva RF, Carmona JU, Rezende CM. Intra-articular injections of autologous platelet concentrates in dogs with surgical reparation of cranial cruciate ligament rupture: a pilot study. *Vet Comp Orthop Traumatol.* 2013;26(4):285–290.

27. Smith JJ, Ross MW, Smith RK. Anabolic effects of acellular bone marrow, platelet rich plasma, and serum on equine suspensory ligament fibroblasts *in vitro*. *Vet Comp Orthop Traumatol.* 2006;19(1):43–47.

28. Souza TF, Andrade AL, Ferreira GT, et al. Healing and expression of growth factors (TGF-ß and PDGF) in canine radial ostectomy gap containing platelet-rich plasma. *Vet Comp Orthop Traumatol.* 2012;25(6):445–452.

29. van Buul GM, Koevoet WL, Kops N, et al. Platelet-rich plasma releasate inhibits inflammatory processes in osteoarthritic chondrocytes. *Am J Sports Med.* 2011;39(11):2362–2370.

30. Xie X, Wu H, Zhao S, et al. The effect of platelet-rich plasma on patterns of gene expression in a dog model of anterior cruciate ligament reconstruction. *J Surg Res.* 2013;180(1):80–88.

31. Xie X, Wang Y, Zhao C, et al. Comparative evaluation of MSCs from bone marrow and adipose tissue seeded in PRP-derived scaffold for cartilage regeneration. *Biomaterials.* 2012;33(29):7008–7018.

32. Broeckx S, Zimmerman M, Crocetti S, et al. Regenerative therapies for equine degenerative joint disease: a preliminary study. *PLOS ONE.* 2014;9(1):e85917. doi:10.1371/journal.pone.0085917

33. Cho HS, Song IH, Park SY, et al. Individual variation in growth factor concentrations in platelet-rich plasma and its influence on human mesenchymal stem cells. *Korean J Lab Med.* 2011;31(3):212–218.

34. Del Bue M, Riccò S, Ramoni R, et al. Equine adipose-tissue derived mesenchymal stem cells and platelet concentrates: their association *in vitro* and in vivo. *Vet Res Commun.* 2008;32(Suppl 1):S51–S55.

35. Drengk A, Zapf A, Stürmer EK, et al. Influence of platelet-rich plasma on chondrogenic differentiation and proliferation of chondrocytes and mesenchymal stem cells. *Cells Tissues Organs (Print).* 2009;189(5):317–326.

36. Dohan Ehrenfest DM, Rasmusson L, Albrektsson T. Classification of platelet concentrates: from pure platelet-rich plasma (P-PRP) to leucocyte- and platelet-rich fibrin (L-PRF). *Trends Biotechnol.* 2009;27(3):158–167.

37. Mishra A, Tummala P, King A, et al. Buffered platelet-rich plasma enhances mesenchymal stem cell proliferation and chondrogenic differentiation. *Tissue Eng Part C Methods.* 2009;15(3):431–435.

38. Schnabel LV, Lynch ME, van der Meulen MC, et al. Mesenchymal stem cells and insulin-like growth factor-I gene-enhanced mesenchymal stem cells improve structural aspects of healing in equine flexor digitorum superficialis tendons. *J Orthop Res.* 2009;27(10):1392–1398.

39. Torricelli P, Fini M, Filardo G, et al. Regenerative medicine for the treatment of musculoskeletal overuse injuries in competition horses. *Int Orthop.* 2011;35(10):1569–1576.

40. Braun HJ, Kim HJ, Chu CR, et al. The effect of platelet-rich plasma formulations and blood products on human synoviocytes: implications for intra-articular injury and therapy. *Am J Sports Med.* 2014;42(5):1204–1210.

41. Sundman EA, Cole BJ, Fortier LA. Growth factor and catabolic cytokine concentrations are influenced by the cellular composition of platelet-rich plasma. *Am J Sports Med.* 2011; 39(10): 2135–2140.

42. Sundman EA, Boswell SG, Schnabel LV, et al. Increasing platelet concentrations in leukocyte-reduced platelet-rich plasma decrease collagen gene synthesis in tendons. *Am J Sports Med.* 2013;42(1):35–41.

43. Castillo TN, Pouliot MA, Kim HJ, et al. Comparison of growth factor and platelet concentration from commercial platelet-rich plasma separation systems. *Am J Sports Med.* 2011;39(2):266–271.

44. Stief M, Gottschalk J, Ionita JC, et al. Concentration of platelets and growth factors in canine autologous conditioned plasma. *Vet Comp Orthop Traumatol.* 2011;24(2):122–125.

45. Boswell SG, Schnabel LV, Mohammed HO, et al. Increasing platelet concentrations in leukocyte-reduced platelet-rich plasma decrease collagen gene synthesis in tendons. *Am J Sports Med.* 2014;42(1):42–49.

46. Cavallo C, Filardo G, Mariani E, et al. Comparison of platelet-rich plasma formulations for cartilage healing: an *in vitro* study. *J Bone Joint Surg Am.* 2014;96(5):423–429.

47. Naldini A, Morena E, Fimiani M, et al. The effects of autologous platelet gel on inflammatory cytokine response in human peripheral blood mononuclear cells. *Platelets.* 2008;19(4):268–274.

48. Yoshida R, Murray MM. Peripheral blood mononuclear cells enhance the anabolic effects of platelet-rich plasma on anterior cruciate ligament fibroblasts. *J Orthop Res.* 2013;31(1):29–34.

49. Franklin SP, Garner BC, Cook JL. Characteristics of canine platelet-rich plasma prepared with five commercially available systems. *Am J Vet Res.* 2015;76(9):822–827.

50. Carr BJ, Canapp SO Jr, Mason DR, et al. Canine platelet-rich plasma systems: a prospective analysis. *Front Vet Sci.* 2015;2:73. doi:10.3389/fvets.2015.00073

51. Bozynski CC, Stannard JP, Smith P, et al. Acute management of anterior cruciate ligament injuries using novel canine models. *J Knee Surg.* 2016;29(7):594–603.

52. Cook JL, Smith PA, Bozynski CC, et al. Multiple injections of leukoreduced platelet rich plasma reduce pain and functional impairment in a canine model of ACL and meniscal deficiency. *J Orthop Res.* 2016;34(4):607–615. doi:10.1002/jor.23054

53. Xie X, Zhao S, Wu H, et al. Platelet-rich plasma enhances autograft revascularization and reinnervation in a dog model of anterior cruciate ligament reconstruction. *J Surg Res.* 2013;183(1): 214–222.

54. Xie X, Wu H, Zhao S, et al. The effect of platelet-rich plasma on patterns of gene expression in a dog model of anterior cruciate ligament reconstruction. *J Surg Res.* 2013;180(1):80–88.

55. Ho LK, Baltzer WI, Nemanic S, et al. Single ultrasound-guided platelet-rich plasma injection for treatment of supraspinatus tendinopathy in dogs. *Can Vet J.* 2015;56(8):845–849.

56. Kazemi D, Fakhrjou A. Leukocyte and platelet rich plasma (L-PRP) versus leukocyte and platelet rich fibrin (L-PRF) for articular cartilage repair of the knee: a comparative evaluation in an animal model. *Iran Red Crescent Med J.* 2015;17(10):e19594. doi:10.5812/ircmj.19594

57. Schippinger G, Prüller F, Divjak M, et al. Autologous platelet-rich plasma preparations: influence of nonsteroidal anti-inflammatory drugs on platelet function. *Orthop J Sports Med.* 2015;3(6). doi:10.1177/2325967115588896

58. Kiefer K, Wucherer KL, Pluhar GE, et al. Autologous and allogeneic stem cells as adjuvant therapy for osteoarthritis caused by spontaneous fragmented coronoid process in dogs. *VOS Symposium Proc.* 2013, Canyons Resort, UT.

59. Black LL, Gaynor J, Adams C, et al. Effect of intraarticular injection of autologous adipose-derived mesenchymal stem and regenerative cells on clinical signs of chronic osteoarthritis of the elbow joint in dogs. *Vet Ther.* 2008;9(3):192–200.

60. Guercio A, Di Marco P, Casella S, et al. Production of canine mesenchymal stem cells from adipose tissue and their application in dogs with chronic osteoarthritis of the humeroradial joints. *Cell Biol Int.* 2012;36(2):189–194.

61. Cuervo B, Rubio M, Sopena J, et al. Hip osteoarthritis in dogs: a randomized study using mesenchymal stem cells from adipose tissue and plasma rich in growth factors. *Int J Mol Sci.* 2014;15(8): 13437–13460.

62. Black LL, Gaynor J, Gahring D, et al. Effect of adipose-derived mesenchymal stem and regenerative cells on lameness in dogs with chronic osteoarthritis of the coxofemoral joints: a randomized, double-blinded, multicenter, controlled trial. *Vet Ther.* 2007;8(4):272–284.

63. Vilar JM, Morales M, Santana A, et al. Controlled, blinded force platform analysis of the effect of intraarticular injection of autologous adipose-derived mesenchymal stem cells associated to PRGF-Endoret in osteoarthritic dogs. *BMC Vet Res.* 2013;9:131. doi:10.1186/1746-6148-9-131

64. Vilar JM, Batista M, Morales M, et al. Assessment of the effect of intraarticular injection of autologous adipose-derived mesenchymal stem cells in osteoarthritic dogs using a double blinded force

platform analysis. *BMC Vet Res.* 2014;10:143. doi:10.1186/1746-6148-10-143

65. Yun S, Ku SK, Kwon YS. Adipose-derived mesenchymal stem cells and platelet-rich plasma synergistically ameliorate the surgical-induced osteoarthritis in Beagle dogs. *J Orthop Surg Res.* 2016;11:9. doi:10.1186/s13018-016-0342-9

66. Tsai SY, Huang YC, Chueh LL, et al. Intra-articular transplantation of porcine adipose-derived stem cells for the treatment of canine osteoarthritis: a pilot study. *World J Transplant.* 2014;4(3): 196–205.

67. Case JB, Palmer R, Valdes-Martinez A, et al. Gastrocnemius tendon strain in a dog treated with autologous mesenchymal stem cells and a custom orthosis. *Vet Surg.* 2013;42(4):355–360.

68. Canapp SO Jr, Canapp DA, Ibrahim V, et al. The use of adipose-derived progenitor cells and platelet-rich plasma combination for the treatment of supraspinatus tendinopathy in 55 dogs: a retrospective study. *Front Vet Sci.* 2016;3:61. doi:10.3389/fvets.2016.00061

69. Canapp SO, Leasure CL, Cox C, Ibrahim V, Carr BJ. Partial cranial cruciate ligament tears treated with stem cell and platelet-rich plasma combination therapy in 36 dogs: a retrospective study. *Vet Regen Med.* 2016. doi:10.3389/fvets.2016.00112

70. Martinello T, Bronzini I, Maccatrozzo L, et al. Canine adipose-derived-mesenchymal stem cells do not lose stem features after a long-term cryopreservation. *Res Vet Sci.* 2011;91(1):18–24.

71. Carvalho Ade M, Badial PR, Álvarez LE, et al. Equine tendonitis therapy using mesenchymal stem cells and platelet concentrates: a randomized controlled trial. *Stem Cell Res Ther.* 2013;4(4):85. doi:10.1186/scrt236

72. Del Bue M, Riccò S, Ramoni R, et al. Equine adipose-tissue derived mesenchymal stem cells and platelet concentrates: their association *in vitro* and in vivo. *Vet Res Commun.* 2008;32(Suppl 1):S51–S55.

73. Chen L, Dong SW, Liu JP, et al. Synergy of tendon stem cells and platelet-rich plasma in tendon healing. *J Orthop Res.* 2012;30(6):991–997.

74. Uysal CA, Tobita M, Hyakusoku H, et al. Adipose-derived stem cells enhance primary tendon repair: biomechanical and immunohistochemical evaluation. *J Plast Reconstr Aesthet Surg.* 2012;65(12):1712–1719.

75. Manning CN, Schwartz AG, Liu W, et al. Controlled delivery of mesenchymal stem cells and growth factors using a nanofiber scaffold for tendon repair. *Acta Biomater.* 2013;9(6):6905–6914.

76. Yun JH, Han SH, Choi SH, et al. Effects of bone marrow-derived mesenchymal stem cells and platelet-rich plasma on bone regeneration for osseointegration of dental implants: preliminary study in canine three-wall intrabony defects. *J Biomed Mater Res Part B Appl Biomater.* 2014;102(5):1021–1030.

77. Tobita M, Uysal CA, Guo X, et al. Periodontal tissue regeneration by combined implantation of adipose tissue-derived stem cells and platelet-rich plasma in a canine model. *Cytotherapy.* 2013;15(12):1517–1526.

78. Harting MT, Jimenez F, Xue H, et al. Intravenous mesenchymal stem cell therapy for traumatic brain injury. *J Neurosurg.* 2009;110(6):1189–1197.

79. Caplan AI, Dennis JE. Mesenchymal stem cells as trophic mediators. *J Cell Biochem.* 2006;98:1076–1084.

80. Ahmad Z, Wardale J, Brooks R, et al. Exploring the application of stem cells in tendon repair and regeneration. *Arthroscopy.* 2012;28(7):1018–1029.

81. Gao J, Caplan AI. Mesenchymal stem cells and tissue engineering for orthopaedic surgery. *Chir Organi Mov.* 2003;88(3):305–316.

82. Guest DJ, Smith MR, Allen WR. Monitoring the fate of autologous and allogeneic mesenchymal progenitor cells injected into the superficial digital flexor tendon of horses: preliminary study. *Equine Vet J.* 2008;40(2):178–181.

83. Izadpanah R, Trygg C, Patel B, et al. Biologic properties of mesenchymal stem cells derived from bone marrow and adipose tissue. *J Cell Biochem.* 2006;99(5):1285–1297.

84. Zhang J, Wang JH. Platelet-rich plasma releasate promotes differentiation of tendon stem cells into active tenocytes. *Am J Sports Med.* 2010;38(12):2477–2486.

85. Chen L, Dong SW, Liu JP, et al. Synergy of tendon stem cells and platelet-rich plasma in tendon healing. *J Orthop Res.* 2012;30(6):991–997.

86. Richardson LE, Dudhia J, Clegg PD, et al. Stem cells in veterinary medicine—attempts at regenerating equine tendon after injury. *Trends Biotechnol.* 2007;25(9):409–416.

87. Ginani F, Soares DM, Barreto MP, et al. Effect of low-level laser therapy on mesenchymal stem cell proliferation: a systematic review. *Lasers Med Sci.* 2015;30(8):2189–2194.

88. Echigo R, Mochizuki M, Nishimura R, et al. Suppressive effect of hyaluronan on chondrocyte apoptosis in experimentally induced acute osteoarthritis in dogs. *J Vet Med Sci.* 2006;68(8): 899–902.

89. Greenberg DD, Stoker A, Kane S, et al. Biochemical effects of two different hyaluronic acid products in a co-culture model of osteoarthritis. *Osteoarthr Cartil*. 2006;14(8):814–822.

90. Kuroki K, Cook JL, Kreeger JM. Mechanisms of action and potential uses of hyaluronan in dogs with osteoarthritis. *J Am Vet Med Assoc*. 2002;221(7):944–950.

91. Hellström LE, Carlsson C, Boucher JF, et al. Intra-articular injections with high molecular weight sodium hyaluronate as a therapy for canine arthritis. *Vet Rec*. 2003;153(3):89–90.

92. Chen CP, Hsu CC, Pei YC, et al. Changes of synovial fluid protein concentrations in supra-patellar bursitis patients after the injection of different molecular weights of hyaluronic acid. *Exp Gerontol*. 2014;52:30–35.

93. Migliore A, Procopio S. Effectiveness and utility of hyaluronic acid in osteoarthritis. *Clin Cases Miner Bone Metab*. 2015;12(1):31–33.

94. Ozkan FU, Uzer G, Türkmen I, et al. Intra-articular hyaluronate, tenoxicam and vitamin E in a rat model of osteoarthritis: evaluation and comparison of chondroprotective efficacy. *Int J Clin Exp Med*. 2015;8(1):1018–1026.

95. Wang CT, Lin YT, Chiang BL, et al. High molecular weight hyaluronic acid down-regulates the gene expression of osteoarthritis-associated cytokines and enzymes in fibroblast-like synoviocytes from patients with early osteoarthritis. *Osteoarthr Cartil*. 2006;14(12):1237–1247.

96. Yan CH, Chan WL, Yuen WH, et al. Efficacy and safety of hylan G-F 20 injection in treatment of knee osteoarthritis in Chinese patients: results of a prospective, multicentre, longitudinal study. *Hong Kong Med J*. 2015;21(4):327–332.

97. Strand V, McIntyre LF, Beach WR, et al. Safety and efficacy of US-approved viscosupplements for knee osteoarthritis: a systematic review and meta-analysis of randomized, saline-controlled trials. *J Pain Res*. 2015;8:217–228.

98. Petrella RJ, Petrella M. A prospective, randomized, double-blind, placebo controlled study to evaluate the efficacy of intraarticular hyaluronic acid for osteoarthritis of the knee. *J Rheumatol*. 2006;33(5):951–956.

99. Rivera F. Single intra-articular injection of high molecular weight hyaluronic acid for hip osteoarthritis. *J Orthop Traumatol*. 2016;17(1):21–26.

100. Franklin SP, Cook JL. Prospective trial of autologous conditioned plasma versus hyaluronan plus corticosteroid for elbow osteoarthritis in dogs. *Can Vet J*. 2013;54(9):881–884.

101. Pashuck TD, Kuroki K, Cook CR, et al. Hyaluronic acid versus saline intra-articular injections for amelioration of chronic knee osteoarthritis: a canine model. *J Orthop Res*. 2016;34(10):1772–1779.

102. American Kennel Club Canine Health Foundation. Managing canine arthritis. http://www.akcchf .org/canine-health/your-dogs-health/caring-for -your-dog/managing-canine-arthritis.html

103. Clayton RA, Court-Brown CM. The epidemiology of musculoskeletal tendinous and ligamentous injuries. *Injury*. 2008;39(12):1338–1344.

104. Cullen KL, Dickey JP, Bent LR, et al. Internet-based survey of the nature and perceived causes of injury to dogs participating in agility training and competition events. *J Am Vet Med Assoc*. 2013;243(7):1010–1018.

105. Baltzer W. Sporting dog injuries. *Veterinary Med*. 2012;4:166–177.

106. Carr BJ. *BMAC vs SVF: What's in the Soup*. Proceedings ACVS Symposium 2015, Nashville, TN: American College of Veterinary Surgeons.

107. Arend CF, Arend AA, da Silva TR. Diagnostic value of tendon thickness and structure in the sonographic diagnosis of supraspinatus tendinopathy: room for a two-step approach. *Eur J Radiol*. 2014;83(6):975–979.

108. Lafuente MP, Fransson BA, Lincoln JD, et al. Surgical treatment of mineralized and nonmineralized supraspinatus tendinopathy in twenty-four dogs. *Vet Surg*. 2009;38(3):380–387.

109. Lewis JS. Rotator cuff tendinopathy. *Br J Sports Med*. 2009;43(4):236–241.

110. Arrington ED, Miller MD. Skeletal muscle injuries. *Orthop Clin North Am*. 1995;26(3):411–422.

111. Kujat R. The microangiographic pattern of the rotator cuff of the dog. *Arch Orthop Trauma Surg*. 1990;109(2):68–71.

112. Rees JD, Maffulli N, Cook J. Management of tendinopathy. *Am J Sports Med*. 2009;37(9):1855–1867.

113. Almekinders LC, Temple JD. Etiology, diagnosis, and treatment of tendonitis: an analysis of the literature. *Med Sci Sports Exerc*. 1998;30(8):1183–1190.

114. Hurt G, Baker CL Jr. Calcific tendinitis of the shoulder. *Orthop Clin North Am*. 2003;34(4):567–575.

115. Hashimoto T, Nobuhara K, Hamada T. Pathologic evidence of degeneration as a primary cause of rotator cuff tear. *Clin Orthop Relat Res*. 2003;415:111–120.

116. Dean BJ, Franklin SL, Carr AJ. A systematic review of the histological and molecular changes in rotator cuff disease. *Bone Joint Res.* 2012;1(7):158–166.

117. Garcia GM, McCord GC, Kumar R. Hydroxyapatite crystal deposition disease. *Semin Musculoskelet Radiol.* 2003;7(3):187–193.

118. Soslowsky LJ, Thomopoulos S, Tun S, et al. Neer Award 1999. Overuse activity injures the supraspinatus tendon in an animal model: a histologic and biomechanical study. *J Shoulder Elbow Surg.* 2000;9(2):79–84.

119. Fransson BA, Gavin PR, Lahmers KK. Supraspinatus tendinosis associated with biceps brachii tendon displacement in a dog. *J Am Vet Med Assoc.* 2005;227(9):1429–33, 1416.

120. Chung CB, Gentili A, Chew FS. Calcific tendinosis and periarthritis: classic magnetic resonance imaging appearance and associated findings. *J Comput Assist Tomogr.* 2004;28(3):390–396.

121. Rupp S, Seil R, Kohn D. Tendinosis calcarea of the rotator cuff. *Orthopade.* 2000;29(10):852–867.

122. Kriegleder H. Mineralization of the supraspinatus tendon: clinical observations in seven dogs. *Vet Comp Orthop Traumatol.* 1995;8:91–97.

123. Long CD, Nyland TG. Ultrasonographic evaluation of the canine shoulder. *Vet Radiol Ultrasound.* 1999;40(4):372–379.

124. Kramer M, Gerwing M. The importance of sonography in orthopedics for dogs. *Berl Munch Tierarztl Wochenschr.* 1996;109(4):130–135.

125. Kramer M, Gerwing M, Sheppard C, et al. Ultrasonography for the diagnosis of diseases of the tendon and tendon sheath of the biceps brachii muscle. *Vet Surg.* 2001;30(1):64–71.

126. Mistieri ML, Wigger A, Canola JC, et al. Ultrasonographic evaluation of canine supraspinatus calcifying tendinosis. *J Am Anim Hosp Assoc.* 2012;48(6):405–410.

127. Iannotti JP, Ciccone J, Buss DD, et al. Accuracy of office-based ultrasonography of the shoulder for the diagnosis of rotator cuff tears. *J Bone Joint Surg Am.* 2005;87(6):1305–1311.

128. Ottenheijm RPG, van Klooster IGM, Starmans, LMM, et al. Ultrasound-diagnosed disorders in shoulder patients in daily general practice: a retrospective observational study. *BMC Family Practice.* 2014;15:115. doi:10.1186/1471-2296-15-115

129. Smith TO, Back T, Toms AP, et al. Diagnostic accuracy of ultrasound for rotator cuff tears in adults: a systematic review and meta-analysis. *Clin Radiol.* 2011;66(11):1036–1048.

130. Teefey SA, Rubin DA, Middleton WD, et al. Detection and quantification of rotator cuff tears. Comparison of ultrasonographic, magnetic resonance imaging, and arthroscopic findings in seventy-one consecutive cases. *J Bone Joint Surg Am.* 2004;86-A(4):708–716.

131. Brose SW, Boninger ML, Fullerton B, et al. Shoulder ultrasound abnormalities, physical examination findings, and pain in manual wheelchair users with spinal cord injury. *Arch Phys Med Rehabil.* 2008;89(11):2086–2093.

132. Canapp SO. *Supraspinatus Tendinopathy in Dogs.* Proceedings ACVS Symposium 2013, San Antonio, TX: American College of Veterinary Surgeons.

133. Isaac C, Gharaibeh B, Witt M, et al. Biologic approaches to enhance rotator cuff healing after injury. *J Shoulder Elbow Surg.* 2012;21(2):181–190.

134. Lorbach O, Baums MH, Kostuj T, et al. Advances in biology and mechanics of rotator cuff repair. *Knee Surg Sports Traumatol Arthrosc.* 2015;23(2):530–541.

135. Ahmad Z, Wardale J, Brooks R, et al. Exploring the application of stem cells in tendon repair and regeneration. *Arthroscopy.* 2012;28(7):1018–1029.

136. Ho LK, Baltzer WI, Nemanic S, et al. Single ultrasound-guided platelet-rich plasma injection for treatment of supraspinatus tendinopathy in dogs. *Can Vet J.* 2015;56(8):845–849.

137. Carmichael S, Marshall W. Muscle and tendon disorders. In: Tobias KM, Johnston SA, eds. *Veterinary Surgery: Small Animal.* St. Louis, MO: Elsevier; 2012:1127–1134.

138. Canapp SO Jr. The canine stifle. *Clin Tech Small Anim Pract.* 2007;22(4):195–205.

139. Anderson K, Strickland SM, Warren R. Hip and groin injuries in athletes. *Am J Sports Med.* 2001;29(4):521–533.

140. Johnston CA, Wiley JP, Lindsay DM, et al. Iliopsoas bursitis and tendinitis. A review. *Sports Med.* 1998;25(4):271–283.

141. Nielsen C, Pluhar GE. Diagnosis and treatment of hind limb muscle strain injuries in 22 dogs. *Vet Comp Orthop Traumatol.* 2005;18(4):247–253.

142. Ragetly GR, Griffon DJ, Johnson AL, et al. Bilateral iliopsoas muscle contracture and spinous process impingement in a German Shepherd dog. *Vet Surg.* 2009;38(8):946–953.

143. Cabon Q, Bolliger C. Iliopsoas muscle injury in dogs. *Compend Contin Educ Vet.* 2013;35(5):E1–E7.

144. Adrega Da Silva C, Bernard F, Bardet JF, et al. Fibrotic myopathy of the iliopsoas muscle in a dog. *Vet Comp Orthop Traumatol.* 2009;22(3): 238–242.

145. Rossmeisl JH Jr, Rohleder JJ, Hancock R, et al. Computed tomographic features of suspected traumatic injury to the iliopsoas and pelvic limb musculature of a dog. *Vet Radiol Ultrasound.* 2004;45(5):388–392.

146. Bui KL, Ilaslan H, Recht M, et al. Iliopsoas injury: an MRI study of patterns and prevalence correlated with clinical findings. *Skeletal Radiol.* 2008;37(3):245–249.

147. Cannon MS, Puchalski SM. Ultrasonographic evaluation of normal canine iliopsoas muscle. *Vet Radiol Ultrasound.* 2008;49(4):378–382.

148. Agten CA, Rosskopf AB, Zingg PO, et al. Outcomes after fluoroscopy-guided iliopsoas bursa injection for suspected iliopsoas tendinopathy. *Eur Radiol.* 2015;25(3):865–871.

149. Anderson K, Strickland SM, Warren R. Hip and groin injuries in athletes. *Am J Sports Med.* 2001; 29(4):521–533.

150. Blankenbaker DG, De Smet AA, Keene JS. Sonography of the iliopsoas tendon and injection of the iliopsoas bursa for diagnosis and management of the painful snapping hip. *Skeletal Radiol.* 2006;35(8):565–571.

151. Johnston CA, Wiley JP, Lindsay DM, et al. Iliopsoas bursitis and tendinitis. A review. *Sports Med.* 1998;25(4):271–283.

152. Laor T. Hip and groin pain in adolescents. *Pediatr Radiol.* 2010;40(4):461–467.

153. Mahler SP. Ultrasound guidance to approach the femoral nerve in the iliopsoas muscle: a preliminary study in the dog. *Vet Anaesth Analg.* 2012;39(5):550–554.

154. Mogicato G, Layssol-Lamour C, Mahler S, et al. Anatomical and ultrasonographic study of the femoral nerve within the iliopsoas muscle in beagle dogs and cats. *Vet Anaesth Analg.* 2015;42(4):425–432.

155. Carmichael S, Marshall W. Tarsus and metatarsus. In: Tobias KM, Johnston SA, eds. *Veterinary Surgery Small Animal.* 1st ed. St. Louis: Elsevier Saunders, 2012:1014–1028.

156. Corr SA, Draffan D, Kulendra E, et al. Retrospective study of Achilles mechanism disruption in 45 dogs. *Vet Rec.* 2010;167(11):407–411.

157. Nielsen C, Pluhar GE. Outcome following surgical repair of achilles tendon rupture and comparison between postoperative tibiotarsal immobilization methods in dogs: 28 cases (1997-2004). *Vet Comp Orthop Traumatol.* 2006;19(4): 246–249.

158. Aspenberg P, Virchenko O. Platelet concentrate injection improves Achilles tendon repair in rats. *Acta Orthop Scand.* 2004;75(1):93–99.

159. Çirci E, Akman YE, Sükür E, et al. Impact of platelet-rich plasma injection timing on healing of Achilles tendon injury in a rat model. *Acta Orthop Traumatol Turc.* 2016;50(3):366–372.

160. Xu K, Al-ani MK, Sun Y, et al. Platelet-rich plasma activates tendon-derived stem cells to promote regeneration of Achilles tendon rupture in rats. *J Tissue Eng Regen Med.* 2017;11(4):1173–1184. doi:10.1002/term.2020

161. Yüksel S, Adanir O, Gültekin MZ, et al. Effect of platelet-rich plasma for treatment of Achilles tendons in free-moving rats after surgical incision and treatment. *Acta Orthop Traumatol Turc.* 2015;49(5):544–551.

162. Hernández-Martínez JC, Vásquez CR, Ceja CB, et al. Comparative study on animal model of acute Achilles tendon rupture with surgical treatment using platelet-rich plasma. *Acta Ortop Mex.* 2012;26(3):170–173.

163. Filardo G, Kon E, Di Matteo B, et al. Platelet-rich plasma injections for the treatment of refractory Achilles tendinopathy: results at 4 years. *Blood Transfus.* 2014;12(4):533–540.

164. Sadoghi P, Rosso C, Valderrabano V, et al. The role of platelets in the treatment of Achilles tendon injuries. *J Orthop Res.* 2013;31(1):111–118.

165. Chiou GJ, Crowe C, McGoldrick R, et al. Optimization of an injectable tendon hydrogel: the effects of platelet-rich plasma and adipose-derived stem cells on tendon healing in vivo. *Tissue Eng Part A.* 2015;21(9–10):1579–1586.

166. Al-Ani MKh, Xu K, Sun Y, et al. Study of bone marrow mesenchymal and tendon-derived stem cells transplantation on the regenerating effect of Achilles tendon ruptures in rats. *Stem Cells Int.* 2015;2015:984146. doi:10.1155/2015/984146

167. Yuksel S, Guleç MA, Gultekin MZ, et al. Comparison of the early period effects of bone marrow-derived mesenchymal stem cells and platelet-rich plasma on the Achilles tendon ruptures in rats. *Connect Tissue Res.* 2016;57(5):360–373.

168. Vieira MH, Oliveira RJ, Eça LP, et al. Therapeutic potential of mesenchymal stem cells to

treat Achilles tendon injuries. *Genet Mol Res.* 2014;13(4):10434–10449.

169. Case JB, Palmer R, Valdes-Martinez A, et al. Gastrocnemius tendon strain in a dog treated with autologous mesenchymal stem cells and a custom orthosis. *Vet Surg.* 2013;42(4):355–360.

170. Stein BE, Stroh DA, Schon LC. Outcomes of acute Achilles tendon rupture repair with bone marrow aspirate concentrate augmentation. *Int Orthop.* 2015;39(5):901–905.

171. Piermattei DL, Flo GL, DeCamp CE. Chapter 18—the stifle joint. In: Piermattei DL, Flo GL, DeCamp CE, eds. *Brinker, Piermattei, and Flo's Handbook of Small Animal Orthopedics and Fracture Repair.* Philadelphia, PA: Saunders; 2006:562–632.

172. Johnson JA, Austin C, Breur GJ. Incidence of canine appendicular musculoskeletal disorders in 16 veterinary teaching hospitals from 1980 through 1989. *Vet Comp Orthop Traumatol.* 1994;7:56–69.

173. Korvick DL, Pijanowski GJ, Schaeffer DJ. Three-dimensional kinematics of the intact and cranial cruciate ligament-deficient stifle of dogs. *J Biomech.* 1994;27(1):77–87.

174. Böddeker J, Drüen S, Meyer-Lindenberg A, et al. Computer-assisted gait analysis of the dog: comparison of two surgical techniques for the ruptured cranial cruciate ligament. *Vet Comp Orthop Traumatol.* 2012;25(1):11–21.

175. Slocum B, Slocum TD. Tibial plateau leveling osteotomy for repair of cranial cruciate ligament rupture in the canine. *Vet Clin North Am Small Anim Pract.* 1993;23:777–795. doi:10.1016/S0195-5616(93)50082-7

176. Mölsä SH, Hyytiäinen HK, Hielm-Björkman AK, et al. Long-term functional outcome after surgical repair of cranial cruciate ligament disease in dogs. *BMC Vet Res.* 2014;10:266. doi:10.1186/s12917-014-0266-8

177. Nelson SA, Krotscheck U, Rawlinson J, et al. Long-term functional outcome of tibial plateau leveling osteotomy versus extracapsular repair in a heterogeneous population of dogs. *Vet Surg.* 2013;42(1):38–50.

178. Cook JL, Luther JK, Beetem J, et al. Clinical comparison of a novel extracapsular stabilization procedure and tibial plateau leveling osteotomy for treatment of cranial cruciate ligament deficiency in dogs. *Vet Surg.* 2010;39(3):315–323.

179. Christopher SA, Beetem J, Cook JL. Comparison of long-term outcomes associated with three surgical techniques for treatment of cranial cruciate ligament disease in dogs. *Vet Surg.* 2013;42(3):329–334.

180. DeLuke AM, Allen DA, Wilson ER, et al. Comparison of radiographic osteoarthritis scores in dogs less than 24 months or greater than 24 months following tibial plateau leveling osteotomy. *Can Vet J.* 2012;53(10):1095–1099.

181. Ledecky V, Hluchy M, Freilichman R, et al. Clinical comparison and short-term radiographic evaluation of tight rope and lateral suture procedures for dogs after cranial cruciate ligament rupture. *Veterinarni Medicina.* 2014;59:502–505.

182. Wolf RE, Scavelli TD, Hoelzler MG, et al. Surgical and postoperative complications associated with tibial tuberosity advancement for cranial cruciate ligament rupture in dogs: 458 cases (2007–2009). *J Am Vet Med Assoc.* 2012;240:1481–1487. doi:10.2460/javma.240.12.1481

183. Molsa SH, Hielm-Bjorkman AK, Laitinen-Vapaavuori OM. Use of an owner questionnaire to evaluate long-term surgical outcome and chronic pain after cranial cruciate ligament repair in dogs: 253 cases (2004–2006). *J Am Vet Med Assoc.* 2013;243:689–695. doi:10.2460/javma.243.5.689

184. Au KK, Gordon-Evans WJ, Dunning D, et al. Comparison of short- and long-term function and radiographic osteoarthrosis in dogs after postoperative physical rehabilitation and tibial plateau leveling osteotomy or lateral fabellar suture stabilization. *Vet Surg.* 2010;39(2):173–180.

185. Vasseur PB, Berry CR. Progression of stifle osteoarthrosis following reconstruction of the cranial cruciate ligament in 21 dogs. *J Am Anim Hosp Assoc.* 1992;28:129–136.

186. Rayward RM, Thomson DG, Davies JV, et al. Progression of osteoarthritis following TPLO surgery: a prospective radiographic study of 40 dogs. *J Small Anim Pract.* 2004;45(2):92–97.

187. Innes JF, Costello M, Barr FJ, et al. Radiographic progression of osteoarthritis of the canine stifle joint: a prospective study. *Vet Radiol Ultrasound.* 2004;45(2):143–148.

188. Lazar TP, Berry CR, deHaan JJ, et al. Long-term radiographic comparison of tibial plateau leveling osteotomy versus extracapsular stabilization for cranial cruciate ligament rupture in the dog. *Vet Surg.* 2005;34(2):133–141.

189. Lineberger JA, Allen DA, Wilson ER, et al. Comparison of radiographic arthritic changes

associated with two variations of tibial plateau leveling osteotomy. *Vet Comp Orthop Traumatol.* 2005;18(1):13–17.

190. Van Eijk F, Saris DB, Riesle J, et al. Tissue engineering of ligaments: a comparison of bone marrow stromal cells, anterior cruciate ligament, and skin fibroblasts as cell source. *Tissue Eng.* 2004;10(5–6):893–903.

191. Chen J, Altman GH, Karageorgiou V, et al. Human bone marrow stromal cell and ligament fibroblast responses on RGD-modified silk fibers. *J Biomed Mater Res A.* 2003;67(2):559–570.

192. Agung M, Ochi M, Yanada S, et al. Mobilization of bone marrow-derived mesenchymal stem cells into the injured tissues after intraarticular injection and their contribution to tissue regeneration. *Knee Surg Sports Traumatol Arthrosc.* 2006;14(12):1307–1314.

193. Linon E, Spreng D, Rytz U, et al. Engraftment of autologous bone marrow cells into the injured cranial cruciate ligament in dogs. *Vet J.* 2014;202(3):448–454.

194. Kanaya A, Deie M, Adachi N, et al. Intra-articular injection of mesenchymal stromal cells in partially torn anterior cruciate ligaments in a rat model. *Arthroscopy.* 2007;23(6):610–617.

195. Oe K, Kushida T, Okamoto N, et al. New strategies for anterior cruciate ligament partial rupture using bone marrow transplantation in rats. *Stem Cells Dev.* 2011;20(4):671–679.

196. Centeno CJ, Pitts J, Al-Sayegh H, et al. Anterior cruciate ligament tears treated with percutaneous injection of autologous bone marrow nucleated cells: a case series. *J Pain Res.* 2015;8:437–447.

197. Centeno CJ, Schultz JR, Cheever M, et al. Safety and complications reporting update on the re-implantation of culture-expanded mesenchymal stem cells using autologous platelet lysate technique. *Curr Stem Cell Res Ther.* 2011;6(4):368–378.

198. Chen L, Dong SW, Liu JP, et al. Synergy of tendon stem cells and platelet-rich plasma in tendon healing. *J Orthop Res.* 2012;30(6):991–997.

199. Molloy T, Wang Y, Murrell G. The roles of growth factors in tendon and ligament healing. *Sports Med.* 2003;33(5):381–394.

200. Zhang J, Wang JH. Platelet-rich plasma releasate promotes differentiation of tendon stem cells into active tenocytes. *Am J Sports Med.* 2010;38(12):2477–2486.

201. Smith JJ, Ross MW, Smith RK. Anabolic effects of acellular bone marrow, platelet rich plasma, and serum on equine suspensory ligament fibroblasts *in vitro. Vet Comp Orthop Traumatol.* 2006;19(1):43–47.

202. Richardson LE, Dudhia J, Clegg PD, et al. Stem cells in veterinary medicine: attempts at regenerating equine tendon after injury. *Trends Biotechnol.* 2011;25:409–416. doi:10.1016/j.tibtech.2007.07.009

203. Cook JL, Smith PA, Bozynski CC, et al. Multiple injections of leukoreduced platelet rich plasma reduce pain and functional impairment in a canine model of ACL and meniscal deficiency. *J Orthop Res.* 2016;34(4):607–615.

204. Fetto JF, Marshall JL. Medial collateral ligament injuries of the knee: a rationale for treatment. *Clin Orthop.* 1978;132:206–218.

205. Peterson L, Junge A, Chomiak J, et al. Incidence of football injuries and complaints in different age groups and skill-level groups. *Am J Sports Med.* 2000;28(5 Suppl):S51–S57.

206. Lorentzon R, Wedrèn H, Pietilä T. Incidence, nature, and causes of ice hockey injuries. A three-year prospective study of a Swedish elite ice hockey team. *Am J Sports Med.* 1988;16(4):392–396.

207. Eirale C, Mauri E, Hamilton B. Use of platelet rich plasma in an isolated complete medial collateral ligament lesion in a professional football (soccer) player: a case report. *Asian J Sports Med.* 2013;4(2):158–162.

208. Nishimori M, Matsumoto T, Ota S, et al. Role of angiogenesis after muscle derived stem cell transplantation in injured medial collateral ligament. *J Orthop Res.* 2012;30(4):627–633.

209. Saether EE, Chamberlain CS, Leiferman EM, et al. Enhanced medial collateral ligament healing using mesenchymal stem cells: dosage effects on cellular response and cytokine profile. *Stem Cell Rev.* 2014;10(1):86–96.

210. Saether EE, Chamberlain CS, Aktas E, et al. Primed mesenchymal stem cells alter and improve rat medial collateral ligament healing. *Stem Cell Rev.* 2016;12(1):42–53.

CHAPTER 6

PRINCIPLES OF PLATELET-RICH PLASMA AND STEM CELLS: FROM PLATELETS TO CYTOKINES

Ricardo E. Colberg and Ariane Maico

The classic approach for treating musculoskeletal conditions has historically included the use of nonsteroidal anti-inflammatory medications and treatment modalities that block the inflammatory cascade to decrease pain and provide the patient with symptom relief. This approach has typically been applied to both acute and chronic injuries, regardless of the histopathology of the injury, whether the injured tissue has an actual active inflammatory process or not (1). For example, chronic tendon injuries have been reported to lack biochemical markers for inflammation and lack inflammatory cells (2,3). If the injured tissue lacks an inflammatory process, then using antiinflammatory medications seems illogical; although the medications may provide the patient short-term relief, there is no evidence for their long-term benefits (4).

Based on this concept, the use of corticosteroid injections would not be supported in a condition that lacks true markers of inflammation. A randomized controlled trial on tendon injuries showed that blocking the inflammatory process with a corticosteroid injection was not superior to the "wait and see" treatment or to physiotherapy

(5). Coombes et al. conducted a meta-analysis, which included 41 randomized controlled trials of the efficacy and safety of corticosteroid injection versus other injections including placebo (saline or local anesthetic), observation, nonsteroidal anti-inflammatory drugs (NSAIDs), physiotherapy, electrotherapy, orthotic devices, or other injections (hyaluronate, botulinum toxin, and platelet-rich plasma [PRP]). Overall, it showed that cortisone injections for tendinopathies provide short-term benefits, but have negative effects on pain and function at greater than 12 weeks (6). Repeated doses (average 4.3 injections, range 3–6 injections, 18-month period) were associated with increased long-term pain as compared to single injection in lateral epicondylitis (7). There is also a well-known severe, yet rare (0.1%), adverse event of tendon rupture reported in the Achilles tendon, as well as relative risk of Achilles and patellar tendon atrophy (6,8). These cannot be ignored given additional negative long-term outcomes and higher recurrence rates compared to no intervention. The exact biological basis for the effect of the corticosteroid injection on tendons is unclear; however, it is known that

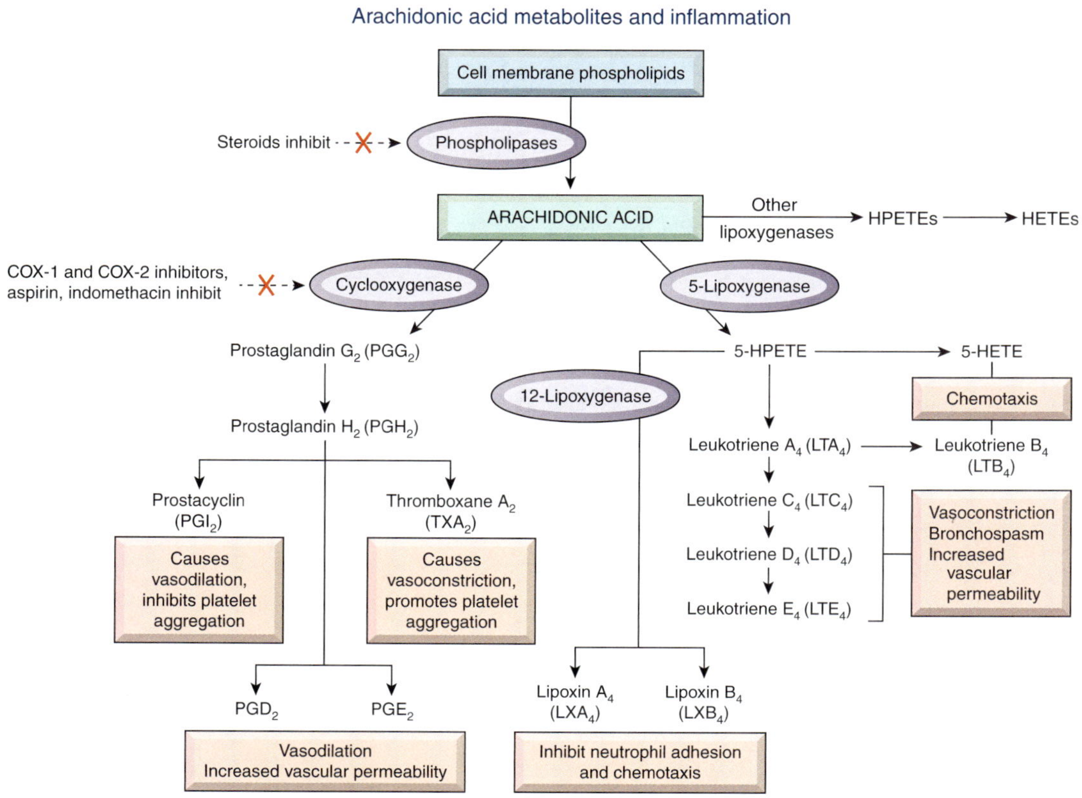

Arachidonic acid metabolites and inflammation

Cell membrane phospholipids

Steroids inhibit ✗→ Phospholipases

ARACHIDONIC ACID

Other lipoxygenases → HPETEs → HETEs

COX-1 and COX-2 inhibitors, aspirin, indomethacin inhibit ✗→ Cyclooxygenase

5-Lipoxygenase

Prostaglandin G_2 (PGG_2)

12-Lipoxygenase

5-HPETE → 5-HETE

Chemotaxis

Prostaglandin H_2 (PGH_2)

Leukotriene A_4 (LTA_4) → Leukotriene B_4 (LTB_4)

Prostacyclin (PGI_2)

Thromboxane A_2 (TXA_2)

Leukotriene C_4 (LTC_4)

Causes vasodilation, inhibits platelet aggregation

Causes vasoconstriction, promotes platelet aggregation

Leukotriene D_4 (LTD_4)

Vasoconstriction Bronchospasm Increased vascular permeability

Leukotriene E_4 (LTE_4)

PGD_2 PGE_2

Lipoxin A_4 (LXA_4)   Lipoxin B_4 (LXB_4)

Vasodilation Increased vascular permeability

Inhibit neutrophil adhesion and chemotaxis

FIGURE 6.1: The inflammatory cascade is affected by steroids by inhibiting phospholipases as opposed to NSAIDs inhibit COX-1 and/or COX-2.

COX-1, cyclooxygenase 1; COX-2, cyclooxygenase 2; NSAID, nonsteroidal anti-inflammatory drug.

Source: From Ref. (9). Kumar V, Abbas AK, Fausto N. *Robbins and Cotran Pathologic Basis of Disease,* 7th ed. Philadelphia, PA: Elsevier Saunders 2005.

corticosteroids inhibit the inflammatory cascade, including the formation of collagen, extracellular matrix molecules, and granulation tissue (6) (Figure 6.1).

The inflammatory cascade has a physiologic purpose of stimulating and orchestrating the healing process of the injured tissue. When this process is inhibited with medications, the body cannot heal the injured site appropriately and a reactive upregulation of the expression of matrix metalloproteinases occurs (10). For example, blocking the inflammatory cascade of an acute tendon strain can lead to impaired healing, which in turn causes progressive degeneration of the extracellular matrix and weakness of the tendon, in some cases resulting in a degenerative tendon tear (11). In other cases, the tendon develops scar tissue fibrosis, pathologic neovessels, and

degenerated collagen that hinder the normal tissue function (12) (Figure 6.2).

The same detrimental effects of antiinflammatory medications can be seen in joint pathology, in which the patient may achieve short-term symptom relief, but the intra-articular degeneration progresses (13). Since the introduction of cortisone injections in the 1950s, intra-articular steroids have been widely used and studied for their short-term pain relief, improvement in the range of motion, and increased functional mobility (14). However, their long-term effects and unpredictable duration have been controversial. The survival of articular chondrocytes is essential for cartilage and joint health. A study on in vitro chondrocyte cell cultures and ex vivo (osteochondral specimens) glucocorticoids showed apoptosis of the cells after exposing the

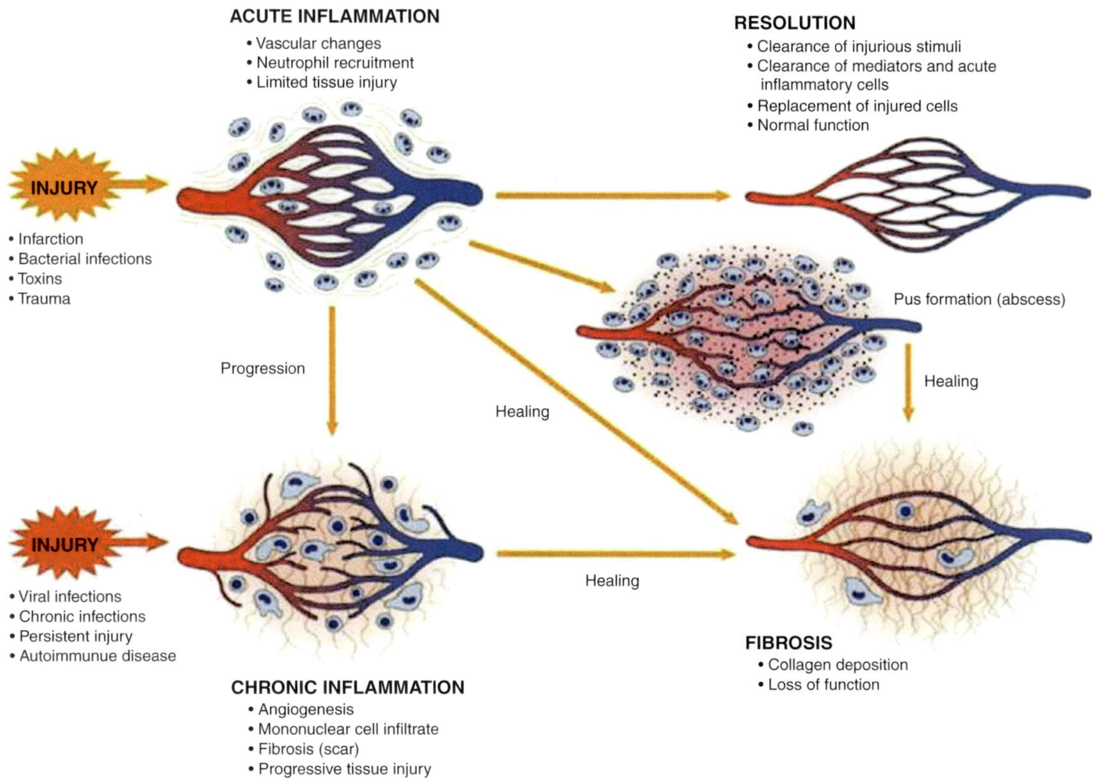

FIGURE 6.2: The inflammatory pathway of tissues is altered in chronic inflammation, which leads to impaired healing and loss of normal function.

Source: From Ref. (9). Kumar V, Abbas AK, Fausto N. *Robbins and Cotran Pathologic Basis of Disease*, 7th ed. Philadelphia, PA: Elsevier Saunders; 2005.

chondrocytes to the steroid. The percentage of cell death in these chondrocytes was noted to also increase at a synergistic rate when glucocorticoids were combined with local anesthetics, which is frequently done in clinical practice (15). A systematic review performed by Wernecke et al. on the effects of corticosteroids on intra–articular cartilage confirmed a dose and time dependent chondrocyte cytotoxicity and gross cartilage damage (16).

PHASES OF TISSUE HEALING VERSUS PATHOLOGIC DEGENERATION

To understand tissue regeneration, it is important to discuss the body's process of healing after suffering an injury, which is broken down into three stages: the inflammatory, proliferative (repair), and maturation (remodeling) stages (Figure 6.3) (17). The inflammatory stage is when the injured site becomes filled with blood products used to remove injured cells and necrotic debris, including the granulocytes discussed later. During the proliferative phase, the native tissue cells replicate to replace the injured or damaged tissues. This initial tissue proliferation is disorganized and physiologically unstable, and may frequently lead to scar tissue formation. The remodeling stage is when the disorganized tissue cells rearrange into more organized structures and recover the physiologic properties. If the tissue maturation phase is suboptimal or impaired, the scar tissue contracts and becomes imbedded

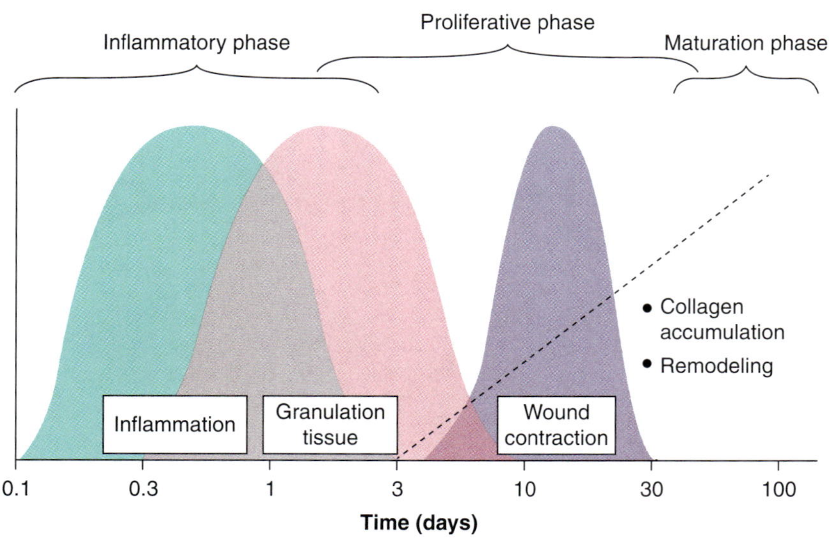

FIGURE 6.3: The three stages of tissue healing.

Source: From Ref. (17). Mautner K, Malanga G, Colberg R. Optimization of ingredients, procedures and rehabilitation for platelet-rich plasma injections for chronic tendinopathy. *Pain Manag*. 2011;1(6):523–532.

in the native tissue. Scar tissue is often functionally weaker and less physiologically capable compared to the native tissue. The potential of the body to heal with regenerated native tissue, without scarring, has become possible with the use of orthobiologics, followed by an appropriate rehabilitation program (17).

Healing potential is determined by the tissue location in the body. During the inflammatory phase, blood serves as the medium to deliver the nutrients and growth factors required for the healing process to begin. Different organs of the body are found to have varying levels of blood supply. Some structures have very little vascular supply, such as articular surfaces and tendons. For example, tendons have minimal blood vessels, nerve supply, or lymphatic system to facilitate cellular regeneration after puberty. This leads to poor healing potential; but with PRP and stem cell therapy, studies have shown the ability to augment the body's natural healing processes of injured tendons (17,18).

Most tissues in the human body have the common thread of the acute inflammatory cascade. However, with the initiation of the body's natural healing process, each organ has its unique intrinsic healing mechanism that modulates the

proliferative and maturation phases (19). For example, bone fractures aim for achieving early restoration of strength and stability through the fracture site (20). During the proliferative phase, the cells of the periosteum in the proximal edge of the fracture and the fibroblasts in the granulation tissue convert into chondroblasts and form hyaline cartilage. During this time, the periosteal cells in the distal edge of the fracture convert into osteoblasts. These two different cellular tissues merge over the fracture gap and convert into the lamellar bone, which is commonly described as the early callus formation. This provides early stabilization of the fracture site. During the maturation phase, the lamellar bone converts to trabecular bone, and later to compact bone, which ultimately restores the bone's full strength (21).

Contrary to this, tendon strains and tears undergo a similar inflammatory phase but have different cells regulating the proliferation and maturation phase to achieve goals oriented toward restoring the tissues' native properties. After a tendon strain or tear, the tendon cellularity increases, fibroblasts infiltrate, and a large quantity of type III collagen is laid down (20%–30%) during the proliferative phase to fill in the residual defect in the injured tendon (22). These

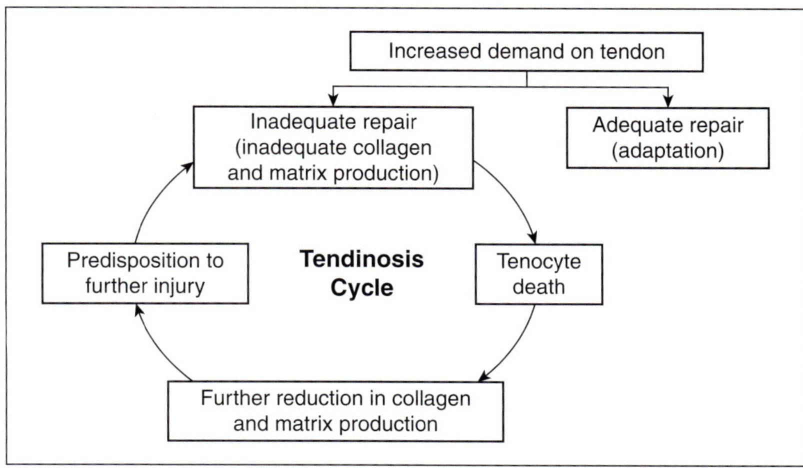

FIGURE 6.4: Development of a chronic tendinopathy due to inadequate tendon repair and restoration of healthy tissue architecture. The theoretical tendinosis cycle. An increased demand on the tendon leads to inadequate collagen repair, tenocyte death, reduction of collagen production, and further injury.

Source: Adapted from Ref. (23). Leadbetter WB. Cell-matrix response in tendon injury. *Clin Sports Med.* 1992;11(3):533–578.

changes in the tendon allow for increased elasticity in the tendon to allow early movement. At the same time, type III collagen has decreased strength, so the tendon is susceptible to a retear (24). Eventually, during the maturation phase, the tendon decreases the type III collagen to less than 1% and replaces it with type I collagen to reestablish its native physiologic properties to withstand tensile loading (25). Impaired progress in the maturation phase leads to a chronic tendinopathy as shown in Figure 6.4.

The healing cascade may be impaired if the injured tissue remains in the inflammatory and proliferative stages, as seen in osteoarthritis, which promotes persistent cartilage breakdown by chronically releasing free radicals and activating proinflammatory mediators, such as matrix metalloproteinases and cytokines, and cannot enter the maturation phase to restore the joint intrinsic physiologic properties. The joint is not able to enter the maturation phase typically because of detrimental biomechanical properties such as joint instability and excessive weight-bearing pressure as seen with obesity. This leads to persistent synovial hypertrophy with neovascularization, among the other changes, which clinically manifests as joint pain, synovial joint effusion, loss of range of motion, and impaired function.

Tissue Regeneration and Orthobiologics

The concept of tissue regeneration with orthobiologics refers to treatments that facilitate the healing of degenerated tissue using biologic products that stimulate regenerating the native tissue back to a fully functional healthy tissue, as opposed to stimulating wound repair with fibrotic scar tissue that does not have the physiologic properties of the native tissue. For example, a tendon tear treated with orthobiologic products would be optimally stimulated to regenerate the tenocytes and extracellular matrix, so that it can recover its physiologic properties and be able to withstand full tensile loading (26). Similarly, a degenerated disc could be stimulated to rehydrate the nucleus pulposus and strengthen the annulus fibrosus, so that it can restore its compressible properties (27). In other cases, orthobiologic treatments are used to reverse degenerative processes, even if the new tissue cannot be stimulated to fully regenerate, as is the case with cartilage in osteo-arthritis (28,29). Biologic products harvested from the patient's own body have been studied the most.

PRP has been applied as a treatment to improve pain and the function of chronic tendinopathies and cartilage pathology for more than a decade. It was first used in the United States in 1987 to facilitate wound healing after cardiac surgery (30). The early successful applications included periodontal and wound healing. During the 1990s, the machines were large and expensive, and were used mainly in hospital operating rooms. Later in the 2000s, smaller machines were introduced making use of PRP more practical for the outpatient office setting. In 2006, Mishra and Pavelko published a study on the efficacy of PRP in recalcitrant lateral epicondylitis and since then, the role of PRP in sports medicine has increased (31). More recently, mesenchymal stem cells (MSCs) have been introduced for the treatment of joint and other pathologies because of their higher concentration of various tissue-healing components such as progenitor cells, growth factors, and cytokines (28,32). These biologic treatments provide great hope for a new standard for orthopedic management centered on enhanced tissue healing by facilitating the body's own healing response, as opposed to surgically replacing the injured tissue with artificial prosthetics, such as joint replacements (18).

BASICS OF PRP THERAPY

PRP therapy aims to provide a favorable environment to recruit progenitor cells to orchestrate the interaction of cytokines and growth factors to stimulate the natural healing response for the successful healing and return of normal strength, range of motion, and function of the injured tissue (19). PRP is defined as any sample of autologous blood that is processed to obtain a plasma sample with platelet concentrations more than the baseline blood values (33). PRP therapy involves the injection of this platelet concentrate, rich in growth factors and nutrients,

to enhance the natural healing response of an injured tissue (34).

Platelets are formed from megakaryocytes that originate in the bone marrow. They contain 30 bioactive proteins that play a role in hemostasis and tissue healing. Platelets initiate all wound healing by actively secreting seven fundamental protein growth factors: insulin-like growth factor-I (IGF-I), transforming growth factor beta (TGFβ), vascular endothelial growth factor (VEGF), platelet-derived growth factor (PDGF), basic fibroblast growth factor (bFGF), epidermal growth factor (EGF), and connective tissue growth factor (CTGF). The first five listed play an essential role in the healing of injured musculoskeletal tissue (35,36) (Table 6.1). These growth factors are found within the platelets in alpha and dense granules that fuse to the cell membrane and secrete these growth factors, which then activate to their bioactive state (35,37).

These growth factors are involved in the different stages of the inflammatory process and are influenced by signaling proteins of the affected tissues. Early in the inflammatory process, IGF-1 is important in the anabolic effects including protein synthesis, enhancing collagen, and matrix synthesis. TGFβ is a proinflammatory immunosuppressant that aids in cell migration, expression of collagen, and helps control angiogenesis and fibrosis. The role of PDGF is to help the proliferation of other growth factors by attracting stem cells and white blood cells to facilitate tissue remodeling (Figure 6.5). PDGF-ββ is not found in extracellular plasma, and therefore is a useful biomarker of how effectively platelets are activated and release their cytokines (38). Later in the inflammatory phase, VEGF and FGF promote angiogenesis and neovascularization. Basic FGF also appears to help in the regulation of cell migration and stimulate endothelial cells to produce granulation tissue. All these growth factors work together as the chemical mediators that influence the cell migration and proliferation vital to regenerative tissue repair (39).

TABLE 6.1 Fundamental Growth Factors of the Healing

Growth Factor	Biological Actions
IGF-I	Anabolic effects including protein synthesis, enhancing collagen, and matrix synthesis in the early inflammatory phase
PDGF (αβ)	Assists in the proliferation of growth factors by attracting stem cells and progenitor cells to stimulate tissue remodeling
TGF (α-β)	A pro-inflammatory immunosuppressant that aids in cell migration, expression of collagen, and helps control angiogenesis and fibrosis
VEGF	Promotes angiogenesis and neovascularization in the late inflammatory phase
FGF	Promotes angiogenesis and neovascularization, and appears to help in the regulation of cell migration and stimulate endothelial cells to produce granulation tissue during the late inflammatory phase

FGF, fibroblast growth factor; IGF-I, insulin-like growth factor-I; PDGF, platelet-derived growth factor; TGF, transforming growth factor; VEGF, vascular endothelial growth factor;

Source: Adapted from Refs. (35,38).

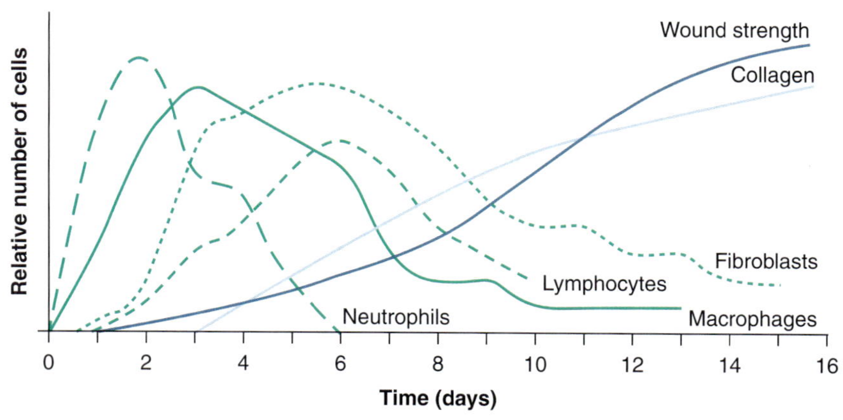

FIGURE 6.5: White blood cells' activity during the inflammatory phase.

Source: From Ref. (17). Mautner K, Malanga G, Colberg R. Optimization of ingredients, procedures and rehabilitation for platelet-rich plasma injections for chronic tendinopathy. *Pain Manag.* 2011;1(6):523–532.

Preparation of PRP

There are various methods of preparing the PRP, and they differ mainly in the technique used to separate the blood components, the number of platelets in the final product, and the concentration of other blood components in the PRP concentrate. First, the technique used to separate the blood components and produce the PRP varies between machines and PRP kits. Depending on the manufacturer, different machines use a syringe or a container to mix the whole blood at ambient temperature. In addition, each manufacturer has specific recommendations with regards to which anticoagulant to use, such as sodium citrate, or anticoagulant citrate dextrose (ACD), or other anticoagulants that bind to calcium, to prevent the initiation of the coagulation cascade and clotting during the preparation process. There is no conclusive evidence that one anticoagulant is superior than the others (19).

Blood drawn from the patient is centrifuged until the various cellular components separate according to their cellular weight, with the red blood cells (RBC) precipitating to the bottom, the white blood cells (WBC) and platelets in the middle ("buffy coat"), and the remaining acellular plasma (platelet poor plasma) on top (Figure 6.6). The middle level of the plasma in which the platelet cells concentrate is called the "PRP layer," constituting a concentration of platelets and their growth factors. This layer is removed and then injected into the target tissue. Depending on the centrifugation machine and its centrifugation properties, different concentrations of the various cellular components are obtained (38).

There are variations in the centrifugal acceleration of the machine and the maximum speed obtained in each machine, referred to as the "relative centrifugal force" (RCF). There is no

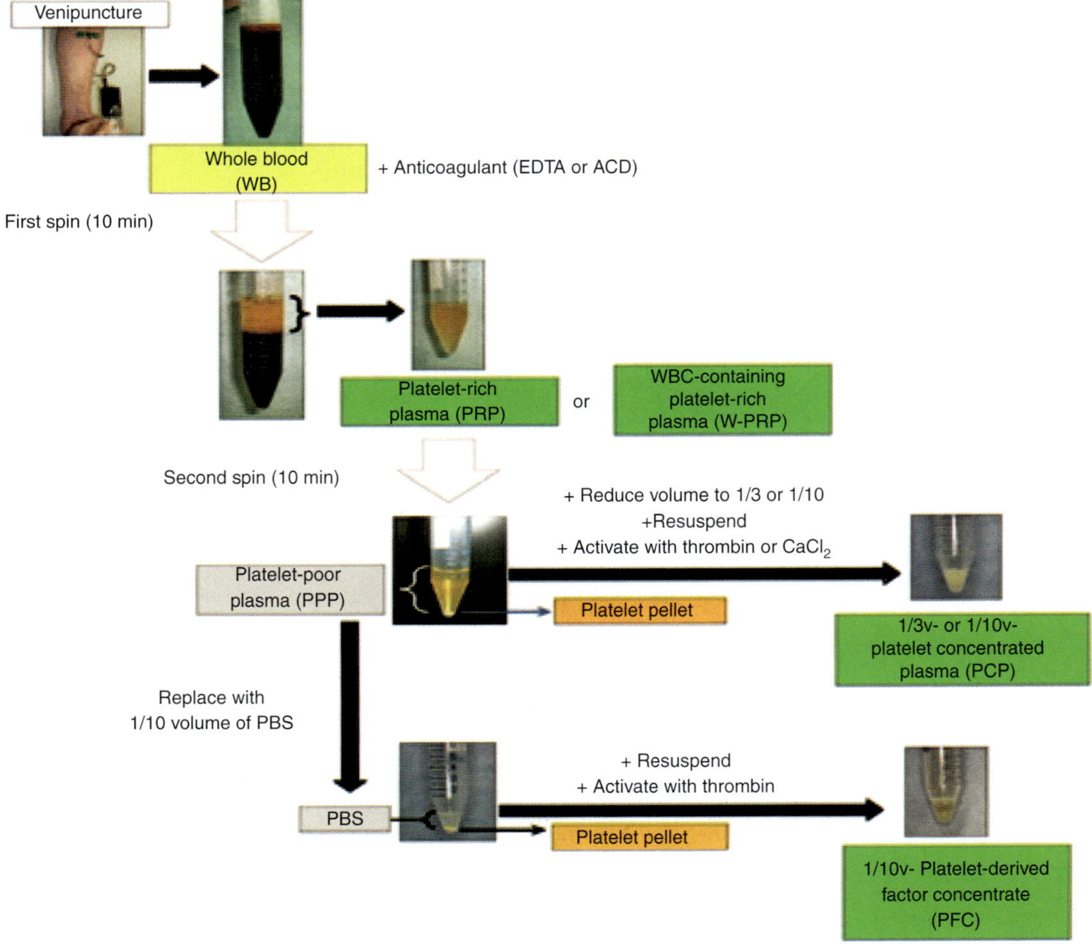

FIGURE 6.6: Flow chart for the preparation process of PRP using the plasma-based method.

PBS, phosphate buffered saline; PCP, platelet concentrated plasma; PFC, platelet-derived factor concentrate; PPP, platelet-poor plasma; W-PRP, WBC and plasma-rich plasma.

Source: Adapted from Ref. (38). Araki J , Jona M , Eto H , et al. Optimized preparation method of platelet-concentrated plasma and noncoagulating platelet-derived factor concentrates: maximization of platelet concentration and removal of fibrinogen. *Tissue Eng Part C Methods*. 2012;18(3):176–185.

consensus to the ideal RCF for obtaining the optimal PRP product, with machines creating a centrifugal force ranging from 70 × g to 3,000 × g (×g = multiples of the Earth's gravitational field). The RCF is directly dependent on the centrifugation speed created by the machine, measured in revolutions per minute (rpm), which ranges from 1,200 to 6,300 rpm, and averages 3,600 rpm in most commercial machines (35,38).

Araki showed that the most efficient collection of leukocyte-rich PRP containing the greatest amount of WBC and platelets was at 70 g for 10 minutes (38). Centrifugation at a slow speed separates the RBC from the rest of the blood product. However, to obtain the optimum recovery of platelets in a leukocyte poor preparation, a second spin at greater than 3,000 g for 10 minutes is performed to separate the WBC from the platelets. Some machines simply do one centrifugation at a higher speed and separate all the blood components at the same time. The main limitation to a single spin technique is that it is less effective in separating the platelets and white blood cells; hence, a leukocyte-rich PRP product is typically obtained with higher platelet concentrations. Average platelet yields from single spin kits and double-spin kits are listed in Table 6.2 (38,40).

Although directly related to the centrifugation speed and the number of spins, there is a difference in the concentration of platelets in the final PRP product obtained from various machines (40). Average platelet concentrations in the blood ranges from 150,000 to 450,000 µL. Normal variations may occur even in the same patient depending on his or her hydration status, time of day, and normal physiologic variations (41). Some machines produce a low concentration (two to three times the baseline concentration), and other machines produce a higher concentration (five to nine times the baseline concentration), depending on the amount of blood obtained and the shape of the container used to centrifuge the blood (Table 6.2). On an average, 1 mL of PRP is obtained for every 8 to 10 mL of WB (33).

There is a debate about what the optimal platelet concentration should be. Early studies suggested that a low platelet concentration was optimal, ranging at around 2.5×, and that higher

TABLE 6.2 Comparison of Commercial PRP Manufacturers

Lower Yield Platelet Count (2.5–3× Baseline)	Higher Yield Platelet Count (4–9× Baseline)
Arthrex ACP (2–3×)	Biomet GPS II and III (3–8×)
Cascade PRP therapy (1.0–1.5×)	Harvest SmartPrep 2 APC + (4–6×)
PRGF by Boitech Institute Spain (2–3×)	ArterioCyte-Medtronic Magellan (3–7×)
Regen PRP Switzerland	Emcyte Pure PRP II 2015 (~7×)
	Arthrex Angel (4×)
	Clear PRP Harvest Terumo with SmartPrep System (5×)

Counts are based off multiples from baseline platelet blood counts.

ACP, autologous conditioned plasma; GPS, gravitational platelet separation; PRP, platelet-rich plasma.

Source: From Ref. (33). Mazzocca AD, McCarthy MB, Chowaniec DM, et al. The positive effects of different platelet-rich plasma methods on human muscle, bone, and tendon cells. *Am J Sports Med.* 2012;40(8):1742–1749.

concentrations would be detrimental to the healing process (42,43). Further studies that were looking in depth into the optimal platelet concentration determined that a platelet concentration of at least 1.2 million (4× baseline) is required for an accelerated wound healing. This effect on soft tissue wound healing was initially demonstrated by Giusti on cultured endothelial cells where less than 1.5 million/µL produced less growth in vitro and a platelet concentration greater than 3 million (10× baseline) showed inhibition (44). These results were later duplicated by Kevy et al. in 2010 (45). In addition, work by Haynesworth showed that an accelerated wound healing was reached around this level of 4 to 5× baseline, and was correlated with an exponential recruitment of MSCs (46). Of note, a stand-alone machine cannot make a platelet concentration so high that the activated growth factors would cause inhibition of the wound healing. Giusti did demonstrate that platelet counts greater than 2 million/μL were detrimental to tenocyte behavior; therefore it has been proposed that 1 to1.5 million platelets per μL would be ideal in the treatment of wounds and chronic tendinopathies (17).

Platelet concentrations that are favorable for intra-articular treatments have lower yield platelet counts; this is most likely because these PRP products also typically have low leukocyte and RBC counts (40,47). It has been shown in cultured synoviocytes that leukocyte-rich PRP causes increased inflammatory markers compared to leukocyte poor PRP (48,49). Although there continues to be a paucity of high-quality clinical studies of intra-articular PRP applications, there is sufficient data to suggest leukocyte poor PRP is most suitable for these injections (47).

As implied earlier, platelets and WBC are found subsequent to each other after centrifuging the WB, with WBC being only slightly heavier than platelets and with an overlap of their specific gravities. Hence, a PRP device that harvests a higher concentration of platelets inevitably obtains part of the WBC concentrate and produces a leukocyte rich PRP, and a technique that yields a lower platelet concentrate produces a leukocyte poor PRP.

The therapeutic value of the presence versus absence of leukocytes in the PRP remains unclear. It is important to recognize the different types of WBCs including neutrophils, monocytes/macrophages, and lymphocytes, and their role in tissue healing and inflammation. The arguments in favor of leukocyte poor PRP are centered on the fact that granulocytes such as neutrophils contain tissue–degenerating enzymes like matrix metalloproteinases (MMPs), interleukins, and other proinflammatory mediators that may be detrimental to the healing response of the injured tissue (50–53).

On the other hand, granulocytes are present at a lower percentage in PRP versus WB (24.46% vs 65.22%), and their presence may be outweighed by the beneficial effects of other leukocyte types for chronic, uncontrolled inflammatory conditions (17,40). In chronic tendinopathy, the phagocytic properties of macrophages may be beneficial in removing debris. The M1 versus M2 properties of macrophages can also assist with balancing the proinflammatory versus the antiinflammatory aspects of healing. Lymphocytes modulate cell-to-cell interactions and modulate healing (54). Nonetheless, the healing process is so complex that it seems that WBCs are more beneficial in soft tissue injuries such as chronic tendinosis, but detrimental in intra-articular pathologies such as arthritis (19).

Some PRP preparation systems are not effective in fully removing all RBCs. RBCs significantly alter the inflammatory process, potentially causing a detrimental effect in the tissue injected. For example, RBCs are believed to be chondrotoxic and potentially lead to cartilage death and advancement of degenerative joint disease (55,56). The best example for the negative effects of whole blood on cartilage is the significant arthropathy experienced by patients with hemophilia who have suffered recurrent hemarthrosis (57,58). Similar findings have been seen in patients with traumatic joint injuries with secondary hemarthrosis (55). Mazzocca in 2012 showed that all PRP preparations had far lower RBCs than whole blood (4.1 ± 0.4 ×106), but the single spin low platelet concentration (378.3 ± 58.64 ×103/μL platelets) and double spin PRP (447.7 ± 44.0 103/μL platelets) preparation had significantly lower RBCs than the single spin high platelet concentration PRP (1.0 ± 1.4 ×106/μL RBC, 873.8 ±207.82 ×103/μL platelets) (40).

Activators also influence the PRP product and are highly debated. The common activators that are used include: thrombin, calcium, and collagen, ordered from fastest to slowest. Activators differ in the extent of platelet activation. The argument in favor of activators is based on the concept that activating the alpha and the dense granules in platelets to quickly release the growth factors may lead to a quicker healing response (59,60). On the contrary, a slow and sustained release of growth factors as the injected platelets interact with the patient's own collagen creates a more physiologic and "normal" healing response. In addition, there is concern that the extrinsic activators may cause the platelets to release all the growth factors before the injured tissue is stimulated to begin its healing response and lead to a weaker effect (61). Sustained release of growth factors may be achieved with synthetic peptides and include recombinant human thrombin that are now available (62).

Finally, the pH of the environment and anticoagulant used in the PRP preparation may influence the healing process. Medications such as the sodium citrate or ACD that are used as anticoagulant, and lidocaine or bupivacaine used for local anesthesia may create a slightly more acidic environment (63,64). Sodium bicarbonate may be used to buffer the solution to a more neutral pH (31). However, wounds are thought to develop an acidic environment themselves, which later balances toward a neutral pH (65,66). In addition, platelets release higher concentrations of platelet-derived growth factors in an acidic environment (67). Sodium citrate is considered the optimal anticoagulant as it has the highest platelet recovery as well as mesenchymal stromal cell proliferation when compared to ACD and EDTA (68). Therefore, PRP may benefit from the slightly more acidic environment created with the injected additional medications.

In summary, various factors may influence the effectiveness of the final PRP product. Mautner et al. proposed that the ideal PRP concentrate should include a leukocyte-rich product with a slightly acidic pH; however, no activators should be included. In addition, the injection should be performed under ultrasound guidance to ensure placement of the PRP in the correct tissue. In addition, an appropriate rehabilitation protocol should be prescribed together with the PRP therapy to enhance the healing process, stimulate the tissue to progress from the proliferative to the maturation phases efficiently, and ultimately restore the normal physiologic function (17) (Table 6.3).

Multiple PRP preparation methods are currently marketed and used in clinical practice with different machines and PRP preparation kits, as mentioned previously (Table 6.2).

This has led to individual differences between methods and kits that have resulted in preparations with varying volumes and concentrations of platelets and leukocytes, which has caused inconsistent clinical results in the clinical trials and difficulty in creating a consensus about the benefits of PRP and the optimal preparation (69–71). This discrepancy in the preparation methods led to the necessity of standardizing the PRP preparations and concentrations when analyzing both clinical and research outcomes.

There have been various classification systems put forward that center around the volume and activation of PRP, as well as the actual concentration of platelets, WBCs, and RBCs (72–74). In 2015, Mautner et al. introduced in the *PM&R* journal the PLRA classification system, which stands for platelet count, leukocyte count, RBC count, and use of the activation factor (75). PLRA helps clearly describe the four main components to characterize PRP. The platelet count is the absolute number of platelets per μL, which accounts for both the patient's baseline cell count and volume obtained or injected into the tissue. Leukocyte concentration, which includes neutrophils, is delineated by being greater or lesser than 1%. RBC concentration is also distinguished by being greater or lesser than 1%. Finally, it is important to state the use of any exogenous activating agents such as calcium chloride, synthetic peptides, or thrombin at the time of the PRP injection. The classification of PRP has become necessary in clinical and laboratory studies to standardize the exact orthobiologic product used so that the researchers can compare outcomes among the various studies, as well as among the various subjects included within a same study.

Basics of Stem Cell Therapy

The therapeutic and regenerative possibilities of stem cell treatments have great potential and have garnered significant media attention in the last decade. The definition of a stem cell is an undifferentiated cell of a multicellular organism

TABLE 6.3 Rehabilitation Protocol After PRP Therapy

Phase	Time	Restrictions	Rehabilitation
Phase I: Tissue protection	Days 0–3	Consider NWB or protected WB for lower extremity procedures, especially if in pain. No weight training, avoid NSAIDs and use limited ice	Relative rest. Activities as tolerated; avoid excess loading or stress to treated area. Gentle AROM
Phase II: Early tissue healing; facilitation of collagen deposition	Days 4–14	Progress to FWB without protective device. Avoid NSAIDs	Light activities to provide motion to tendon; aerobic exercise that avoids loading of the treated tendon. Gentle prolonged stretching. Begin treatment on kinetic chain/adjacent regions. Glutei strengthening and core strengthening
	Weeks 2–6	Avoid eccentric exercises. Avoid NSAIDs. Avoid ice	Progress to WB activities. Low weight, high repetition isometrics (pain scale <3/10). OKC activities. Soft tissue work to tendon with CFM, IASTM, and "dynamic" stretching
Phase III: Collagen strengthening	Weeks 6–12	–	Eccentric exercises (keep pain scale <3/10). Two sets of 15 repetitions. CKC activities. Plyometrics; proprioceptive training, and other sport-specific exercises. Progress to WB activities and consider return to sport, if pain scale is less than 3/10
	Months 3+	Reassess improvement; if not more than 75% improved consider repeat injection and return to phase I	Progress back to functional sport-specific activities with increasing load on tendon as pain allows

AROM, active range of motion; CFM, cross-frictional massage; CKC, closed kinetic chain; FWB, full weight bearing; IASTM, instrument-assisted soft tissue mobilization; NWB, non-weight bearing; OKC, open kinetic chain; PRP, platelet-rich plasma; WB, weight bearing.

Source: Republished with permission of Future Medicine Ltd., from Ref. (17). Mautner K, Malanga G, Colberg R. Optimization of ingredients, procedures and rehabilitation for platelet-rich plasma injections for chronic tendinopathy. *Pain Manag*. 2011;1(6):523–532; permission conveyed through Copyright Clearance Center, Inc.

that can give rise to more cells of a particular differentiated cell type (Webster's). Stem cell biologic products arise from many sources including: aborted fetal brains, human embryos created in laboratories or left over in clinics while performing in vitro fertilization, amniotic membrane or chorion from donated placentas, spinal cord tissue, hematopoetic cells, immortalized stem cell lines (from human teratocarcinoma), adipose tissue, umbilical cord blood, and harvested autologous cells from bone marrow and adipose tissue.

The unparalleled interest in research comes from its pluripotency, or the ability to differentiate from undifferentiated cells into specific cells from all three germ layers. This unique property gives hope to restore function to all major organ systems. However, the source of these cells and applications are highly controversial.

Multipotent stem cells are derived from adult cells, and unlike the pluripotent cells, have a limited capacity to differentiate into preferred cell types. They are found in bone marrow, hair follicle, adipose tissue, and intestinal villus crypt. Despite their limitations compared to pluripotent cells, they retain an affinity to differentiate into cartilage, adipose tissue, and bone cells. The examples of multipotent stem cells are bone marrow-derived MSCs, hematopoietic cells, adipose cells, and umbilical cord blood cells (76).

Mesenchymal Stem Cells

MSC treatments have certainly come a long way since the time of Aristotle when the use of bone marrow was described for restorative treatments (77). Applications in orthopedics have garnered much interest since the late 1980s, much like PRP. There have been high hopes for the potential of stem cell treatments given that, in stem cell therapy, the progenitor cells are directly injected into the damaged tissue and they could potentially differentiate into the native tissue. This differs from PRP where the platelets are injected in order for the high concentration of growth factors to stimulate the injured tissue to heal. Throughout the 1990s, Connolly and others identified the value of autologous bone marrow harvesting and injecting into the treated tissue to optimize the outcomes of surgical treatments such as spinal fusions (78). In addition, bone marrow transplants have been used by hematologists for more than 50 years after studies showed that patients with hematologic diseases could recover by getting donated healthy bone marrow (79). Autologous bone marrow stem cells have been thought of in three different classifications for research: nucleated cell isolates, isolated MSC, and isolated MSC with culture expansion (80).

Adult stem cells have two classifications: hematopoietic stem cells that give rise to blood products and MSCs that give rise to nearly all other peripheral tissues including bone, marrow, brain, dermis, periosteum, skeletal muscle, synovium, and trabecular bone (81,82). The mesengenic process, initially proposed in the 1980s, suggested a path through which MSCs differentiate into these mesodermal cell types (Figure 6.7). It was thought that MSCs differentiate into mesodermal cell types that fabricated bone, cartilage, and muscle. However, it is now clear that pericytes and perivascular cells give rise to MSCs that can be isolated from many different tissues.

Bone marrow–derived MSCs are commonly called "bone marrow aspirate concentrate" (BMAC). BMAC stem cells are heterogeneous, but differentiate into two main categories: osteogenic pathway and immunomodulatory/trophic pathway. At the site of a broken or inflamed blood vessel, a pericyte detaches from the vascular wall and becomes an activated MSC. An example of the MSCs' immunomodulatory effects is in the treatment of graft-versus-host disease where they help dampen an aggressive immune response by secreting bioactive agents (84). MSCs also exhibit "trophic" effects at the damaged site. They do this in several ways including: inhibiting apoptosis due to ischemia, inhibiting scar formation, secreting large amounts of VEGF to promote angiogenesis that stimulates some MSCs to transform back to pericytes to support capillary walls, and secreting tissue progenitor specific mitogens to regenerate tissue (85). Through these mechanisms, the body has the potential to regenerate tissue and heal itself (84). As the body ages, the quantity of MSCs in the bone marrow naturally drops. There is an approximate 10-fold decrease between birth and adolescence, with another 10-fold drop before middle age (80).

In addition to bone marrow-derived MSCs, adipose-derived MSCs and peripheral blood stem cells (PBSCs) have also been studied in orthopedic treatments (84). Adipose-derived MSCs lack TGFβ type 1 receptor and have reduced bone morphogenetic protein (BMP)-2, BMP-4, and BMP-6, when compared to bone marrow derived MSCs. To stimulate chondrogenic differentiation

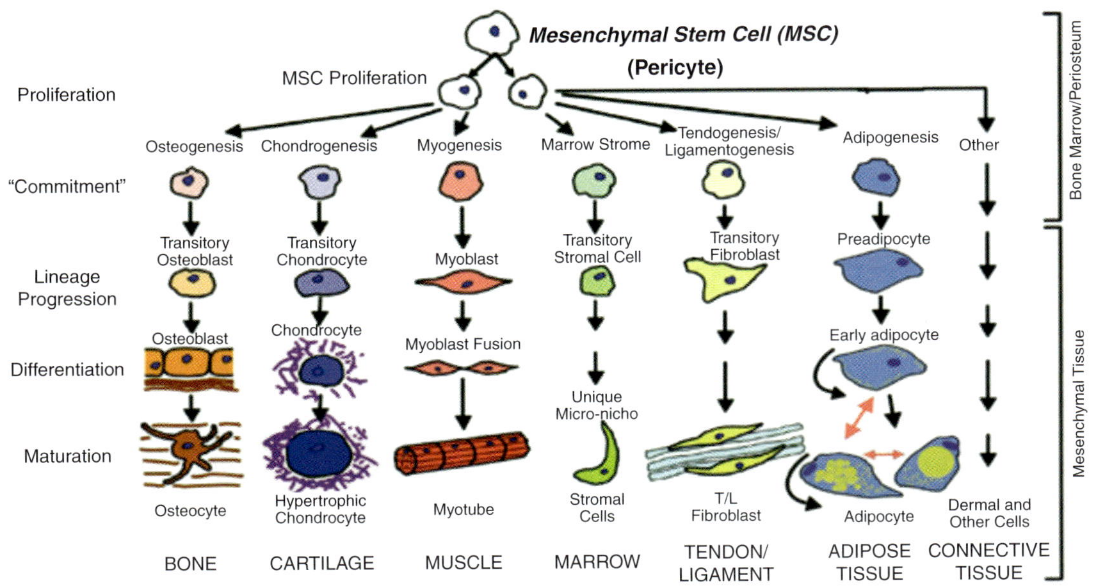

FIGURE 6.7: The Mesengenic process.

Source: From Ref. (83). DiMarino AM, Caplan AI, Bonfield TL. Mesenchymal stem cells in tissue repair. *Front Immunol.* 2013;4,201.

in adipose-derived MSCs, it is necessary to increase BMP-6, which is more potent than TGFβ in this transformation (86). Proponents of using adipose stem cell tissue over bone marrow favor its relative ease of harvest, higher cell yield, increased angiogenic capability, and resistance to age-related decline in proliferative potential and cellular function (87,88). However, the process to separate the stem cells from the adipose cells is difficult and requires enzymatic digestion of the aspirated adipose tissue. Currently, this enzymatic digestion is prohibited by the FDA (U.S. Food and Drug Administration) because it is considered "more than minimal" manipulation of the cells (89,90).

The harvesting process for obtaining autologous MSCs carries less ethical debate than the embryonic stem cell sources, and is obtained by relatively safe procedures. Hematology-oncology specialists have long used bone marrow aspiration for the diagnosis and treatment of multiple conditions. The technical issues regarding bone marrow aspiration are covered in detail in another chapter in this textbook (89).

Adipose-derived stem cells have also been used for a variety of orthopedic conditions. To obtain adipose stem cells, a low volume liposuction procedure is performed with the goal of obtaining 12 to 20 mL of liquefied adipose (traditional liposuction yields 100 mL to >3 L). Specific technical issues regarding obtaining and processing adipose tissue for orthopedic conditions are also discussed in the chapter by Bowen et al. (Chapter 12).

As previously discussed, the FDA tightly regulates the process of bone marrow and adipose aspiration, and even scrutinizes the number of steps performed under the "minimal manipulation" standards, which excludes separation with collagenase. Specific brands have different processing techniques (Table 6.4). To date, there have been no high-quality studies that support the use of one kit over the others (89).

PBSCs obtained through apheresis have been used by the hematology-oncology specialists for more than 20 years for stem cell transplantation (91). Comparison of bone-marrow MSCs and PBSCs demonstrate similar trophic and proliferative abilities, but also hold promise in that they

TABLE 6.4 Bone Marrow Aspiration Spin Rates

Company/ Product	Volume	Spin No.1 × Time	Spin No. 2 × Time
-	60 mL	3,600 rpm × 10 min	N/A
PureBMC	75 mL	3,800 rpm × 2.5 min	3,800 rpm × 5 min
Arteriocyte	30–60 mL	2,800 (610 g) × 4 min	3,800 rpm × 6 min
Celling Technologies	Not stated	3,200 rpm × 12 min	N/A

G force is consistent among centrifuges, but RPMs vary based on radius of centrifuge.

Source: From Ref. (89). Bowen JE . Technical issues in harvesting and concentrating stem cells (bone marrow and adipose). *PMR*. 2015;7(4 Suppl):S8–S18, with permission from Elsevier.

share more similarities with embryonic stem cells. In this way, they are more immature than bone-marrow MSCs so they can differentiate into more cells types as well as express transcription factors like embryonic stem cells (92,93).

The capacity of stem cells to differentiate into the native injured tissue treated remains a topic of debate. In muscle injuries treated with stems cells, there is a sparse amount of studies, of which most are on animal models (19). Bacou showed that 3-month-old white rabbits had significant improvement in the force generated and cross sectional area in the injured tibialis anterior muscle 2 months after an injection of adipose tissue stromal cells compared to placebo (94). Winkler showed promising results in muscular dystrophy models where dystrophin improved after the systemic delivery of stem cells (95). Specifically, basic fibroblast growth factor, insulin-like growth factor, and nerve growth factors have been identified as cytokines capable of enhancing muscle regeneration (96).

Despite ligament injuries being quite common, there is limited knowledge on the basic science of cell differentiation toward developing ligamentous tissue. Therefore, the studies that are investigating orthobiologics on ligaments are extremely limited (19). Thus the most promising results, so far, have been with a process called "coculture." This is where stem cells are cultured together with the targeted mature cells. In New Zealand, white rabbits' anterior cruciate ligament (ACL) fibroblasts were successfully cocultured with MSCs on a bio-scaffold that could differentiate after 2 weeks (97). This area of research continues to be important given the rate of ligament injuries in sports. For example, ACL reconstructions can be complicated by ligament laxity with the use of allograft or autograft (98). Developing a technique in which stem cells could regenerate an ACL to repair a tear would be a major "game changer" in the treatment of these injuries.

Stem cell treatment trials for tendinopathies are relatively numerous as compared to muscle, ligament, and bone (19). In 2013, an equine model where bone marrow-derived MSCs were injected into the superficial digital flexor tendon (similar to Achilles tendon) of 12 horses that had sustained natural injuries compared to a placebo injection of saline demonstrated that those treated with bone marrow-derived MSCs had greater elasticity, reduced cross sectional area, and improved collagen organization (99).

Skin-derived fibroblast have also been used for chronic tendinopathy. In a study of 12 patients with refractory lateral epicondylitis, a prospective pilot study was performed with collagen-producing tenocyte-like cells derived from skin fibroblasts that were injected under ultrasound guidance. At 6 months, there were no adverse events with any patients, and 11 out of 12 of them had notable improvement on tissue structure that could be seen on ultrasound (81). Another study showed that skin-derived tenocyte-like cells suspended in autologous plasma after culture for 4 weeks were more effective in treatment of patellar tendinopathies as compared to autologous blood alone (n = 40). The metrics studied were the rate of improvement in pain and functional mobility at up to 6 months (100).

With regards to cartilage disorders, stem cell therapy is a hot topic as researchers seek to understand the role of stem cells in regulating the pathomechanics of acute and chronic cartilage injuries. Articular cartilage lesions, including degenerative joint disease, show impaired healing by catabolic reactions, as described earlier (Figure 6.2). The chronic inflammatory state causes chondrocyte apoptosis by the persistent activation of proteolytic enzymes secondary to an increase in the activity of pro-inflammatory cytokines (interleukin [IL] 1a, IL-1, and tumor necrosis factor-α) and a decrease in the activity of the antiinflammatory cytokines (IL-4, IL-10, and IL-1ar) (102–104). Stem cells are believed to have an antiinflammatory effect, as well as a proliferative effect, given their secretory, immunomodulatory, pro-angiogenic, antiapoptotic, and antifibrotic properties (13,28).

Case series studies have shown promising outcomes in patients treated with bone marrow-derived MSCs for chondral lesions as well as osteoarthritis, specifically with regards to improvement in pain scores and function (28,104). For example, a case series on 41 patients with osteoarthritis treated with MSCs from the bone marrow and the adipose tissue combined and followed for 1 year after the injection showed an average 50% improvement in pain scores and functional scales, with better outcomes in the mild to moderate osteoarthritis cases, as defined by the radiographic Kellgren Lawrence Grading system (105). A systematic review of the literature published from 1980 to 2015 reported overall "good" to "excellent" outcomes with BMAC injections for the treatment of knee osteoarthritis and chondral defects, and low complications rates (106). Randomized controlled trials and further meta-analysis studies are needed to fully understand the potential of MSCs as a treatment option for patients with cartilage disorders.

ETHICAL CONSIDERATIONS

Over the last few decades, the field of regenerative medicine has become intertwined with ethical controversy, increasing FDA regulations, and significant media hype. Ethical considerations became evident when life itself was questioned with a study that used 3-day-old embryos in the blastocyst stage as the source for pluripotent stem cells (76). In 2006, Takahashi and Yamanaka discovered how to make induced pluripotent stem cells (iPSCs) from adult autologous skin cells (107). This study put an end to the major ethical dilemma around stem cells by proving that pluripotent cells can be harvested from a patient's own body. Furthermore, the growing body of knowledge of the benefits of other forms of stem cells has given hope to many patients. For example, orthopedic applications have relatively hushed the ethical discussions by showing promising results with the use of autologous bone marrow-derived MSCs. Yet, the lack of understanding of the full potential, as well as the concern of the unknown complications that may arise from stimulating a human tissue to regenerate with PRP, MSCs or amniotic stem cells, among others, clearly show that the field of regenerative medicine needs to fully mature with further research studies.

Autologous stem cells avoid the complication of graft versus host disease and were treated as a medical procedure till late 2006 under the 21 CFR 1271 regulation. At this point the FDA changed subtle wording ("another" to "a") to encompass even autologous cells treatment as a drug, and thus subject to undergoing costly, multiphase clinical drug trials. In 2006, "minimal manipulation" regulation under 1271 further limited treatment prospects in the United States, as this vague definition not only prohibited cell expansion, but added stringent guidelines on clinical trials regarding the time and number of steps taken to isolate progenitor cells (108).

Internationally, some countries have reduced the regulatory restrictions of stem cell therapies. For example, Japan permits trials as their version of the FDA has set up a regenerative medicine classification to avoid restrictions that fall upon drug therapies. In the Unites States, "stem cell tourism" is also of concern in given situations such as a child who visited a Moscow stem cell therapy clinic and developed multiple tumors in his brain and spinal cord after treatment. Fortunately, when properly performed, the risks appear to be quite low. For example, Centeno et al. reported that there were no neoplastic complications after the treatment for orthopedic conditions with mesenchymal autologous culture-expanded stem cells in 2011, and no significant treatment related adverse events in 2015 (103,108). Safety concerns and a limited number of high-quality studies among all regenerative therapies warrant extensive patient education and detailed informed consent before considering regenerative treatments (76).

CONCLUSION

The field of regenerative medicine holds much promise for effectively treating acute and chronic musculoskeletal injuries. Important considerations regarding these treatments were reviewed in this chapter. As discussed, conventional therapies such as nonsteroidal antiinflammatories, local analgesics, and corticosteroids offer short-term benefit, but potential long-term detrimental effects. Overall, PRP studies have reported significant benefits for treating muscle, ligament, joint, and especially chronic tendinopathies that have failed conservative treatment. Recently there has been a call to action to standardize PRP research using the PLRA format (19). Autologous stem cell studies are also reporting promising results, especially for treating degenerative conditions. Given the ethical concerns, all regenerative therapy cases warrant thorough patient education and detailed informed consent (76).

ACKNOWLEDGMENT

We would like to thank Isaac Miller, MD, for his contribution to this chapter with the literature review on mesenchymal stem cells.

REFERENCES

1. Khan KM, Cook JL, Bonar F, et al. Histopathology of common tendinopathies: update and implications for clinical management. *Sports Med.* 1999;27(6):393–408.
2. Alfredson H, Lorentzon R. Chronic tendon pain: no signs of chemical inflammation but high concentrations of the neurotransmitter glutamate. Implications for treatment? *Curr Drug Targets.* 2002;3(1):43–54.
3. Rees JD, Wilson AM, Wolman RL. Current concepts in the management of tendon disorders. *Rheumatology (Oxford).* 2006;45(5):508–521.
4. Smidt N, Assendelft WJ, van der Windt DA, et al. Corticosteroid injections for lateral epicondylitis: a systematic review. *Pain.* 2002;96(1–2):23–40.
5. Smidt N, van der Windt DA, Assendelft WJ, et al. Corticosteroid injections, physiotherapy, or a wait-and-see policy for lateral epicondylitis: a randomised controlled trial. *Lancet.* 2002;359(9307):657–662.
6. Coombes BK, Bisset L, Vicenzino B. Efficacy and safety of corticosteroid injections and other injections for management of tendinopathy: a systematic review of randomised controlled trials. *Lancet.* 2010;376(9754):1751–1767.
7. Okcu G, Yercan H, Ozic U. The comparison of single dose versus multi-dose local corticosteroid injections for tennis elbow. *Clin Res.* 2002;13:158–163.
8. Linke E. Achilles tendon ruptures following direct cortisone injection. *Hefte Unfallheilkd.* 1975;(121):302–303.
9. Kumar V, Abbas AK, Fausto N. *Robbins and Cotran Pathologic Basis of Disease,* 7th ed. Philadelphia, PA: Elsevier Saunders 2005.
10. Tsai WC, Hsu CC, Chang HN, et al. Ibuprofen upregulates expressions of matrix metalloproteinase-1, -8, -9, and -13 without affecting expressions of types I and III collagen in tendon cells. *J Orthop Res.* 2010;28(4):487–491.
11. Kleinman M, Gross AE. Achilles tendon rupture following steroid injection. Report of three cases. *J Bone Joint Surg Am.* 1983;65(9):1345–1347.
12. Rees JD, Maffulli N, Cook J. Management of tendinopathy. *Am J Sports Med.* 2009;37(9):1855–1867.
13. Gupta PK, Das AK, Chullikana A, et al. Mesenchymal stem cells for cartilage repair in osteoarthritis. *Stem Cell Res Ther.* 2012;3(4):25.

14. Hollander JL. Intra-articular hydrocortisone in arthritis and allied conditions; a summary of two years' clinical experience. *J Bone Joint Surg Am.* 1953;35-A(4):983–990.

15. Farkas B, Kvell K, Czömpöly T, et al. Increased chondrocyte death after steroid and local anesthetic combination. *Clin Orthop Relat Res.* 2010;468(11):3112–3120.

16. Wernecke C, Braun HJ, Dragoo JL. The effect of intra-articular corticosteroids on articular cartilage: a systematic review. *Orthop J Sports Med.* 2015;3(5). doi:10.1177/2325967115581163

17. Mautner K, Malanga G, Colberg R. Optimization of ingredients, procedures and rehabilitation for platelet-rich plasma injections for chronic tendinopathy. *Pain Manag.* 2011;1(6):523–532.

18. Malanga GA. Regenerative treatments for orthopedic conditions. *PM R.* 2015;7(4 Suppl):S1–S3.

19. Mautner K, Blazuk J. Where do injectable stem cell treatments apply in treatment of muscle, tendon, and ligament injuries? *PM R.* 2015;7(4 Suppl):S33–S40.

20. Tamas N, Scamell BE. Principles of bone and joint injuries and their healing. *Surgery.* 2015;33(1):7–14.

21. Jahagirdar R, Scammell BE. Principles of fracture healing and disorders of bone union. *Surgery.* 2008;27(2):63–69.

22. Sharma P, Maffulli N. Biology of tendon injury: healing, modeling and remodeling. *J Musculoskelet Neuronal Interact.* 2006;6(2):181–190.

23. Leadbetter WB. Cell-matrix response in tendon injury. *Clin Sports Med.* 1992;11(3):533–578.

24. Williams IF, Heaton A, McCullagh KG. Cell morphology and collagen types in equine tendon scar. *Res Vet Sci.* 1980;28(3):302–310.

25. Sharma P, Maffulli N. Tendon injury and tendinopathy: healing and repair. *J Bone Joint Surg Am.* 2005;87(1):187–202.

26. Nguyen RT, Borg-Stein J, McInnis K. Applications of platelet-rich plasma in musculoskeletal and sports medicine: an evidence-based approach. *PM R.* 2011;3(3):226–250.

27. Pettine K, Suzuki R, Sand T, et al. Treatment of discogenic back pain with autologous bone marrow concentrate injection with minimum two year follow-up. *Int Orthop.* 2016;40(1):135–140.

28. Sampson S, Botto-van Bemden A, Aufiero D. Stem cell therapies for treatment of cartilage and bone disorders: osteoarthritis, avascular necrosis, and non-union fractures. *PM R.* 2015;7(4 Suppl):S26–S32.

29. Wang-Saegusa A, Cugat R, Ares O, et al. Infiltration of plasma rich in growth factors for osteoarthritis of the knee: short-term effects on function and quality of life. *Arch Orthop Trauma Surg.* 2011;131(3):311–317.

30. Ferrari M, Zia S, Valbonesi M, et al. A new technique for hemodilution, preparation of autologous platelet-rich plasma and intraoperative blood salvage in cardiac surgery. *Int J Artif Organs.* 1987;10(1):47–50.

31. Mishra A, Pavelko T. Treatment of chronic elbow tendinosis with buffered platelet-rich plasma. *Am J Sports Med.* 2006;34(11):1774–1778.

32. Centeno CJ. Clinical challenges and opportunities of mesenchymal stem cells in musculoskeletal medicine. *PM R.* 2014;6(1):70–77.

33. Mazzocca AD, McCarthy MB, Chowaniec DM, et al. The positive effects of different platelet-rich plasma methods on human muscle, bone, and tendon cells. *Am J Sports Med.* 2012;40(8):1742–1749.

34. Foster TE, Puskas BL, Mandelbaum BR, et al. Platelet-rich plasma: from basic science to clinical applications. *Am J Sports Med.* 2009;37(11):2259–2272.

35. Dhurat R, Sukesh M. Principles and methods of preparation of platelet-rich plasma: a review and author's perspective. *J Cutan Aesthet Surg.* 2014;7(4):189–197.

36. Molloy T, Wang Y, Murrell G. The roles of growth factors in tendon and ligament healing. *Sports Med.* 2003;33(5):381–394.

37. Alsousou J, Thompson M, Hulley P, et al. The biology of platelet-rich plasma and its application in trauma and orthopaedic surgery: a review of the literature. *J Bone Joint Surg Br.* 2009;91(8):987–996.

38. Araki J, Jona M, Eto H, et al. Optimized preparation method of platelet-concentrated plasma and noncoagulating platelet-derived factor concentrates: maximization of platelet concentration and removal of fibrinogen. *Tissue Eng Part C Methods.* 2012;18(3):176–185.

39. Vora A, Borg-Stein J, Nguyen RT. Regenerative injection therapy for osteoarthritis: fundamental concepts and evidence-based review. *PM R.* 2012;4(5 Suppl):S104–S109.

40. Mazzocca AD, McCarthy MB, Chowaniec DM, et al. Platelet-rich plasma differs according to preparation method and human variability. *J Bone Joint Surg Am.* 2012;94(4):308–316.

41. Kevy SV, Jacobson MS. Comparison of methods for point of care preparation of autologous platelet gel. *J Extra Corpor Technol.* 2004;36(1): 28–35.

42. Graziani F, Ivanovski S, Cei S, et al. The *in vitro* effect of different PRP concentrations on osteoblasts and fibroblasts. *Clin Oral Implants Res.* 2006;17(2):212–219.

43. Weibrich G, Hansen T, Kleis W, et al. Effect of platelet concentration in platelet-rich plasma on peri-implant bone regeneration. *Bone.* 2004;34(4):665–671.

44. Giusti I, Rughetti A, D'Ascenzo S, et al. Identification of an optimal concentration of platelet gel for promoting angiogenesis in human endothelial cells. *Transfusion.* 2009;49(4):771–778.

45. Kevy S, Jacobson M, Mandle R. *Defining the Composition and Healing Effect of Platelet-Rich Plasma.* Presented at Platelet-Rich Plasma Symposium, Hospital for Special Surgery, NY, August 5, 2010.

46. Haynesworth S, Bruder SP. Mitogenic stimulation of human mesenchymal stem cells by platelet releasate. Poster Presentation, American Academy of Orthopedic Surgery. 2001 Mar.

47. Riboh JC, Saltzman BM, Yanke AB, et al. Human amniotic membrane–derived products in sports medicine: basic science, early results, and potential clinical applications. *Am J Sports Med.* 2016 Sep;44(9):2425–2434.

48. Braun HJ, Kim HJ, Chu CR, et al. The effect of platelet-rich plasma formulations and blood products on human synoviocytes: implications for intra-articular injury and therapy. *Am J Sports Med.* 2014;42(5):1204–1210.

49. Chang KV, Hung CY, Aliwarga F, et al. Comparative effectiveness of platelet-rich plasma injections for treating knee joint cartilage degenerative pathology: a systematic review and meta-analysis. *Arch Phys Med Rehabil.* 2014;95(3):562–575.

50. Tidball JG. Inflammatory processes in muscle injury and repair. *Am J Physiol Regul Integr Comp Physiol.* 2005;288(2):R345–R353.

51. Pizza FX, McLoughlin TJ, McGregor SJ, et al. Neutrophils injure cultured skeletal myotubes. *Am J Physiol, Cell Physiol.* 2001;281(1):C335–C341.

52. Pizza FX, Peterson JM, Baas JH, et al. Neutrophils contribute to muscle injury and impair its resolution after lengthening contractions in mice. *J Physiol (Lond).* 2005;562(Pt 3):899–913.

53. Schneider LA, Korber A, Grabbe S, et al. Influence of pH on wound-healing: a new perspective for wound-therapy? *Arch Dermatol Res.* 2007;298(9):413–420.

54. El-Sharkawy H, Kantarci A, Deady J, et al. Platelet-rich plasma: growth factors and pro- and anti-inflammatory properties. *J Periodontol.* 2007;78(4):661–669.

55. Hooiveld M, Roosendal G, Wenting M, et al. Short term exposure of cartilage to blood results in apoptosis. *American Journal of Pathology.* 2003;162:943–951.

56. Roosendaal G, Vianen ME, Marx JJ, et al. Blood-induced joint damage: a human *in vitro* study. *Arthritis Rheum.* 1999;42(5):1025–1032.

57. Jansen NW, Roosendaal G, Bijlsma JW, et al. Exposure of human cartilage tissue to low concentrations of blood for a short period of time leads to prolonged cartilage damage: an *in vitro* study. *Arthritis Rheum.* 2007;56(1):199–207.

58. Stein H, Duthie RB. The pathogenesis of chronic haemophilic arthropathy. *J Bone Joint Surg Br.* 1981;63B(4):601–609.

59. Fufa D, Shealy B, Jacobson M, et al. Activation of platelet-rich plasma using soluble type I collagen. *J Oral Maxillofac Surg.* 2008;66(4):684–690.

60. Roussy Y, Bertrand Duchesne MP, Gagnon G. Activation of human platelet-rich plasmas: effect on growth factors release, cell division and *in vivo* bone formation. *Clin Oral Implants Res.* 2007;18(5):639–648.

61. Han B, Woodell-May J, Ponticiello M, et al. The effect of thrombin activation of platelet-rich plasma on demineralized bone matrix osteoinductivity. *J Bone Joint Surg Am.* 2009;91(6):1459–1470.

62. Tsay RC, Vo J, Burke A, Eisig SB, et al. Differential growth factor retention by platelet-rich plasma composites. *J Oral Maxillofac Surg.* 2005;63(4): 521–528.

63. Nilsson E, Wendeberg B. Effect of local anaesthetics on wound healing. An experimental study with special reference to carbocain. *Acta Anaesth. Scandinav.* 1957, 2, 87–99. *Acta Anaesthesiol Scand.* 2007;51(8):991–1003; discussion 1004.

64. Scherb MB, Han SH, Courneya JP, et al. Effect of bupivacaine on cultured tenocytes. *Orthopedics.* 2009;32(1):26. doi:10.3928/01477447-20090101-19

65. Edlow DW, Sheldon WH. The pH of inflammatory exudates. *Proc Soc Exp Biol Med.* 1971;137(4):1328–1332.

66. Leveen HH, Falk G, Borek B, et al. Chemical acidification of wounds: an adjuvant to healing and

the unfavorable action of alkalinity and ammonia. *Ann Surg*. 1973;178(6):745–753.

67. Liu Y, Kalén A, Risto O, et al. Fibroblast proliferation due to exposure to a platelet concentrate *in vitro* is pH dependent. *Wound Repair Regen*. 2002;10(5):336–340.

68. do Amaral RJ, da Silva NP, Haddad NF, et al. Platelet-rich plasma obtained with different anticoagulants and their effect on platelet numbers and mesenchymal stromal cells behavior *in vitro*. *Stem Cells Int*. 2016;2016:7414036. doi:10.1155/2016/7414036

69. Colberg R, Mautner K. Platelet-rich plasma, an option for tendinopathy. *Lower Extremity Review*. Oct 2013:53–60.

70. Mautner K, Colberg RE, Malanga G, et al. Outcomes after ultrasound-guided platelet-rich plasma injections for chronic tendinopathy: a multicenter, retrospective review. *PM R*. 2013;5(3):169–175.

71. de Vos RJ, van Veldhoven PL, Moen MH, et al. Autologous growth factor injections in chronic tendinopathy: a systematic review. *Br Med Bull*. 2010;95:63–77.

72. Dohan Ehrenfest DM, Rasmusson L, Albrektsson T. Classification of platelet concentrates: from pure platelet-rich plasma (P-PRP) to leucocyte- and platelet-rich fibrin (L-PRF). *Trends Biotechnol*. 2009;27(3):158–167.

73. Dohan Ehrenfest DM, Bielecki T, Mishra A, et al. In search of a consensus terminology in the field of platelet concentrates for surgical use: platelet-rich plasma (PRP), platelet-rich fibrin (PRF), fibrin gel polymerization and leukocytes. *Curr Pharm Biotechnol*. 2012;13(7):1131–1137.

74. DeLong JM, Russell RP, Mazzocca AD. Platelet-rich plasma: the PAW classification system. *Arthroscopy*. 2012;28(7):998–1009.

75. Mautner K, Malanga GA, Smith J, et al. A call for a standard classification system for future biologic research: the rationale for new PRP nomenclature. *PM R*. 2015;7(4 Suppl):S53–S59.

76. Banja JD. Ethical considerations in stem cell research on neurologic and orthopedic conditions. *PM R*. 2015;7(4 Suppl):S66–S75.

77. Connolly J, Guse R, Lippiello L, et al. Development of an osteogenic bone-marrow preparation. *J Bone Joint Surg Am*. 1989;71(5):684–691.

78. Connolly JF. Clinical use of marrow osteoprogenitor cells to stimulate osteogenesis. *Clin Orthop Relat Res*. 1998;(355 Suppl):S257–S266.

79. Santos GW. History of bone marrow transplantation. *Clin Haematol*. 1983;12(3):611–639.

80. Alison MR. Stem cells in pathobiology and regenerative medicine. *J Pathol*. 2009;217(2):141–143.

81. Connell D, Datir A, Alyas F, et al. Treatment of lateral epicondylitis using skin-derived tenocyte-like cells. *Br J Sports Med*. 2009;43(4):293–298.

82. Bruder SP, Fink DJ, Caplan AI. Mesenchymal stem cells in bone development, bone repair, and skeletal regeneration therapy. *J Cell Biochem*. 1994;56(3):283–294.

83. DiMarino AM, Caplan AI, Bonfield TL. Mesenchymal stem cells in tissue repair. *Front Immunol*. 2013;4,201.

84. Murrell WD, Anz AW, Badsha H, et al. Regenerative treatments to enhance orthopedic surgical outcome. *PM R*. 2015;7(4 Suppl):S41–S52.

85. Caplan AI, Dennis JE. Mesenchymal stem cells as trophic mediators. *J Cell Biochem*. 2006;98(5):1076–1084.

86. Kock L, van Donkelaar CC, Ito K. Tissue engineering of functional articular cartilage: the current status. *Cell Tissue Res*. 2012;347(3):613–627.

87. Onishi K, Jones DL, Riester SM, et al. Human adipose-derived mesenchymal stromal/stem cells remain viable and metabolically active following needle passage. *PM R*. 2016;8(9):844–854.

88. Nakao N, Nakayama T, Yahata T, et al. Adipose tissue–derived mesenchymal stem cells facilitate hematopoiesis *in vitro* and in vivo: advantages over bone marrow-derived mesenchymal stem cells. *Am J Pathol*. 2010;177(2):547–554.

89. Bowen JE. Technical issues in harvesting and concentrating stem cells (bone marrow and adipose). *PMR*. 2015;7(4 Suppl):S8–S18.

90. Casteilla L, Planat-Benard V, Laharrague P, et al. Adipose-derived stromal cells: Their identity and uses in clinical trials, an update. *World J Stem Cells*. 2011;3(4):25–33.

91. Hölig K, Kramer M, Kroschinsky F, et al. Safety and efficacy of hematopoietic stem cell collection from mobilized peripheral blood in unrelated volunteers: 12 years of single-center experience in 3928 donors. *Blood*. 2009;114(18):3757–3763.

92. Cesselli D, Beltrami AP, Rigo S, et al. Multipotent progenitor cells are present in human peripheral blood. *Circ Res*. 2009;104(10):1225–1234.

93. Saw KY, Anz A, Siew-Yoke Jee C, et al. Articular cartilage regeneration with autologous peripheral

blood stem cells versus hyaluronic acid: a randomized controlled trial. *Arthroscopy.* 2013;29(4): 684–694.

94. Bacou F, el Andalousi RB, Daussin PA, et al. Transplantation of adipose tissue–derived stromal cells increases mass and functional capacity of damaged skeletal muscle. *Cell Transplant.* 2004;13(2):103–111.

95. Quintero AJ, Wright VJ, Fu FH, Huard J. Stem cells for the treatment of skeletal muscle injury. *Clin Sports Med.* 2009;28(1):1–11.

96. Kasemkijwattana C, Menetrey J, Bosch P. Use of growth factors to improve muscle healing after strain injury. *Clin Orthop Relat Res.* 2000;(370):272–285.

97. Fan H, Liu H, Toh SL, et al. Enhanced differentiation of mesenchymal stem cells co-cultured with ligament fibroblasts on gelatin/silk fibroin hybrid scaffold. *Biomaterials.* 2008;29(8):1017–1027.

98. Miller SL, Gladstone JN. Graft selection in anterior cruciate ligament reconstruction. *Orthop Clin North Am.* 2002;33(4):675–683.

99. Smith RKW. Stem cell therapy for tendinopathy: lessons learned from a large animal model. *British Journal of Sports Medicine.* 2013;47:e2. doi:10.1136/bjsports-2013-092459.42

100. Clarke AW, Alyas F, Morris T, et al. Skin-derived tenocyte-like cells for the treatment of patellar tendinopathy. *Am J Sports Med.* 2011;39(3):614–623.

101. Frazer A, Bunning RA, Thavarajah M, et al. Studies on type II collagen and aggrecan production in human articular chondrocytes *in vitro* and effects of transforming growth factor-beta and interleukin-1beta. *Osteoarthr Cartil.* 1994;2(4):235–245.

102. Goldring MB. The role of the chondrocyte in osteoarthritis. *Arthritis Rheum.* 2000;43(9): 1916–1926.

103. Centeno CJ, Schultz JR, Cheever M, et al. Safety and complications reporting update on the re-implantation of culture-expanded mesenchymal stem cells using autologous platelet lysate technique. *Curr Stem Cell Res Ther.* 2011;6(4):368–378.

104. Davatchi F, Abdollahi BS, Mohyeddin M, et al. Mesenchymal stem cell therapy for knee osteoarthritis: preliminary report of four patients. *Int J Rheum Dis.* 2011;14(2):211–215.

105. Kim JD, Lee GW, Jung GH, et al. Clinical outcome of autologous bone marrow aspirates concentrate (BMAC) injection in degenerative arthritis of the knee. *Eur J Orthop Surg Traumatol.* 2014;24(8):1505–1511.

106. Chahla J, Dean CS, Moatshe G, et al. Concentrated bone marrow aspirate for the treatment of chondral injuries and osteoarthritis of the knee: a systematic review of outcomes. *Orthop J Sports Med.* 2016;4(1). doi:10.1177/2325967115625481

107. Takahashi K, Yamanaka S. Induction of pluripotent stem cells from mouse embryonic and adult fibroblast cultures by defined factors. *Cell.* 2006;126(4):663–676.

108. Centeno CJ, Bashir J. Safety and regulatory issues regarding stem cell therapies: one clinic's perspective. *PM R.* 2015;7(4 Suppl):S4–S7.

CHAPTER 7

SCIENTIFIC EVIDENCE OF PLATELET-RICH PLASMA FOR ORTHOPEDIC CONDITIONS: BASIC SCIENCE TO CLINICAL RESEARCH AND APPLICATION

Peter I-Kung Wu, Robert Diaz, and Joanne Borg-Stein

The clinical application of platelet-rich plasma (PRP) and other regenerative therapies in sports, spine, and musculoskeletal medicine has soared in the last decade. During this period, many factors have converged to fuel this development. Advances in scientific understanding of tendinopathy as a degenerative cellular and connective tissue process; lack of long-term efficacy of steroid injection therapies, which has prompted the need for alternative therapies; advances in musculoskeletal ultrasound (US) to facilitate diagnosis and guide interventions; as well as translation of treatment paradigms from our colleagues in oral and veterinary surgery have all contributed to the advancement of this regenerative field.

This chapter provides the latest clinically relevant information on the basic science of PRP and practical considerations for its use, evidence for PRP use in musculoskeletal medicine, and recommendations for PRP preparation. We identify the limitations in current knowledge of this regenerative therapy and recommend critical areas for future research.

BASIC SCIENCE

In musculoskeletal and sports medicine, PRP therapy has become highly attractive for its potential benefit and influence on repairing injured tissue, treating a wide range of degenerative disorders, and accelerating return to sport, finding its role as an injectable biologic used to augment healing of the tendon, ligament, muscle, and cartilage (1). Early and ongoing basic science investigations have identified the therapeutic mechanisms of PRP and its key components and have begun to elucidate the parameters for its use.

Wound Healing

The value of PRP in accelerating wound healing by providing angiogenic and tissue growth factors is especially significant for damaged tendons, ligaments, and cartilage, whose baseline healing response can be sluggish and poor due to slow cell turnover and limited blood supply (2,3). In general, wound healing can be separated into three phases: inflammation, proliferation, and remodeling (4). The initial inflammation phase is characterized by hemostasis, with platelets producing clot formation, and the release of growth factors that aid in the activation and attraction of inflammatory cells like neutrophils and macrophages to the site of injury. The proliferation phase is characterized by the establishment of an extracellular matrix associated with granulation, contraction, and epithelialization (1,4). Finally, the remodeling phase is associated with the production of collagen and scar tissue. Blood components in PRP can release and modulate not only many of the growth factors and cytokines that govern progression through these phases of wound healing, but also angiogenic growth factors that can increase blood and nutrient supply to further facilitate tissue repair (2).

Components of PRP

Platelets

Although platelets are known to play an essential role in hemostasis, they are crucial to orchestrating the regenerative effects of PRP by releasing growth factors contained in their alpha granules. In the early phases of wound healing, activated platelets attract and facilitate cell migration into damaged tissue by aggregating and forming a fibrin matrix. This matrix serves as a tissue scaffold for sustained release of platelet growth factors and cytokines, which stimulate cell recruitment, differentiation, and communication (5). Both angiogenic and anti-angiogenic factors are contained within platelets; however, their release kinetics differ (5,6). Noteworthy growth factors involved in the healing cascade that are released from platelets include

platelet-derived growth factor (PDGF), transforming growth factor (TGF-β), vascular endothelial growth factor (VEGF), epidermal growth factor (EGF), basic fibroblast growth factor (bFGF), and insulin-like growth factor (IGF-1) (2). See Table 7.1.

Regarding platelet content, the clinical literature has commonly suggested using platelet concentrations four to six times greater than that in the whole blood for PRP. Concentrations greater than an optimal amount may provide no additional effect or even inhibit healing (9). In vitro studies have shown that 1.5×10 (6) platelets (PLT)/μL was optimal to promote human umbilical vein endothelial cell proliferation, motility, and morphology, with greater concentrations causing inhibition (10). A range of 0.5 to 1.5×10 (6) PLT/μL was optimal for normal human dermal fibroblast proliferation, motility, and wound healing (11). In vitro treatment with a platelet-rich preparation containing 0.494×10 (6) PLT/μL was able to significantly enhance hyaluronic acid secretion in synovial fibroblasts from osteoarthritic patients (12). Tenocyte function plateaued by a concentration of 2.0×10 (6) platelets (PLT)/μL, beyond which no greater benefit to function was achieved (13).

Leukocytes

Leukocytes are key coordinators of the host defense against infectious organisms, inflammatory response, and wound healing (2). Neutrophils are involved in the inflammation phase of wound healing. Monocytes and macrophages facilitate tissue repair through debriding and phagocytosing damaged tissue. Macrophages also secrete growth factors that are vital in tissue repair and have been shown to aid in subchondral bone regeneration (7,14). The pro-inflammatory and immunologic functions of leukocytes are critical in protecting against infectious organisms; however, these same inflammatory effects can also provoke unwanted local cell and tissue damage that can counteract the therapeutic effects of PRP.

The superiority of leukocyte-poor or leukocyte-rich PRP has been investigated and given concern over the pro-inflammatory effects of leukocytes and their inhibitory effect on tissue

TABLE 7.1 Key Regenerative Growth Factors Stored in Platelet Alpha Granules and Their Functions

Growth Factor	Function
PDGF	Stimulates cell proliferation, chemotaxis, and differentiation Stimulates angiogenesis
TGF-β	Stimulates production of collagen type I and type III, angiogenesis, reepithelialization, and synthesis of protease inhibitors to inhibit collagen breakdown
VEGF	Stimulates angiogenesis by regulating endothelial cell proliferation and migration
EGF	Influences cell proliferation and cytoprotection Accelerates reepithelialization Increases tensile strength in wounds Facilitates organization of granulation tissue
bFGF	Stimulates angiogenesis Promotes stem cell differentiation and cell proliferation Promotes collagen production and tissue repair
IGF-1	Regulates cell proliferation and differentiation Influences matrix secretion from osteoblasts and production of proteoglycan, collagen, and other non-collagen proteins

EGF, epidermal growth factor; bFGF, basic fibroblast growth factor; IGF-1, insulin-like growth factor; PDGF, platelet-derived growth factor; TGF-β, transforming growth factor-β; VEGF, vascular endothelial growth factor.
Source: From Refs. (2,6–8).

healing (15–19). Although leukocyte-poor PRP releasate inhibited inflammatory processes in human osteoarthritic chondrocytes (20), leukocyte-rich PRP resulted in greater pro-inflammatory mediator and cytokine production and greater cell death in human synoviocytes (16,17). Despite a synergistic interaction between mononuclear cells and platelets to result in greater anabolic growth factor release and cellular effect (21,22), high leukocyte concentrations (greater than 21,000/μL) (18), especially of neutrophils, result in greater release of pro-inflammatory and catabolic substances (23,24), that is independent of the ratio of platelets to leukocytes (19), produce an acute inflammatory response (18), and increase synoviocyte cell death (17,18), suggesting that leukocyte-poor (less than 1,000/μL) PRP is a better option. Studies in tendon models showed that reducing leukocyte concentrations, and thus decreasing the inflammatory response, may be more important than maximizing platelet concentrations to optimize PRP efficacy (25). A survey of various preclinical studies involving leukocyte concentration in PRP is provided in Table 7.2. Further preclinical studies are needed to clarify the optimal concentration of leukocytes and the ratio of leukocytes to platelets to have in PRP in order to enhance healing without inducing undesirable tissue damage.

TABLE 7.2 Findings From Preclinical Studies of Leukocyte Concentration in PRP

Tissue of Interest	Findings
Human synoviocytes (17)	Treatment with leukocyte-rich PRP and RBC concentrates resulted in significant cell death and pro-inflammatory mediator production. Consider using leukocyte-poor and RBC-free preparations of PRP for intra-articular therapy.
Rabbit patellar tendons (18)	Leukocyte-rich PRP resulted in significantly greater inflammatory response 5 days after intra-tendinous injection compared with leukocyte-poor PRP. There was no difference in inflammatory response 14 days after injection between leukocyte-rich and leukocyte-poor PRP.
Human synoviocytes (16)	Leukocyte-rich PRP is able to maintain long-term up-regulation of pro-inflammatory factors and down-regulation of anti-catabolic mediators in cartilage compared with leukocyte-poor PRP and platelet-poor plasma.
Equine flexor digitorum superficialis tendons (14)	High leukocyte concentrations in PRP can contribute to the expression of inflammatory cytokines in flexor digitorum superficialis tendon explants. Leukocyte-poor PRP may be the preferred preparation to stimulate healing without scar tissue formation.

PRP, platelet-rich plasma; RBC, red blood cells.

Red Blood Cells

Red blood cells (RBCs) use hemoglobin to perform their chief function of delivering oxygen, metabolic gases, nutrients, and regulatory molecules like nitric oxide to tissues throughout the body. Although nitric oxide is known to stimulate vasodilation, it has also been implicated in rendering insensitivity in diseased cartilage to the anabolic effects of IGF-1 (2). During oxidative stress, heme molecules that contain iron can release cytotoxic oxygen-free radicals that induce apoptosis of host cells (2). This harmful process is thought to take place in human synoviocytes treated with RBC concentrates, leading to significantly greater cell death and cartilage destruction (17,26–29). Such results suggest that RBC concentrations should be reduced or eliminated in PRP formulations used for intra-articular applications. RBC content is typically reduced or absent in PRP due to the centrifugation process during preparation, with concentrations of more than 1,000/μL reported (18).

Considerations for Use of PRP

Variability Among PRP Products

There continues to be a large variability in PRP products used for regenerative therapy. Presently, there is no general consensus on the optimal method of preparation or the ideal concentration of each blood component. From reported studies, investigators have used an assortment of PRP preparation protocols, differing by preparation kit, centrifugation system, number of centrifugation steps, activation method with or without thrombin and/or calcium, and resulting PRP component concentration (platelets, leukocytes, RBCs) (30,31). The numerous names and preparation methods used in studies for this biologic treatment, such as "platelet-rich plasma," "autologous-conditioned plasma," and "platelet lysate," as well as newer methods of production, such as a preparation rich in growth factors (32), platelet-rich fibrin matrix (33), simplified buffy coat method, and platelet-rich fibrin (34), reflect the complexity and diversity of this therapy (7). Each PRP formulation has its own exclusive biologic properties and effects, which has contributed to the mixed results of PRP's clinical efficacy from human trials. The large variability in PRP formulations further creates challenges to accurately draw conclusions from the literature to guide PRP production, determine indications for use, and translate findings from clinical trials to clinical practice, prompting the development of PRP classification schemes to facilitate the reporting of clinical investigations (35–38).

Validation studies have shown that PRP cellular composition and biomolecular characteristics vary according to the preparation protocol (39,40) and the system used (33,41–46). Preclinical investigations suggest that PRP-preparation methods additionally affect growth factor release kinetics and efficacy, with significant differences between classic PRP and second-generation preparations like platelet-rich fibrin (47–54). Furthermore, PRP biologic activity is known to diminish with storage time (55). Ongoing efforts strive to elucidate the influence of PRP-preparation methods and formulation characteristics on growth factor release, biologic effect, and therapeutic outcomes.

Activated Versus Nonactivated PRP

PRP preparations are commonly activated with the addition of thrombin and/or calcium before the administration in order to induce the release of a highly concentrated bolus of growth factors to the target tissue. Up to 70% of growth factor content from activated PRP can be released over 10 minutes (56). Roy et al. showed that PRP activated with a low dose mixture of thrombin and calcium significantly increased growth factor release over 7 days compared to nonactivated PRP (57). As a result, activation has been shown to lower the platelet concentration required to reach a plateau in tenocyte proliferation from $2.0 \times 10\,(6)$ PLT/µL to $4.0 \times 10\,(5)$ PLT/µL (13). However, both the amount and the kinetics of growth factor release induced by activation also vary and depend on the means of activation.

Thrombin and calcium have a dose-response effect on growth factor release from platelets, with higher concentrations leading to immediate and significantly greater anabolic growth factor release, and lower concentrations leading to delayed and reduced release (58). Compared with thrombin, collagen activation results in a more sustained growth factor release (59).

Uncertainty exists as to whether a rapid bolus of growth factors is ideal for PRP therapy. The literature reveals conflicting results supporting PRP activation, with activated preparations resulting in less efficient fibroblast differentiation and wound healing but providing equivalent bony regeneration compared with nonactivated preparations (5,60). Debate continues on whether activated PRP produces superior results compared to nonactivated formulations, but it is understood that activation alters the properties and the effects of PRP and must be considered when comparing results from clinical studies.

Drug Interactions

The application of PRP has generally not been recommended in individuals who take or cannot suspend taking antiplatelet therapy, which may inhibit platelet degranulation and the release of growth factors and bioactive molecules, thereby significantly diminishing the healing properties of PRP formulations. Such antiplatelet agents act by various mechanisms of action and come from drug classes that include reversible and irreversible cyclooxygenase inhibitors, adenosine diphosphate receptor inhibitors, adenosine reuptake inhibitors, phosphodiesterase inhibitors, and glycoprotein IIB/IIIA inhibitors (61). Autologous PRP produced from subjects taking nonsteroidal anti-inflammatory drugs (NSAIDs), reversible cyclooxygenase inhibitors that are commonly taken for anti-inflammation and pain management, was shown to have significantly impaired platelet aggregation, and thus potentially diminished therapeutic effect (62).

Other medications may also interfere with platelet function. Pioglitazone, an antihyperglycemic agent, has been shown to both directly inhibit platelet release of thromboxane (an inducer of platelet aggregation), and enhance aspirin inhibition of platelet aggregation and adenosine triphosphate (ATP) release (63). Furthermore, lidocaine and ropivacaine anesthetics, often used concomitantly with PRP injection for local analgesia, have been shown to inhibit platelet aggregation in response to activation by collagen or adenosine diphosphate (64).

EVIDENCE FOR MUSCULOSKELETAL DISORDERS

PRP therapies are used increasingly for treating musculoskeletal soft tissue injuries, including tendinopathies and tendon tears, ligament, muscle, and cartilage injuries (65). Therapies have been used as both principal treatment and augmentative therapy alongside surgical repair. A most recent 2014 Cochrane review of single-centered, randomized controlled trials (RCTs) of PRP in the literature reveals that the evidence for the primary outcomes of function and pain are of low quality and at high risk of bias. Overall results showed that PRP provides no clinically significant improvement in short- and long-term function but only a small reduction in short-term pain compared with control. Adverse effects were associated with concerns about persisting pain. Difficulty in drawing clear conclusions from this collection of studies stems from using heterogeneous PRP-preparation methods, application techniques, and outcome measures; treating disparate musculoskeletal disorders; and conducting underpowered studies. The current evidence also comprises a collection of earlier, smaller studies, many with nonrandomized or uncontrolled methodology, that demonstrate variable results for the effectiveness of PRP to treat musculoskeletal injuries. The review presented here emphasizes findings spanning early case reports and cohort studies to the most recent RCTs.

Tendon

Lateral Epicondyle Tendinopathy

The results for PRP treatment of lateral epicondyle tendinopathy (LET) have been promising, as showed in early case series and cohort studies (66–70). RCTs have demonstrated the efficacy of PRP for treating chronic LET, with superior 1-year (71) and 2-year (72) improvements in function and pain compared with steroid injection. However, more recent RCTs have demonstrated variable efficacy of PRP compared with saline, steroid, autologous whole blood, and bupivacaine (73–77):

- PRP was superior at reducing pain at 6 weeks (74) but no better at improving the function by 6 months compared with autologous blood injection (73).

- PRP was no different than steroid or saline at reducing pain and improving the function at 3 months, was inferior to steroid at improving pain and function at 1 month, and was associated with greater postinjection pain (75). Another RCT found PRP to provide no difference in pain reduction or functional improvement compared with steroid at 6 weeks (77).

- PRP was superior to bupivacaine at improving pain at 6 months (76), and pain and function at 1 year (78).

A study by Wolf et al. comparing autologous blood, steroid, and saline control injections for lateral epicondylitis showed no significant difference among groups for pain and function up to 6 months (79). A further RCT by Raeissadat et al. comparing the efficacy of PRP to that of autologous whole blood injection showed that both methods are comparably effective in treating LET, with no significant difference among groups in pain reduction and functional improvement in 12 months of follow-up (80). Although results from Raeissadat et al.'s study suggest that there may be no need to have platelet concentrations greater than in whole blood to obtain therapeutic effects, limitations of this study included a relatively small number of cases and the absence of a placebo control group. Factoring in results from both studies, however, would suggest neither autologous blood nor PRP is superior to saline control or the natural course of recovery.

Results are pending from a multicenter RCT comparing autologous PRP, autologous whole blood, dry needle tendon fenestration, and physical therapy (PT) alone on pain and quality of life in patients with LET (IMpact of Platelet Rich Plasma Over Alternative Therapies in Patients with Lateral Epicondylitis: IMPROVE Trial) (81). See Table 7.3.

Achilles Tendinopathy

Results for PRP treatment of Achilles tendinopathy have been mixed. Earlier return to sport by 7 weeks has been observed after local application of plasma rich in growth factors at the time of open repair of complete Achilles tendon tear (3). However, PRP injection did not improve mechanical properties or functional performance of Achilles tendon up to 1 year after surgical repair of an acute rupture compared with no PRP injection (82).

For chronic Achilles tendinopathy, case series (83–89), pilot studies (90), and retrospective studies (91–93) have reported promising results for the efficacy of PRP injection, with lasting improvements in functional outcomes at 4 years (94). RCTs, however, demonstrated no significant difference in the outcomes of clinical function, tendon healing, or return-to-sport times at either 6 months (95) or 1 year between PRP and saline control (96). Nor did PRP injection provide a significantly different neovascularization response or ultrasonographically assessed change in tendon structure over 6 months than saline injection did for chronic Achilles tendinopathy (97).

Meta-analyses comparing various injection therapies for lateral epicondylitis (98,99) and noninsertional Achilles tendinosis (100) revealed no strong evidence for selecting one injectable over another and indicated that large-scale studies are needed before the treatment recommendations can be made. See Table 7.4.

Patellar Tendinopathy

Results from case series (85,87,101–104) and retrospective studies (93) have shown promise for PRP injection to improve healing and function (105) in patients with chronic patellar tendinopathy, with lasting effects in functional outcomes at 4 years (106).

Comparative studies showed that PRP therapy may be more effective for those who have not received earlier infiltrative or surgical treatments (107). Trials comparing the efficacy of a single PRP injection to that of two closely timed PRP injections have not consistently shown that two injections significantly improve efficacy over 1 to 2 years of follow-up (108,109). Although another comparative study did not find the addition of PRP injection to rehabilitation to provide greater pain reduction at 6 months (110), an RCT demonstrated the efficacy of PRP for treating patellar tendinopathy, with superior 1-year outcomes in pain and function compared with extracorporeal shock-wave therapy (111).

In an RCT, US-guided PRP injection administered with dry needling accelerated recovery from patellar tendinopathy relative to dry needling alone, but benefits to pain and function dissipated after 3 months, occurring without any significant improvement in the quality of life (112).

The application of PRP to patellar tendon harvest sites for anterior cruciate ligament (ACL) reconstruction was found in RCTs to provide significant reduction in postoperative pain (113), greater donor patellar tendon healing at 6 months (114), and greater function at 12 months (115). See Table 7.5.

Rotator Cuff Tendinopathy

Studies of augmentative PRP used alongside rotator cuff repair have been of variable quality and have shown mixed results:

- Following initial safety studies (116), early, underpowered studies demonstrated no significant benefit to pain or function of PRP

TABLE 7.3 Studies of Lateral Epicondyle Tendinopathy

Study	Type of Study	Intervention	Main Results
Edwards and Calandruccio (66) (2003)	Case series (level IV evidence)	28 patients injected with 2 mL of autologous blood under extensor carpi radialis brevis	79% of patients with resolution of pain at 9.5 months; reduction of pain score from 7.8 to 2.3 and reduction of Nirschl score from 6.5 to 2.0 at last follow-up
Connell et al. (67) (2006)	Case series (level IV evidence)	35 patients underwent dry needling and injection of 2 mL of autologous blood	Reduction of Nirschl scores from 6 to 4 at 4 weeks and to 0 at 6 months; reduction of pain scores from 9 to 6 at 4 weeks and to 0 at 6 months. Significant reduction in US-assessed tendon thickness, hypoechoic change, and neovascularity
Chaudhury et al. (68) (2013)	Case series (level IV evidence)	6 patients received 3 mL PRP injection	Improved extensor tendon morphology on US
Hechtman et al. (69) (2011)	Cohort study (level III evidence)	31 patients received a 3 mL PRP injection with peppering technique	Patient satisfaction score improved from 5.1 ± 2.5 to 9.1 ± 1.9. Significant reduction of worst pain from 7.2 ± 1.6 at baseline to 1.1 ± 1.7 after 6 or more months
Mishra and Pavelko (70) (2006)	Cohort (level II evidence)	3 mL PRP (15 patients) vs. 3 mL Bupivacaine (5 patients)	60% improvement in VAS with PRP vs. 16% improvement in Bupivacaine at 8 weeks
Peerbooms et al. (71) (2010)	RCT (level I evidence)	1 mL PRP injection (51 patients) vs. 1 mL Corticosteroid triamcinolone injection (49 patients)	73% in PRP group vs. 49% in corticosteroid group had successful outcome based on VAS reduction of >25% at 1 year; 73% in PRP group vs. 51% in corticosteroid group had successful outcome based on DASH score reduction >25% at 1 year
Gosens et al. (72) (2011)	RCT (level I evidence)	1 mL PRP injection (51 patients) vs. 1 mL Corticosteroid triamcinolone injection (49 patients)	77% in PRP group vs. 43% in corticosteroid group had successful outcome based on VAS reduction of >25% at 2 years; 73% in PRP group vs. 39% in corticosteroid group had successful outcome based on DASH score reduction >25% at 2 years
Omar et al. (77) (2012)	RCT (level I evidence)	PRP injection (15 patients) vs. Steroid injection (15 patients)	PRP was no different from steroid at reducing pain and improving function at 6 weeks

(continued)

TABLE 7.3 Studies of Lateral Epicondyle Tendinopathy   (*continued*)

Study	Type of Study	Intervention	Main Results
Krogh et al. (75) (2013)	RCT (level I evidence)	3 mL PRP (20 patients) vs. 3 mL glucocorticoid — triamcinolone + lidocaine (20 patients) vs. 3 mL isotonic saline (20 patients)	PRP was no different than steroid or saline at reducing pain and improving function at 3 months; PRP was inferior to steroid at improving pain and function at 1 month
Creaney et al. (73) (2011)	RCT (level I evidence)	1.5 mL PRP injection (70 patients) vs. 1.5 mL ABI (60 patients)	No significant difference in successful outcome, as defined by improvement in PRTEE score >25 points by final follow-up, between PRP and ABI groups at 6 months
Thanasas et al. (74) (2011)	RCT (level I evidence)	3 mL PRP injection (14 patients) vs. 3 mL ABI (14 patients)	PRP group had significantly greater reduction in pain at 6 weeks compared with ABI group, but no significant difference in pain at 3 and 6 months
Raeissadat et al. (80) (2014)	RCT (level I evidence)	2 mL PRP (33 patients) vs. 2 mL ABI (31 patients)	Significant improvement in both groups in pain compared to baseline at 4 and 8 weeks, 6 and 12 months. No significant differences between ABI and PRP groups at any follow-up
Mishra et al. (76) (2014)	RCT (level II evidence)	3 mL PRP (116 patients) vs. 3 mL Bupivacaine (114 patients)	83.9% in PRP group vs. 68.3% in bupivacaine group had successful outcome based on VAS reduction of >25% with resisted wrist extension at 24 weeks
Behera et al. (78) (2015)	RCT (level I evidence)	3 mL PRP (15 patients) vs. 3 mL bupivacaine (10 patients)	PRP group demonstrated significantly greater improvement in pain and function compared with bupivacaine group at 6 months and 1 year

ABI, autologous blood injection; DASH, disabilities of the arm, shoulder and hand; PRP, platelet-rich plasma; PRTEE, patient-related tennis elbow evaluation; RCT, randomized controlled trial; US, ultrasound; VAS, Visual Analogue Scale.

TABLE 7.4 Studies of Achilles Tendinopathy

Study	Type of Study	Intervention	Main Results
Sanchez et al. (3) (2007)	Case–control study (level III evidence)	6 athletes injected with 4 mL PRGF during operative repair of Achilles tendon rupture	The PRGF group had significantly earlier recovery of ankle range of motion, reduced tendon thickness, and earlier return to sport.
Schepull et al. (82) (2011)	RCT (level II evidence)	PRP + surgical repair of Achilles tendon rupture (16 patients) vs. surgical repair alone (14 patients)	No difference in function between groups at 12 months. Tendon had lower biomechanical performance in PRP group.
Gaweda et al. (83) (2010)	Case series (level IV evidence)	14 patients injected with 3 mL PRP	Significant improvement in clinical and imaging outcomes over 18 months.
Monto et al. (84) (2012)	Case series (level IV evidence)	30 patients with one US-guided injection of 4 mL PRP	Significant clinical improvement over 24 months. US and MRI abnormalities resolved after 6 months.
Ferrero et al. (85) (2012)	Case series (level IV evidence)	30 patients received two US-guided injections of 6mL PRP + percutaneous tenotomy at 3-week interval.	PRP improved pain and function and tendon structure (improved fibrillar echotexture, reduced hypervascularity) at 6 months.
Deans et al. (86) (2012)	Case series (level IV evidence)	26 patients received one injection of 3 mL PRP	Significant improvement in pain, activities of daily living, sport, quality of life at 6 weeks.
Volpi et al. (87) (2010)	Case series (level IV evidence)	Three patients received one injection of PRP	Significant clinical improvement after 3 months, lasting up to 2 years.
Finnoff et al. (88) (2011)	Case series (level IV evidence)	14 patients received 1 injection of 2.5–3.5 mL PRP	Improvement in clinical outcomes at 14 months. Some improvement in sonographic tendon morphology.
Oloff et al. (89) (2015)	Case series (level IV evidence)	One injection of PRP + surgery (13 patients) vs. 1 injection of PRP alone (13 patients)	No significant difference among groups in improving function and tendon morphology on MRI.
Kearney et al. (90) (2013)	RCT (level I evidence)	1 injection of 3–5 mL PRP (10 patients) vs. eccentric exercise (10 patients)	No statistically significant difference among groups in pain or function at 6 months.

(continued)

TABLE 7.4 Studies of Achilles Tendinopathy (*continued*)

Study	Type of Study	Intervention	Main Results
Murawski et al. (91) (2014)	Retrospective study (level IV evidence)	32 patients received one injection of 3 mL PRP	78% of patients had clinical improvement after PRP and avoided surgical intervention at 6 months.
Owens et al. (92) (2011)	Retrospective study (level IV evidence)	10 patients received one injection of 3 mL PRP	PRP led to modest improvement in function and overall health over 24 months, and no change in tendon morphology on MRI.
Mautner et al. (93) (2013)	Retrospective study (level IV evidence)	27 patients with one PRP injection if 80% global improvement, or more injections if poorer results	PRP led to complete resolution of symptoms at 6 months.
Filardo et al. (94) (2014)	Case series (level IV evidence)	27 patients received three US-guided injections of 5 mL PRP at 2-week intervals	PRP led to significant improvements in pain and function, with stable results lasting up to 4.5 years. Longer symptom duration was associated with a more difficult return to sport.
de Vos et al. (95) (2010)	RCT (level I evidence)	One US-guided injection of 4 mL PRP (27 patients) vs. one US-guided injection of 4 mL saline (27 patients)	No significant difference among groups in improvement of pain and activity by 24 weeks.
de Jonge et al. (96) (2011)	RCT (level I evidence)	One US-guided injection of 4 mL PRP (27 patients) vs. one US-guided injection of 4 mL saline (27 patients)	No significant difference among groups in improvement of pain, activity, or ultrasonographic tendon structure at 1 year.
de Vos et al. (97) (2011)	RCT (level I evidence)	One US-guided injection of 4 mL PRP (27 patients) vs. one US-guided injection of 4 mL saline (27 patients)	No significant difference among groups in improvement of tendon structure or increase of neovascularization at 24 weeks.

PRGF, plasma rich in growth factors; PRP, platelet-rich plasma; RCT, randomized controlled trial; US, ultrasound.

TABLE 7.5 Studies of Patellar Tendinopathy

Study	Type of Study	Intervention	Main Results
Ferrero et al. (85) (2012)	Case series (level IV evidence)	28 tendons injected with 6 mL PRP × 2 under US guidance at 3-week interval	PRP-improved pain and function and tendon structure (improved fibrillar echotexture, reduced hypervascularity) at 6 months.
Volpi et al. (87) (2010)	Case series (level IV evidence)	9 patellar tendons injected with 1 US-guided PRP	Significant clinical improvement after 3 months, lasting up to 2 years. Improvement in MRI tendon structure.
Kon et al. (101) (2009)	Case series (level IV evidence)	20 patients injected with 5 mL of PRP × 3 at 2-week intervals	PRP was safe and provided significant improvement in the function and quality-of-life scores across 6 months, allowing return to sport.
Charousset et al. (102) (2014)	Case series (level IV evidence)	28 athletes injected with 3 weekly US-guided, 6 mL of PRP	Improvements in pain and function after 2 years, enabling earlier return to sport. Tendons regained normal MRI architecture.
Dallaudière et al. (105) (2014)	Case series (level IV evidence)	1 US-guided injection of 3 mL PRP	PRP allows significantly improved function and smaller lesions after 6 months.
Filardo et al. (106) (2013)	Case series (level IV evidence)	43 patients with three US-guided 5 mL PRP injections at 2-week intervals	Improvement in clinical outcomes with stable results over 48 months. Bilateral and chronic pathology had poor results.
Kaux et al. (103) (2015)	Case series (level IV evidence)	20 patients with one US-guided 6 mL PRP injection	PRP was associated with decrease in pain during function over 3 months.
Kaux et al. (104) (2015)	Case series (level IV evidence)	20 patients with one US-guided 6 mL PRP injection	Improvement in pain and function up to 1 year.
Mautner et al. (93) (2013)	Retrospective study (level IV evidence)	27 patients with one PRP injection if 80% global improvement, or more injections if poorer results	Moderate (>50%) improvement in symptoms and good satisfaction after 15 months.
Gosens et al. (107) (2012)	Comparative study (level II evidence)	36 patients (14 with previous treatment, 22 without) injected with 3 mL PRP by peppering technique	Improvement in pain and function scores, more significantly in those without previous infiltrative or surgical treatments.
Kaux et al. (108) (2016)	Randomized and comparative study (level II evidence)	6 mL PRP × 1 injection (10 patients) vs. 6 mL PRP × 2 injections at 1-week interval (10 patients)	No significant difference among groups in pain and function over 1 year.

(continued)

TABLE 7.5 Studies of Patellar Tendinopathy *(continued)*

Study	Type of Study	Intervention	Main Results
Zayni et al. (109) (2015)	RCT (level II evidence)	6 mL PRP x 1 injection (20 athletes) vs. 6 mL PRP × 2 injections 2 weeks apart (20 athletes)	2 injections provided significantly greater improvement in pain and function over 2 years.
Filardo et al. (110) (2010)	Comparative study (level II evidence)	3 injections of 5 mL PRP 2 weeks apart + rehabilitation (15 patients) vs. rehabilitation alone (16 patients)	PRP treatment was associated with significant improvement in function and quality of life after 6 months, but improvement was not significantly different from those associated with rehabilitation alone.
Vetrano et al. (111) (2013)	RCT (level I evidence)	Two US-guided injections of 5 mL PRP 1 week apart (23 patients) vs. three sessions of ESWT at 48–72 h interval	PRP showed significantly greater improvement in pain and function compared with ESWT at 6 and 12 months.
Dragoo et al. (112) (2014)	RCT (level I evidence)	One injection of 6 mL PRP + US-guided dry needling (10 patients) vs. US-guided dry needling alone (13 patients)	Faster recovery in PRP group at 12 weeks. No difference in clinical outcomes between PRP group and control at 26 weeks.
Seijas et al. (113) (2016)	RCT (level I evidence)	4 mL of PRGF injected to site of patellar tendon harvest after ACL reconstructive surgery (23 patients) vs. ACL reconstruction alone (23 patients)	PRGF reduced donor site pain in the first 2 months following surgery.
de Almeida et al. (114) (2012)	RCT (level I evidence)	PRP gel added to the site of patellar tendon harvest after ACL reconstructive surgery (12 patients) vs. ACL reconstruction alone (15 patients)	PRP reduced immediate postoperative pain, and led to significantly greater healing at the patellar tendon harvest site on MRI after 6 months.
Cervellin et al. (115) (2012)	RCT (level I evidence)	PRP gel added to the site of patellar tendon harvest after ACL reconstructive surgery (20 patients) vs. ACL reconstruction alone (20 patients)	PRP led to significantly greater functional improvement at 12 months.

ACL, anterior cruciate ligament; ESWT, extracorporeal shock-wave therapy; PRGF, plasma rich in growth factors; PRP, platelet-rich plasma, RCT, randomized controlled trial; US, ultrasound.

augmentation during arthroscopic rotator cuff repair (117,118).

- Intra-operative local application of autologous PRP to the arthroscopic repair site of complete rotator cuff tears has been associated with significantly less pain within the first postoperative month and greater strength within the first 3 months compared with standard repair alone, with benefit more pronounced for less extensive tears (119); however, benefits to pain, function, and healing integrity were not found to endure beyond a year for small, moderate (120), or complete (121–123) rotator cuff tears.

- PRP improved repair integrity for large tears without an associated greater improvement in function (124) and had lower rates of re-tears for small to large tears at 1 year (119,120,124,125).

- Other studies have demonstrated not only no significant benefit of PRP, but also possible negative effects on rotator cuff healing (123,126). The platelet-rich fibrin injection during arthroscopic rotator cuff tendon repair was associated with a greater persistence of rotator cuff tendon defect at 3 months (123). Similarly, the PRP injection with arthroscopic acromioplasty in patients with chronic rotator cuff tendinopathy was associated with reduced cellularity and vascularity and increased levels of apoptosis in tendons at a 12-week follow-up (126).

For principal treatment of chronic rotator cuff tendinopathy, the PRP injection was no more effective than saline by 1 year, but significantly more effective than dry needling by 6 months, in improving pain, disability, and shoulder range of motion (127,128). See Table 7.6.

Plantar Fascia Aponeurosis Pain

Early cohort studies have reported the benefit of PRP injection on improving pain (129), function (130), and tissue structure (131) for chronic plantar fascia pain.

RCTs have compared PRP with conventional treatments. A most recent double-blinded RCT showed that PRP was as effective as or more effective than corticosteroid injection when compared with normal saline control to reduce pain over 3 months of follow-up and improve functional scores for chronic plantar fasciopathy (132).

Multiple earlier studies have compared the efficacy of PRP and corticosteroid without a placebo control and showed variable results, ranging from PRP providing greater early pain reduction and functional improvement (77,133) with lasting effects at 1 (134) and 2 years of follow-up (135), to being equally effective at 3 months (136) and at 6 months (134,137), to being less effective in reducing pain at 3 months (138).

A single-blinded RCT showed that PRP was as effective as prolotherapy (139).

Further trials showed that PRP was as effective as extracorporeal shock-wave therapy at improving pain and functional outcomes beyond conventional therapy for plantar fasciitis (140).

Greater Trochanteric Pain/Gluteus Medius Tendinopathy

A small observational study that evaluated US-guided percutaneous needle tenotomy followed by a PRP injection for treating chronic recalcitrant tendinopathy, including gluteus medius tendinopathy, found that PRP injection was an effective and safe treatment option associated with sonographic improvements in tendon morphology (88). A recent single-blinded, prospective study of patients with greater trochanteric pain syndrome and US findings of gluteal tendinosis or a partial tear (<50% depth) showed that US-guided, intratendinous PRP injection performed equally as effective as US-guided percutaneous tendon fenestration at significantly reducing pain from gluteal tendinosis over 2 weeks (141).

Ligament

Anterior Cruciate Ligament Reconstruction

Several studies of PRP applied during ACL reconstruction demonstrated no benefit to postoperative functional scores. The intraoperative

TABLE 7.6 Studies of Rotator Cuff Tendinopathy

Study	Type of Study	Intervention	Main Results
Randelli et al. (116) (2008)	Case series (level IV evidence)	14 patients received intra-operative PRP injection × 1 during arthroscopic single-row repair of complete rotator cuff tear	PRP application during arthroscopic rotator cuff repair is safe and effective. Patients experienced significant improvement in pain and function, with stable results over 24 months.
Hak et al. (117) (2015)	RCT (level I evidence)	Injection of 6–9 mL PRP (12 patients) vs. 6–9 mL saline control (13 patients) during arthroscopic single-row repair of rotator cuff tear and at 4 weeks	PRP did not provide statistically significantly greater improvement in pain or function at 6 weeks.
Jo et al. (118) (2011)	Cohort trial (level II evidence)	Arthroscopic double-row rotator cuff repair with application of 3 mL PRP gel at tendon-bone interface (19 patients) vs. repair without PRP (23 patients)	No statistically significant greater improvement in pain, strength, function, or satisfaction in PRP group over 16 months.
Randelli et al. (119) (2011)	RCT (level I evidence)	Arthroscopic single-row repair of complete rotator cuff tear with intra-operative injection of 6 mL PRP (26 patients) vs. repair without PRP (27 patients)	PRP treatment significantly reduced pain at 1 month after surgery and provided better clinical score than controls at 3 months. For grade I–II tears, PRP provided better results even at 24 months.
Castrinci et al. (120) (2011)	RCT (level I evidence)	Arthroscopic double-row repair of small to medium rotator cuff tear with intra-operative application of autologous platelet-rich fibrin matrix (PRFM) at the tendon-bone interface (43 patients) vs. repair without PRFM (45 patients)	No statistically significant difference between groups for functional score or MRI tendon structure at 16 months.
Antuna et al. (121) (2013)	RCT (level I evidence)	Arthroscopic repair of massive rotator cuff tear with intraoperative injection of 6 mL platelet-rich fibrin (14 patients) vs. repair without PRP (14 patients)	No statistically significant difference among groups for improvement of function and MRI tendon structure at 2 years.
Malavolta et al. (122) (2014)	RCT (level I evidence)	Arthroscopic single-row repair of complete rotator cuff tear with intra-operative injection of 20 mL PRP at tendon-bone interface (28 patients) vs. repair without PRP (27 patients)	No statistically significant difference between groups for improvement of pain and function at 2 years.

(continued)

TABLE 7.6 Studies of Rotator Cuff Tendinopathy (*continued*)

Study	Type of Study	Intervention	Main Results
Rodeo et al. (123) (2012)	RCT (level I evidence)	Arthroscopic repair of rotator cuff tear with intra-operative application of autologous PRFM at the tendon-bone interface (40 patients) vs. repair without PRFM (39 patients)	No statistically significant difference among groups for tendon-to-bone healing at 12 months. No difference in healing determined by ultrasound at 6 and 12 weeks. Greater persistence of rotator cuff tendon defect at 3 months in PRFM group.
Gumina et al. (124) (2012)	RCT (level I evidence)	Arthroscopic single-row repair of full-thickness rotator cuff tear with intra-operative application of PRP membrane at tendon-bone interface (40 patients) vs. repair without PRP (40 patients)	PRP group was associated with better repair integrity on MRI but not greater improvement in functional outcome at 13 months.
Carr et al. (126) (2015)	RCT (level I evidence)	Arthroscopic acromioplasty for rotator cuff tendinopathy with intra-operative subacromial injection of 6 mL PRP (25 patients) vs. acromioplasty without PRP (23 patients)	No statistically significant difference among groups for function at 2 years. PRP significantly alters tissue characteristics with reduced cellularity and vascularity and increased apoptosis at 12 weeks.
Kesikburun et al. (127) (2013)	RCT (level I evidence)	US-guided injection of 5 mL PRP × 1 (20 patients) vs. 5 mL saline × 1 (20 patients) to the subacromial space for rotator cuff tendinopathy	No statistically significant difference among groups for pain, function, range of motion, quality of life at 1 year.
Rha et al. (128) (2013)	RCT (level I evidence)	US-guided injection of 3 mL PRP × 2 (20 patients) vs. US-guided dry needling × 2 (19 patients) at 4-week interval for tendinosis or partial tear of supraspinatus tendon	PRP group had significantly greater reduction of pain and improvement of function at 6 weeks and 6 months.

PRFM, platelet-rich fibrin matrix; PRP, platelet-rich plasma; RCT, randomized controlled trial.

application of PRP during ACL reconstruction using hamstring tendon grafts improved graft maturation (142,143) and anteroposterior knee stability at 6 months (144) but was ineffective in preventing femoral or tibial bone tunnel enlargement (142,145) or improving postoperative functional scores at 15 months (146). PRP improved maturation of bone-patellar tendon-bone allografts (147), but did not improve clinical function or biomechanical properties of these grafts at 24 months (148). The PRP application has been inconsistently shown to accelerate graft-to-bone incorporation, ranging from being ineffective for osteoligamentous integration (142,149,150), to improving healing (151), reducing edema, increasing vascularity at the bone-graft interface (152,153), and reducing time for the graft to achieve a "ligamentous-like" MRI signal by 48% (154). Significantly less swelling and inflammation have been associated with the use of PRP without leukocytes to augment ACL reconstruction (155).

Medial Collateral Ligament of the Knee

Presently, there is no strong evidence to support the efficacy of PRP injections for treating medial collateral ligament (MCL) lesions in humans. A case report described favorable outcomes in managing a high-grade acute MCL lesion using PRP treatment (156).

Ankle Sprains

A double-blinded RCT comparing the injection of PRP and saline placebo in addition to standard therapy for severe ankle sprains showed no statistically significant difference in pain and function outcomes among groups over 30 days of follow-up (157).

A separate study comparing the addition of US-guided PRP injection to rehabilitation to treat anterior inferior tibiofibular ligament tears from high-ankle sprains in elite athletes showed PRP-accelerated return to sport by nearly 3 weeks, improved joint stability, and reduced residual pain (158).

Ulnar Collateral Ligament of the Elbow

A case series of overhand throwing athletes (i.e., baseball, softball, tennis, and volleyball players) with a partial ulnar collateral ligament (UCL) tear of the elbow who had failed at least 2 months of nonoperative treatment provided level IV evidence of the favorable outcomes of PRP therapy. Theses athletes, who received a single, US-guided, leukocyte-rich PRP injection into the injured UCL followed by a guided post-PRP rehabilitation program, had an average return to play time of 12 weeks, compared with the significant 12-month rehabilitation period commonly associated with surgical repair (159).

Muscle

Following case reports describing the promise of PRP injection for muscle injuries (160), a small, randomized, non-blinded study demonstrated US-guided PRP treatment for acute muscle injuries (thigh, shoulder, foot, and ankle) compared with conservative therapy provided greater reduction of early pain, improvement of range of motion, and earlier return to sport (161).

Hamstring

Acute hamstring injury is one of the most common types of muscle injury affecting athletes, resulting in loss of competition time (162,163). A single-blinded RCT demonstrated PRP significantly reduced pain intensity over 10 weeks and accelerated return to sport by 16 days for acute hamstring partial tears (164).

Larger, double-blinded RCTs, however, showed that PRP injection provided no significant benefit. A single PRP injection in combination with intensive rehabilitation provided no significantly greater benefit when compared with intensive rehabilitation alone to accelerate return to sport, improve muscle strength, or influence reinjury rates after 2 and 6 months in athletes following an acute hamstring injury (165).

Similarly, a US-guided intramuscular injection of PRP compared with saline, both combined with a rehabilitation program, for acute hamstring injury showed no significant difference among groups in reinjury rate at 2 months or 1 year or return to sport at 6 months (166) or 1 year (167).

Gastrocnemius and Rectus Femoris

Injection of autologous PRP in combination with standard conservative care compared with standard care alone for gastrocnemius and rectus femoris muscle tears with hematoma did not significantly improve healing (168).

Cartilage

Although few studies have been published on the use of PRP for management of hip and ankle arthritis, several trials have focused on PRP use for knee arthritis.

Knee

Several trials have suggested the efficacy of PRP to improve functional outcomes for mild knee osteoarthritis (OA) (169–179). Overall findings from RCTs have been unable to consistently demonstrate the superiority of PRP over traditional approaches. Comparative trials have demonstrated that autologous PRP intra-articular injections have greater efficacy than hyaluronic acid injections in reducing pain and recovering articular function (180–182), especially for younger patients and milder knee OA (183–186), with one study showing the benefit of PRP even for grade 3 knee OA (187). Others have shown inconsistent superiority of PRP over viscosupplementation (175). In an RCT with 1-year follow-up, PRP was not superior to viscosupplementation for knee OA, with diminishing benefit beyond 9 months (188,189).

No difference in outcomes for pain and function came from having a single or a double injection of PRP, but both provided superior outcomes compared with saline control (190). Another study demonstrated the superiority of

PRP compared with viscosupplementation only when multiple PRP injections were used (185). PRP was shown to be superior to steroid injection for knee OA (191).

Adverse effects have been minor, with leukocyte-rich PRP associated with increased pain and swelling relative to leukocyte-poor PRP (31). See Table 7.7.

Hip

Two case series demonstrated the safety and promise of PRP injection for treating hip OA (192), but with time-dependent benefit and non-superiority over viscosupplementation (193,194). An RCT demonstrated the superiority of PRP compared with hyaluronic acid injection for hip OA to improve pain and function at 6 months (195).

Ankle

A small, prospective study comparing the efficacy of PRP injection with viscosupplementation for talar osteochondral lesions proved PRP to be significantly more effective in controlling pain and reestablishing function (196). PRP injection was shown, similarly, to provide clinical improvement for low-grade ankle OA (197), and as an adjunct to arthroscopic microfracture surgery for treating osteochondral talus lesions (198).

Meniscus

Few studies have evaluated the use of PRP for meniscal applications. A small retrospective study demonstrated the promise of PRP injection to relieve pain, facilitate return to sport, and halt progression of injury over 6 months for intrasubstance, grade 2, knee meniscal lesions (199). A small study showed that PRP augmentation of arthroscopic meniscal repair did not improve reoperation rates or accelerate return to activity (200). A clinical trial reported that PRP augmentation of open meniscal repair improved outcomes compared with that of open repair alone (201).

Study	Type of Study	Intervention	Main Results
Filardo et al. (169) (2011)	Case series (level IV evidence)	Chronic knee degeneration treated with three intra-articular PRP injections every three weeks; each PRP injection activated with 10% calcium chloride	Favorable results in younger patients and lower degrees of cartilage degeneration. Median duration of improvement was 9 months.
Kon et al. (170) (2010)	Case series (level IV evidence)	Chronic knee degeneration treated with three intra-articular PRP injections every 3 weeks; each PRP injection activated with 10% calcium chloride	Significant improvement in all clinical IKDC scores at 6–12 month follow-up from baseline. PRP injections reduce pain and improve knee function in younger patients and lower degree of articular degeneration.
Napolitano et al. (171) (2012)	Case series (level IV evidence)	Chronic knee degenerative cartilage disease treated with three intra-articular PRP injections at weekly intervals; each PRP injection activated with 10% calcium gluconate	Significant improvement at 6-month follow-up on the Numerical Rating Scale (NRS) for subjective measurement of pain.
Wang-Saegusa et al. (172) (2010)	Case series (level IV evidence)	Patients with knee pathology of more than 3 months treated with plasma rich in growth factors (PRGF) at 2-week intervals following Anitua Technique	Significant improvements in pain, stiffness, and functional capacity in the WOMAC Index, Lequesne Index, SF-36 physical, and VAS pain score at 6 months from baseline.
Sanchez et al. (173) (2008)	Observational Retrospective Cohort Study (level III evidence)	Patients with osteoarthritis of the knee with three weekly PRGF injections vs. hyaluronan injections (control)	Significant improvement in pain and physical function on WOMAC scores in the PRGF group at 5 weeks.
Li et al. (175) (2011)	Randomized Prospective Study (level II evidence)	Patients with knee articular cartilage degeneration injected with PRP or sodium hyaluronate (control) at 3-week intervals	No significant difference in IKDC score, WOMAC score, and Lequesne index between two groups within 4 months but with better improvement of PRP group at 6 months.

(continued)

TABLE 7.7 **Studies of Knee Arthropathy and Arthritis**   (*continued*)

Study	Type of Study	Intervention	Main Results
Raeissadat et al. (176) (2013)	Case series (level IV evidence)	Patients treated with two leukocyte rich PRP (LR-PRP) injections at 4-week intervals	Significant improvements in pain, stiffness, and functional capacity in WOMAC Index at 6 months compared with baseline.
Gobbi et al. (177) (2012)	Case series (level IV evidence)	Patients with knee OA treated with two intra-articular injections of autologous PRP at monthly intervals	Significant improvement at 6 and 12 months in all scores.
Rayegani et al. (178) (2014)	RCT (level I evidence)	Therapeutic exercise plus two injections of PRP at 4-week intervals (31 patients) vs. therapeutic exercise alone (31 patients)	Addition of intra-articular PRP knee injection to therapeutic exercise is more effective in reducing pain and improving range of motion assessed by WOMAC and quality of life assessed by SF-36 compared with therapeutic exercise alone after 6 months.
Sampson et al. (179) (2010)	Case series (level IV evidence)	14 patients with knee OA treated with three injections of PRP at 4-week intervals	Clinical improvement assessed by the Brittberg-Peterson Visual Pain, Activities, and Expectations score and the Knee Injury and Osteoarthritis Outcome Scores after 12 months.
Vaquerizo et al. (180) (2013)	RCT (level I evidence)	14 patients with knee OA treated with three injections of PRGF at 1-week intervals or one injection with Durolane hyaluronic acid (control)	Rate of response was higher in the PRGF group compared with hyaluronic acid group for all scores in the WOMAC, Lequesne index, and OMEERACT-OARSI at 24 and 48 weeks.

(*continued*)

TABLE 7.7 **Studies of Knee Arthropathy and Arthritis** (*continued*)

Study	Type of Study	Intervention	Main Results
Spakova et al. (181) (2012)	Prospective Cohort Study (level II evidence)	Patients with knee OA treated with either three PRP or hyaluronic acid injections at weekly intervals	At 6 months, the PRP group showed improvement in Numerical Rating Scale (NRS) and the WOMAC index compared with hyaluronic acid.
Raeissadat et al. (182) (2015)	Randomized Non-Placebo-Controlled Trial (level II evidence)	Patients with knee OA treated with two PRP or hyaluronic acid injections at 4-week intervals	Significant improvement in WOMAC pain score and bodily pain at 12 months in PRP group.
Sanchez et al. (183) (2012)	RCT (level I evidence)	Patients with knee OA treated with three PRP injections or hyaluronic acid injections at weekly intervals	Significant higher response rate in 50% decrease in WOMAC pain subscale in PRP group at 24 weeks.
Kon et al. (184) (2011)	Prospective Comparative Study (level II evidence)	Cartilage degenerative lesions and early and severe OA treated with three PRP injections or low molecular weight/high molecular weight hyaluronic acid injections; calcium chloride was added to activate PRP	Significant improvement in PRP group in IKDC and EQ VAS scores. No difference in scores between PRP and controls in patients older than 50 years.
Gormeli et al. (185) (2015)	RCT (level I evidence)	Patients with knee OA treated with either three PRP, one PRP, one hyaluronic acid, or saline injections	Significant improvement in IKDC and EQ VAS scores in all treatment groups compared with saline group. Knee scores were better in those with three PRP injections. In early OA, significantly better results in those treated with three PRP injections.
Montanez-Heredia et al. (186) (2016)	RCT (level I Evidence)	Knee OA patients treated with either three PRP or hyaluronic acid injections at 15-day intervals	Improvements in pain scales with either PRP or hyaluronic acid at 3 or 6 months posttreatment. PRP more effective in patients with lower OA grade scales.
Cerza F et al. (187) (2012)	RCT (level I evidence)	Knee gonarthrosis patients treated with either four PRP injections or hyaluronic acid injections at weekly intervals	Significant improvement at 24 weeks in WOMAC scores in PRP group.

(*continued*)

TABLE 7.7 Studies of Knee Arthropathy and Arthritis   (*continued*)

Study	Type of Study	Intervention	Main Results
Filardo et al. (188) (2012)	RCT (level I evidence)	Knee chondropathy or OA treated with either three PRP or hyaluronic acid injections at weekly intervals	No significant difference in clinical improvement in all scores. A trend favorable for PRP was found in those with low-grade articular degeneration.
Filardo et al. (189) (2015)	RCT (level I evidence)	Knee OA treated with either three PRP or hyaluronic acid injections at weekly intervals	No significant difference observed for all clinical scores between PRP and hyaluronic acid.
Patel et al. (190) (2013)	RCT (level I evidence)	Knee OA treated with either one PRP injection, three PRP injections 3 weeks apart, or one normal saline injection	Significant improvement at 6 months in WOMAC in the PRP groups but no difference between single or multiple PRP injection groups from 3 to 6 months.
Forogh et al. (191) (2015)	RCT (level I evidence)	Knee OA treated with one PRP or corticosteroid injection	Pain relief, activities of daily living, and quality of life were better in PRP group at 2 and 6 months.
Filardo et al. (31) (2012)	Comparative Study (level II evidence)	Knee OA treated with three injections of platelet concentrate prepared with a single-spinning procedure–PRGF (72 patients) vs. three injections of PRP obtained with a double-spinning approach	Similar improvements in pain and function between PRGF and PRP over 12 months, but greater swelling and procedural pain reaction with PRP.

IKDC, International Knee Documentation Committee; OA, osteoarthritis; PRGF, plasma rich in growth factors; PRP, platelet-rich plasma; RCT, randomized controlled trial; VAS, Visual Analogue Scale; WOMAC, Western Ontario and McMaster Universities Osteoarthritis Index.

Intervertebral Disc

Early studies have investigated the potential for PRP to treat discogenic low-back pain from degenerative disc disease, with promising benefit (202). A prospective, double-blinded, RCT showed that intradiscal injection of PRP compared with contrast control was shown to significantly improve pain and function at 8 weeks and up to 2 years (203).

Future Work

Studies suggest that the best time for PRP injections is 3 to 6 months after injury, with repeat administrations ranging between 2- and 8-week intervals. The efficacy of multiple injections is under investigation, with some studies showing no significant difference in outcomes between single and double injections for knee OA (190), and others demonstrating the superiority of multiple injections for knee OA (185) and patellar tendinopathy (109). By alleviating pain and increasing activity tolerance, PRP is thought to enable earlier return to sport and activity by 2 to 3 weeks, compared with no PRP injection (1). Questions remain as to the proper preparation, dosing, and timing of PRP. There is need for future studies to have better randomization and blinding procedures, larger sample sizes, subjects with more consistent duration of injuries, adequate and consistent descriptions of preparation and injection techniques, radiographic data to provide additional objective data for analysis, standard postinjection rehabilitation protocols, longer-term follow-up of more than 2 years, and standard functional outcome scores. Further studies comparing leukocyte-rich with leukocyte-poor PRP are also needed.

CONCLUSION

This is an exciting era for regenerative sports medicine. We are beyond infancy and now toddling as we strive to optimize platelet-based therapies. Research on PRP continues to advance.

Presently, moderate quality evidence supports the use of PRP for lateral epicondylosis and knee OA. Low-quality evidence suggests safety and benefit of PRP for ankle and hip OA; patellar and Achilles tendinopathy; and injuries of the UCL of the elbow, ankle ligaments, and possibly medial meniscus. Early results indicate potential for PRP to treat discogenic pain. For the next phase of advancement, further investigations are needed to optimize platelet dosing, cellular composition, and postprocedure rehabilitation protocols for PRP. Patient physiologic and genetic factors that influence response to treatment should also be considered and investigated. Precise outcome measures as well as follow-up over years, not weeks to months, are required to accurately evaluate efficacy. PRP is a therapy for and investment in long-term connective tissue health and should not be regarded as a short-term pain management strategy. Until research consistently accounts for and measures this scope of therapeutic benefit, results will likely continue to mislead and frustrate.

REFERENCES

1. Nguyen RT, Borg-Stein J, McInnis K. Applications of platelet-rich plasma in musculoskeletal and sports medicine: an evidence-based approach. *Pm R* 2011;3(3):226–250.
2. Boswell SG, Cole BJ, Sundman EA, et al. Platelet-rich plasma: a milieu of bioactive factors. *Arthroscopy.* 2012;28(3):429–439.
3. Sánchez M, Anitua E, Azofra J, et al. Comparison of surgically repaired Achilles tendon tears using platelet-rich fibrin matrices. *Am J Sports Med.* 2007;35(2):245–251.
4. Broughton G, 2nd, Janis JE, Attinger CE. Wound healing: an overview. *Plast Reconstr Surg.* 2006; 117(7 Suppl):1e-S–32e-S.
5. Scherer SS, Tobalem M, Vigato E, et al. Nonactivated versus thrombin-activated platelets on wound healing and fibroblast-to-myofibroblast differentiation *in vivo* and *in vitro. Plast Reconstr Surg.* 2012;129(1):46e–54e.
6. Blair P, Flaumenhaft R. Platelet alpha-granules: basic biology and clinical correlates. *Blood Rev.* 2009;23(4):177–189.

7. Davis VL, Abukabda AB, Radio NM, et al. Platelet-rich preparations to improve healing. Part I: workable options for every size practice. *J Oral Implantol*. 2014;40(4):500–510.

8. Malanga GA, Goldin M. PRP: review of the current evidence for musculoskeletal conditions. *Curr Phys Med Rehabil Rep*. 2014;2:1–5.

9. Boswell SG, Schnabel LV, Mohammed HO, et al. Increasing platelet concentrations in leukocyte-reduced platelet-rich plasma decrease collagen gene synthesis in tendons. *Am J Sports Med*. 2014;42(1):42–49.

10. Giusti I, Rughetti A, D'Ascenzo S, et al. Identification of an optimal concentration of platelet gel for promoting angiogenesis in human endothelial cells. *Transfusion*. 2009;49(4):771–778.

11. Giusti I, Rughetti A, D'Ascenzo S, et al. The effects of platelet gel-released supernatant on human fibroblasts. *Wound Repair Regen*. 2013;21(2):300–308.

12. Anitua E, Sánchez M, Nurden AT, et al. Platelet-released growth factors enhance the secretion of hyaluronic acid and induce hepatocyte growth factor production by synovial fibroblasts from arthritic patients. *Rheumatology (Oxford)*. 2007;46(12):1769–1772.

13. Jo CH, Kim JE, Yoon KS, et al. Platelet-rich plasma stimulates cell proliferation and enhances matrix gene expression and synthesis in tenocytes from human rotator cuff tendons with degenerative tears. *Am J Sports Med*. 2012;40(5):1035–1045.

14. Hoemann CD, Chen G, Marchand C, et al. Scaffold-guided subchondral bone repair: implication of neutrophils and alternatively activated arginase-1+ macrophages. *Am J Sports Med*. 2010;38(9):1845–1856.

15. Bielecki T, Dohan Ehrenfest DM, Everts PA, et al. The role of leukocytes from L-PRP/L-PRF in wound healing and immune defense: new perspectives. *Curr Pharm Biotechnol*. 2012;13(7):1153–1162.

16. Assirelli E, Filardo G, Mariani E, et al. Effect of two different preparations of platelet-rich plasma on synoviocytes. *Knee Surg Sports Traumatol Arthrosc*. 2015;23(9):2690–2703.

17. Braun HJ, Kim HJ, Chu CR, et al. The effect of platelet-rich plasma formulations and blood products on human synoviocytes: implications for intra-articular injury and therapy. *Am J Sports Med*. 2014;42(5):1204–1210.

18. Dragoo JL, Braun HJ, Durham JL, et al. Comparison of the acute inflammatory response of two commercial platelet-rich plasma systems in healthy rabbit tendons. *Am J Sports Med*. 2012;40(6):1274–1281.

19. McCarrel TM, Minas T, Fortier LA. Optimization of leukocyte concentration in platelet-rich plasma for the treatment of tendinopathy. *J Bone Joint Surg Am*. 2012;94(19):e1431–e1438.

20. van Buul GM, Koevoet WL, Kops N, et al. Platelet-rich plasma releasate inhibits inflammatory processes in osteoarthritic chondrocytes. *Am J Sports Med*. 2011;39(11):2362–2370.

21. Yoshida R, Murray MM. Peripheral blood mononuclear cells enhance the anabolic effects of platelet-rich plasma on anterior cruciate ligament fibroblasts. *J Orthop Res*. 2013;31(1):29–34.

22. Zimmermann R, Arnold D, Strasser E, et al. Sample preparation technique and white cell content influence the detectable levels of growth factors in platelet concentrates. *Vox Sang*. 2003;85(4):283–289.

23. Pifer MA, Maerz T, Baker KC, et al. Matrix metalloproteinase content and activity in low-platelet, low-leukocyte and high-platelet, high-leukocyte platelet-rich plasma (PRP) and the biologic response to PRP by human ligament fibroblasts. *Am J Sports Med*. 2014;42(5):1211–1218.

24. Sundman EA, Cole BJ, Fortier LA. Growth factor and catabolic cytokine concentrations are influenced by the cellular composition of platelet-rich plasma. *Am J Sports Med*. 2011;39(10):2135–2140.

25. Boswell SG, Schnabel LV, Mohammed HO, et al. Increasing platelet concentrations in leukocyte-reduced platelet-rich plasma decrease collagen gene synthesis in tendons. *Am J Sports Med*. 2014;42(1):42–49.

26. Hooiveld M, Roosendaal G, Wenting M, et al. Short-term exposure of cartilage to blood results in chondrocyte apoptosis. *Am J Pathol*. 2003;162(3):943–951.

27. Madhok R, Bennett D, Sturrock RD, et al. Mechanisms of joint damage in an experimental model of hemophilic arthritis. *Arthritis Rheum*. 1988;31(9):1148–1155.

28. Roosendaal G, Vianen ME, Marx JJ, et al. Blood-induced joint damage: a human *in vitro* study. *Arthritis Rheum*. 1999;42(5):1025–1032.

29. Roosendaal G, Vianen ME, van den Berg HM, et al. Cartilage damage as a result of hemarthrosis in a human *in vitro* model. *J Rheumatol*. 1997;24(7):1350–1354.

30. Castillo TN, Pouliot MA, Kim HJ, et al. Comparison of growth factor and platelet concentration from

commercial platelet-rich plasma separation systems. *Am J Sports Med*. 2011;39(2):266–271.

31. Filardo G, Kon E, Pereira Ruiz MT, et al. Platelet-rich plasma intra-articular injections for cartilage degeneration and osteoarthritis: single- versus double-spinning approach. *Knee Surg Sports Traumatol Arthrosc*. 2012;20(10):2082–2091.

32. Anitua E. The use of plasma-rich growth factors (PRGF) in oral surgery. *Pract Proced Aesthet Dent*. 2001;13(6):487–93; quiz 487.

33. Leitner GC, Gruber R, Neumüller J, et al. Platelet content and growth factor release in platelet-rich plasma: a comparison of four different systems. *Vox Sang*. 2006;91(2):135–139.

34. Dohan DM, Choukroun J, Diss A, et al. Platelet-rich fibrin (PRF): a second-generation platelet concentrate. Part I: technological concepts and evolution. *Oral Surg Oral Med Oral Pathol Oral Radiol Endod*. 2006;101(3):e37–e44.

35. DeLong JM, Russell RP, Mazzocca AD. Platelet-rich plasma: the PAW classification system. *Arthroscopy*. 2012;28(7):998–1009.

36. Dohan Ehrenfest DM, Andia I, Zumstein MA, et al. Classification of platelet concentrates (platelet-rich plasma-PRP, platelet-rich fibrin-PRF) for topical and infiltrative use in orthopedic and sports medicine: current consensus, clinical implications and perspectives. *Muscles Ligaments Tendons J*. 2014;4(1):3–9.

37. Mautner K, Malanga GA, Smith J, et al. A call for a standard classification system for future biologic research: the rationale for new PRP nomenclature. *PM R*. 2015;7(4 Suppl):S53–S59.

38. Mishra A, Harmon K, Woodall J, et al. Sports medicine applications of platelet-rich plasma. *Curr Pharm Biotechnol*. 2012;13(7):1185–1195.

39. Oh JH, Kim W, Park KU, et al. Comparison of the cellular composition and cytokine-release kinetics of various platelet-rich plasma preparations. *Am J Sports Med*. 2015;43(12):3062–3070.

40. Arora S, Doda V, Kotwal U, et al. Quantification of platelets and platelet-derived growth factors from platelet-rich plasma (PRP) prepared at different centrifugal force (g) and time. *Transfus Apher Sci*. 2016;54(1):103–110.

41. Weibrich G, Kleis WK, Hafner G. Growth factor levels in the platelet-rich plasma produced by 2 different methods: curasan-type PRP kit versus PCCS PRP system. *Int J Oral Maxillofac Implants*. 2002;17(2):184–190.

42. Weibrich G, Kleis WK, Buch R, et al. The Harvest Smart PRePTM system versus the Friadent-Schütze platelet-rich plasma kit. *Clin Oral Implants Res*. 2003;14(2):233–239.

43. Weibrich G, Kleis WK, Hafner G, et al. Comparison of platelet, leukocyte, and growth factor levels in point-of-care platelet-enriched plasma, prepared using a modified Curasan kit, with preparations received from a local blood bank. *Clin Oral Implants Res*. 2003;14(3):357–362.

44. Weibrich G, Kleis WK, Hitzler WE, et al. Comparison of the platelet-concentrate collection system with the plasma-rich-in-growth-factors kit to produce platelet-rich plasma: a technical report. *Int J Oral Maxillofac Implants*. 2005;20(1):118–123.

45. Magalon J, Bausset O, Serratrice N, et al. Characterization and comparison of 5 platelet-rich plasma preparations in a single-donor model. *Arthroscopy*. 2014;30(5):629–638.

46. Aydin F, Pancar Yuksel E, Albayrak D. Platelet-collection efficiencies of three different platelet-rich plasma preparation systems. *J Cosmet Laser Ther*. 2015;17(3):165–168.

47. Dohan Ehrenfest DM, de Peppo GM, Doglioli P, et al. Slow release of growth factors and thrombospondin-1 in Choukroun's platelet-rich fibrin (PRF): a gold standard to achieve for all surgical platelet-concentrates technologies. *Growth Factors*. 2009; 27(1):63–69.

48. Dohan Ehrenfest DM, Bielecki T, Jimbo R, et al. Do the fibrin architecture and leukocyte content influence the growth factor release of platelet concentrates? An evidence-based answer comparing a pure platelet-rich plasma (P-PRP) gel and a leukocyte- and platelet-rich fibrin (L-PRF). *Curr Pharm Biotechnol*. 2012;13(7):1145–1152.

49. Dohan DM, Choukroun J, Diss A, et al. Platelet-rich fibrin (PRF): a second-generation platelet concentrate. Part II: platelet-related biologic features. *Oral Surg Oral Med Oral Pathol Oral Radiol Endod*. 2006;101(3):e45–e50.

50. Schär MO, Diaz-Romero J, Kohl S, et al. Platelet-rich concentrates differentially release growth factors and induce cell migration *in vitro*. *Clin Orthop Relat Res*. 2015;473(5):1635–1643.

51. Passaretti F, Tia M, D'Esposito V, et al. Growth-promoting action and growth factor release by different platelet derivatives. *Platelets*. 2014; 25(4): 252–256.

52. Gassling VL, Açil Y, Springer IN, et al. Platelet-rich plasma and platelet-rich fibrin in human cell culture. *Oral Surg Oral Med Oral Pathol Oral Radiol Endod*. 2009;108(1):48–55.

53. Zumstein MA, Berger S, Schober M, et al. Leukocyte- and platelet-rich fibrin (L-PRF) for long-term delivery of growth factor in rotator cuff repair: review, preliminary results and future directions. *Curr Pharm Biotechnol*. 2012;13(7):1196–1206.

54. He L, Lin Y, Hu X, et al. A comparative study of platelet-rich fibrin (PRF) and platelet-rich plasma (PRP) on the effect of proliferation and differentiation of rat osteoblasts *in vitro*. *Oral Surg Oral Med Oral Pathol Oral Radiol Endod*. 2009;108(5): 707–713.

55. Braune S, Walter M, Schulze F, et al. Changes in platelet morphology and function during 24 hours of storage. *Clin Hemorheol Microcirc*. 2014;58(1):159–170.

56. Marx RE, Carlson ER, Eichstaedt RM, et al. Platelet-rich plasma: growth factor enhancement for bone grafts. *Oral Surg Oral Med Oral Pathol Oral Radiol Endod*. 1998;85(6):638–646.

57. Roh YH, Kim W, Park KU, et al. Cytokine-release kinetics of platelet-rich plasma according to various activation protocols. *Bone Joint Res*. 2016;5(2): 37–45.

58. Martineau I, Lacoste E, Gagnon G. Effects of calcium and thrombin on growth factor release from platelet concentrates: kinetics and regulation of endothelial cell proliferation. *Biomaterials*. 2004;25(18):4489–4502.

59. Harrison S, Vavken P, Kevy S, et al. Platelet activation by collagen provides sustained release of anabolic cytokines. *Am J Sports Med*. 2011;39 (4):729–734.

60. Jeon YR, Jung BK, Roh TS, et al. Comparing the effect of nonactivated platelet-rich plasma, activated platelet-rich plasma, and bone morphogenetic protein-2 on calvarial bone regeneration. *J Craniofac Surg*. 2016;27(2):317–321.

61. Varon D, Spectre G. Antiplatelet agents. *Hematology Am Soc Hematol Educ Program*. 2009;1:267–272.

62. Schippinger G, Prüller F, Divjak M, et al. Autologous platelet-rich plasma preparations: influence of non-steroidal anti-inflammatory drugs on platelet function. *Orthop J Sports Med*. 2015;3(6). doi:10.1177/ 2325967115588896

63. Mongan J, Mieszczanska HZ, Smith BH, et al. Pioglitazone inhibits platelet function and potentiates the effects of aspirin: a prospective observation study. *Thromb Res*. 2012;129(6):760–764.

64. Bausset O, Magalon J, Giraudo L, et al. Impact of local anaesthetics and needle calibres used for painless PRP injections on platelet functionality. *Muscles Ligaments Tendons J*. 2014;4(1):18–23.

65. Moraes VY, Lenza M, Tamaoki MJ, et al. Platelet-rich therapies for musculoskeletal soft tissue injuries. *Cochrane Database Syst Rev*. 2014;4: CD010071. doi:10.1002/14651858.CD010071.pub3

66. Edwards SG, Calandruccio JH. Autologous blood injections for refractory lateral epicondylitis. *J Hand Surg Am*. 2003;28(2):272–278.

67. Connell DA, Ali KE, Ahmad M, et al. Ultrasound-guided autologous blood injection for tennis elbow. *Skeletal Radiol*. 2006;35(6):371–377.

68. Chaudhury S, de La Lama M, Adler RS, et al. Platelet-rich plasma for the treatment of lateral epicondylitis: sonographic assessment of tendon morphology and vascularity (pilot study). *Skeletal Radiol*. 2013;42(1):91–97.

69. Hechtman KS, Uribe JW, Botto-vanDemden A, et al. Platelet-rich plasma injection reduces pain in patients with recalcitrant epicondylitis. *Orthopedics*. 2011;34(2):92. doi:10.3928/ 01477447-20101221-05

70. Mishra A, Pavelko T. Treatment of chronic elbow tendinosis with buffered platelet-rich plasma. *Am J Sports Med*. 2006;34(11):1774–1778.

71. Peerbooms JC, Sluimer J, Bruijn DJ, et al. Positive effect of an autologous platelet concentrate in lateral epicondylitis in a double-blind randomized controlled trial: platelet-rich plasma versus corticosteroid injection with a 1-year follow-up. *Am J Sports Med*. 2010;38(2):255–262.

72. Gosens T, Peerbooms JC, van Laar W, et al. Ongoing positive effect of platelet-rich plasma versus corticosteroid injection in lateral epicondylitis: a double-blind randomized controlled trial with 2-year follow-up. *Am J Sports Med*. 2011;39(6):1200–1208.

73. Creaney L, Wallace A, Curtis M, et al. Growth factor-based therapies provide additional benefit beyond physical therapy in resistant elbow tendinopathy: a prospective, single-blind, randomised trial of autologous blood injections versus platelet-rich plasma injections. *Br J Sports Med*. 2011;45(12):966–971.

74. Thanasas C, Papadimitriou G, Charalambidis C, et al. Platelet-rich plasma versus autologous whole blood for the treatment of chronic lateral elbow epicondylitis: a randomized controlled clinical trial. *Am J Sports Med*. 2011;39(10):2130–2134.

75. Krogh TP, Fredberg U, Stengaard-Pedersen K, et al. Treatment of lateral epicondylitis with

platelet-rich plasma, glucocorticoid, or saline: a randomized, double-blind, placebo-controlled trial. *Am J Sports Med.* 2013;41(3):625–635.

76. Mishra AK, Skrepnik NV, Edwards SG, et al. Efficacy of platelet-rich plasma for chronic tennis elbow: a double-blind, prospective, multicenter, randomized controlled trial of 230 patients. *Am J Sports Med.* 2014;42(2):463–471.

77. Omar AS, Ibrahim ME, Ahmed AS, et al. Local injection of autologous platelet-rich plasma and corticosteroid in treatment of lateral epicondylitis and plantar fasciitis: randomized clinical trial. *Egypt Rheumatol.* 2012;34:43–49.

78. Behera P, Dhillon M, Aggarwal S, et al. Leukocyte-poor platelet-rich plasma versus bupivacaine for recalcitrant lateral epicondylar tendinopathy. *J Orthop Surg (Hong Kong).* 2015;23(1):6–10.

79. Wolf JM, Ozer K, Scott F, et al. Comparison of autologous blood, corticosteroid, and saline injection in the treatment of lateral epicondylitis: a prospective, randomized, controlled multicenter study. *J Hand Surg Am.* 2011;36(8):1269–1272.

80. Raeissadat SA, Rayegani SM, Hassanabadi H, et al. Is platelet-rich plasma superior to whole blood in the management of chronic tennis elbow: one year randomized clinical trial. *BMC Sports Sci Med Rehabil.* 2014;6:12.

81. Chiavaras MM, Jacobson JA, Carlos R, et al. IMpact of Platelet Rich plasma OVer alternative therapies in patients with lateral Epicondylitis (IMPROVE): protocol for a multicenter randomized controlled study: a multicenter, randomized trial comparing autologous platelet-rich plasma, autologous whole blood, dry needle tendon fenestration, and physical therapy exercises alone on pain and quality of life in patients with lateral epicondylitis. *Acad Radiol.* 2014;21(9):1144–1155.

82. Schepull T, Kvist J, Norrman H, et al. Autologous platelets have no effect on the healing of human Achilles tendon ruptures: a randomized single-blind study. *Am J Sports Med.* 2011;39(1):38–47.

83. Gaweda K, Tarczynska M, Krzyzanowski W. Treatment of Achilles tendinopathy with platelet-rich plasma. *Int J Sports Med.* 2010;31(8):577–583.

84. Monto RR. Platelet-rich plasma treatment for chronic Achilles tendinosis. *Foot Ankle Int.* 2012;33(5):379–385.

85. Ferrero G, Fabbro E, Orlandi D, et al. Ultrasound-guided injection of platelet-rich plasma in chronic Achilles and patellar tendinopathy. *J Ultrasound.* 2012;15(4):260–266.

86. Deans VM, Miller A, Ramos J. A prospective series of patients with chronic Achilles tendinopathy treated with autologous-conditioned plasma injections combined with exercise and therapeutic ultrasonography. *J Foot Ankle Surg.* 2012;51(6):706–710.

87. Volpi P, Quaglia A, Schoenhuber H, et al. Growth factors in the management of sport-induced tendinopathies: results after 24 months from treatment. A pilot study. *J Sports Med Phys Fitness.* 2010;50(4):494–500.

88. Finnoff JT, Fowler SP, Lai JK, et al. Treatment of chronic tendinopathy with ultrasound-guided needle tenotomy and platelet-rich plasma injection. *PM R.* 2011;3(10):900–911.

89. Oloff L, Elmi E, Nelson J, et al. Retrospective analysis of the effectiveness of platelet-rich plasma in the treatment of Achilles tendinopathy: pretreatment and posttreatment correlation of magnetic resonance imaging and clinical assessment. *Foot Ankle Spec.* 2015;8(6):490–497.

90. Kearney RS, Parsons N, Costa ML. Achilles tendinopathy management: a pilot randomised controlled trial comparing platelet-rich plasma injection with an eccentric loading programme. *Bone Joint Res.* 2013;2(10):227–232.

91. Murawski CD, Smyth NA, Newman H, et al. A single platelet-rich plasma injection for chronic midsubstance Achilles tendinopathy: a retrospective preliminary analysis. *Foot Ankle Spec.* 2014;7(5):372–376.

92. Owens RF Jr, Ginnetti J, Conti SF, et al. Clinical and magnetic resonance imaging outcomes following platelet-rich plasma injection for chronic midsubstance Achilles tendinopathy. *Foot Ankle Int.* 2011;32(11):1032–1039.

93. Mautner K, Colberg RE, Malanga G, et al. Outcomes after ultrasound-guided platelet-rich plasma injections for chronic tendinopathy: a multicenter, retrospective review. *PM R.* 2013;5(3):169–175.

94. Filardo G, Kon E, Di Matteo B, et al. Platelet-rich plasma injections for the treatment of refractory Achilles tendinopathy: results at 4 years. *Blood Transfus.* 2014;12(4):533–540.

95. de Vos RJ, Weir A, van Schie HT, et al. Platelet-rich plasma injection for chronic Achilles tendinopathy: a randomized controlled trial. *JAMA.* 2010;303(2):144–149.

96. de Jonge S, de Vos RJ, Weir A, et al. One-year follow-up of platelet-rich plasma treatment in

chronic Achilles tendinopathy: a double-blind randomized placebo-controlled trial. *Am J Sports Med*. 2011;39(8):1623–1629.

97. de Vos RJ, Weir A, Tol JL, et al. No effects of PRP on ultrasonographic tendon structure and neovascularisation in chronic midportion Achilles tendinopathy. *Br J Sports Med*. 2011;45(5):387–392.

98. Krogh TP, Bartels EM, Ellingsen T, et al. Comparative effectiveness of injection therapies in lateral epicondylitis: a systematic review and network meta-analysis of randomized controlled trials. *Am J Sports Med*. 2013;41(6):1435–1446.

99. Rabago D, Best TM, Zgierska AE, et al. A systematic review of four injection therapies for lateral epicondylosis: prolotherapy, polidocanol, whole blood and platelet-rich plasma. *Br J Sports Med*. 2009;43(7):471–481.

100. Gross CE, Hsu AR, Chahal J, et al. Injectable treatments for noninsertional Achilles tendinosis: a systematic review. *Foot Ankle Int*. 2013;34(5): 619–628.

101. Kon E, Filardo G, Delcogliano M, et al. Platelet-rich plasma: new clinical application: a pilot study for treatment of jumper's knee. *Injury*. 2009;40(6):598–603.

102. Charousset C, Zaoui A, Bellaiche L, et al. Are multiple platelet-rich plasma injections useful for treatment of chronic patellar tendinopathy in athletes? a prospective study. *Am J Sports Med*. 2014;42(4):906–911.

103. Kaux JF, Croisier JL, Bruyere O, et al. One injection of platelet-rich plasma associated to a submaximal eccentric protocol to treat chronic jumper's knee. *J Sports Med Phys Fitness*. 2015;55(9): 953–961.

104. Kaux JF, Bruyere O, Croisier JL, et al. One-year follow-up of platelet-rich plasma infiltration to treat chronic proximal patellar tendinopathies. *Acta Orthop Belg*. 2015;81(2):251–256.

105. Dallaudière B, Pesquer L, Meyer P, et al. Intratendinous injection of platelet-rich plasma under US guidance to treat tendinopathy: a long-term pilot study. *J Vasc Interv Radiol*. 2014;25(5):717–723.

106. Filardo G, Kon E, Di Matteo B, et al. Platelet-rich plasma for the treatment of patellar tendinopathy: clinical and imaging findings at medium-term follow-up. *Int Orthop*. 2013;37(8):1583–1589.

107. Gosens T, Den Oudsten BL, Fievez E, et al. Pain and activity levels before and after platelet-rich plasma injection treatment of patellar tendinopathy: a prospective cohort study and the influence of previous treatments. *Int Orthop*. 2012;36(9): 1941–1946.

108. Kaux JF, Croisier JL, Forthomme B, et al. Using platelet-rich plasma to treat jumper's knees: exploring the effect of a second closely-timed infiltration. *J Sci Med Sport*. 2016;19(3):200–204.

109. Zayni R, Thaunat M, Fayard JM, et al. Platelet-rich plasma as a treatment for chronic patellar tendinopathy: comparison of a single versus two consecutive injections. *Muscles Ligaments Tendons J*. 2015;5(2):92–98.

110. Filardo G, Kon E, Della Villa S, et al. Use of platelet-rich plasma for the treatment of refractory jumper's knee. *Int Orthop*. 2010;34(6):909–915.

111. Vetrano M, Castorina A, Vulpiani MC, et al. Platelet-rich plasma versus focused shock waves in the treatment of jumper's knee in athletes. *Am J Sports Med*. 2013;41(4):795–803.

112. Dragoo JL, Wasterlain AS, Braun HJ, et al. Platelet-rich plasma as a treatment for patellar tendinopathy: a double-blind, randomized controlled trial. *Am J Sports Med*. 2014;42(3):610–618.

113. Seijas R, Cuscó X, Sallent A, et al. Pain in donor site after BTB-ACL reconstruction with PRGF: a randomized trial. *Arch Orthop Trauma Surg*. 2016;136(6):829–835.

114. de Almeida AM, Demange MK, Sobrado MF, et al. Patellar tendon healing with platelet-rich plasma: a prospective randomized controlled trial. *Am J Sports Med*. 2012;40(6):1282–1288.

115. Cervellin M, de Girolamo L, Bait C, et al. Autologous platelet-rich plasma gel to reduce donor-site morbidity after patellar tendon graft harvesting for anterior cruciate ligament reconstruction: a randomized, controlled clinical study. *Knee Surg Sports Traumatol Arthrosc*. 2012;20(1): 114–120.

116. Randelli PS, Arrigoni P, Cabitza P, et al. Autologous platelet-rich plasma for arthroscopic rotator cuff repair. A pilot study. *Disabil Rehabil*. 2008;30(20-22):1584–1589.

117. Hak A, Rajaratnam K, Ayeni OR, et al. A double-blinded placebo randomized controlled trial evaluating short-term efficacy of platelet-rich plasma in reducing postoperative pain after arthroscopic rotator cuff repair: a pilot study. *Sports Health*. 2015;7(1):58–66.

118. Jo CH, Kim JE, Yoon KS, et al. Does platelet-rich plasma accelerate recovery after rotator cuff

repair? A prospective cohort study. *Am J Sports Med.* 2011;39(10):2082–2090.

119. Randelli P, Arrigoni P, Ragone V, et al. Platelet-rich plasma in arthroscopic rotator cuff repair: a prospective RCT study, 2-year follow-up. *J Shoulder Elbow Surg.* 2011;20(4):518–528.

120. Castricini R, Longo UG, De Benedetto M, et al. Platelet-rich plasma augmentation for arthroscopic rotator cuff repair: a randomized controlled trial. *Am J Sports Med.* 2011;39(2): 258–265.

121. Antuña S, Barco R, Martínez Diez JM, et al. Platelet-rich fibrin in arthroscopic repair of massive rotator cuff tears: a prospective randomized pilot clinical trial. *Acta Orthop Belg.* 2013;79(1): 25–30.

122. Malavolta EA, Gracitelli ME, Ferreira Neto AA, et al. Platelet-rich plasma in rotator cuff repair: a prospective randomized study. *Am J Sports Med.* 2014;42(10):2446–2454.

123. Rodeo SA, Delos D, Williams RJ, et al. The effect of platelet-rich fibrin matrix on rotator cuff tendon healing: a prospective, randomized clinical study. *Am J Sports Med.* 2012;40(6):1234–1241.

124. Gumina S, Campagna V, Ferrazza G, et al. Use of platelet-leukocyte membrane in arthroscopic repair of large rotator cuff tears: a prospective randomized study. *J Bone Joint Surg Am.* 2012;94(15):1345–1352.

125. Chahal J, Van Thiel GS, Mall N, et al. The role of platelet-rich plasma in arthroscopic rotator cuff repair: a systematic review with quantitative synthesis. *Arthroscopy.* 2012;28 (11):1718–1727.

126. Carr AJ, Murphy R, Dakin SG, et al. Platelet-rich plasma injection with arthroscopic acromioplasty for chronic rotator cuff tendinopathy: a randomized controlled trial. *Am J Sports Med.* 2015;43(12):2891–2897.

127. Kesikburun S, Tan AK, Yilmaz B, et al. Platelet-rich plasma injections in the treatment of chronic rotator cuff tendinopathy: a randomized controlled trial with 1-year follow-up. *Am J Sports Med.* 2013;41(11):2609–2616.

128. Rha DW, Park GY, Kim YK, et al. Comparison of the therapeutic effects of ultrasound-guided platelet-rich plasma injection and dry needling in rotator cuff disease: a randomized controlled trial. *Clin Rehabil.* 2013;27(2):113–122.

129. Martinelli N, Marinozzi A, Carnì S, et al. Platelet-rich plasma injections for chronic plantar fasciitis. *Int Orthop.* 2013;37(5):839–842.

130. Kumar V, Millar T, Murphy PN, et al. The treatment of intractable plantar fasciitis with platelet-rich plasma injection. *Foot (Edinb).* 2013;23(2-3): 74–77.

131. Ragab EM, Othman AM. Platelet-rich plasma for treatment of chronic plantar fasciitis. *Arch Orthop Trauma Surg.* 2012;132(8):1065–1070.

132. Mahindra P, Yamin M, Selhi HS, et al. Chronic plantar fasciitis: effect of platelet-rich plasma, corticosteroid, and placebo. *Orthopedics.* 2016;39(2): e285–e289.

133. Say F, Gürler D, Inkaya E, et al. Comparison of platelet-rich plasma and steroid injection in the treatment of plantar fasciitis. *Acta Orthop Traumatol Turc.* 2014;48(6):667–672.

134. Jain K, Murphy PN, Clough TM. Platelet-rich plasma versus corticosteroid injection for plantar fasciitis: a comparative study. *Foot (Edinb).* 2015;25(4):235–237.

135. Monto RR. Platelet-rich plasma efficacy versus corticosteroid injection treatment for chronic severe plantar fasciitis. *Foot Ankle Int.* 2014;35(4): 313–318.

136. Shetty VD, Dhillon M, Hegde C, et al. A study to compare the efficacy of corticosteroid therapy with platelet-rich plasma therapy in recalcitrant plantar fasciitis: a preliminary report. *Foot Ankle Surg.* 2014;20(1):10–13.

137. Aksahin E, Dogruyol D, Yüksel HY, et al. The comparison of the effect of corticosteroids and platelet-rich plasma (PRP) for the treatment of plantar fasciitis. *Arch Orthop Trauma Surg.* 2012;132(6):781–785.

138. Lee TG, Ahmad TS. Intralesional autologous blood injection compared to corticosteroid injection for treatment of chronic plantar fasciitis. A prospective, randomized, controlled trial. *Foot Ankle Int.* 2007;28(9):984–990.

139. Kim E, Lee JH. Autologous platelet-rich plasma versus dextrose prolotherapy for the treatment of chronic recalcitrant plantar fasciitis. *PM R.* 2014;6(2):152–158.

140. Chew KT, Leong D, Lin CY, et al. Comparison of autologous conditioned plasma injection, extracorporeal shockwave therapy, and conventional treatment for plantar fasciitis: a randomized trial. *PM R.* 2013;5(12):1035–1043.

141. Jacobson JA, Yablon CM, Henning PT, et al. Greater trochanteric pain syndrome: percutaneous tendon fenestration versus platelet-rich

plasma injection for treatment of gluteal tendinosis. *J Ultrasound Med.* 2016;35(11):2413–2420.

142. Orrego M, Larrain C, Rosales J, et al. Effects of platelet concentrate and a bone plug on the healing of hamstring tendons in a bone tunnel. *Arthroscopy.* 2008;24(12):1373–1380.

143. Sánchez M, Anitua E, Azofra J, et al. Ligamentization of tendon grafts treated with an endogenous preparation rich in growth factors: gross morphology and histology. *Arthroscopy.* 2010;26(4):470–480.

144. Vogrin M, Rupreht M, Crnjac A, et al. The effect of platelet-derived growth factors on knee stability after anterior cruciate ligament reconstruction: a prospective randomized clinical study. *Wien Klin Wochenschr.* 2010;122 Suppl 2:91–95.

145. Mirzatolooei F, Alamdari MT, Khalkhali HR. The impact of platelet-rich plasma on the prevention of tunnel widening in anterior cruciate ligament reconstruction using quadrupled autologous hamstring tendon: a randomised clinical trial. *Bone Joint J.* 2013;95-B(1):65–69.

146. Vadalà A, Iorio R, De Carli A, et al. Platelet-rich plasma: does it help reduce tunnel widening after ACL reconstruction? *Knee Surg Sports Traumatol Arthrosc.* 2013;21(4):824–829.

147. Seijas R, Ares O, Catala J, et al. Magnetic resonance imaging evaluation of patellar tendon graft remodelling after anterior cruciate ligament reconstruction with or without platelet-rich plasma. *J Orthop Surg (Hong Kong).* 2013;21(1):10–14.

148. Nin JR, Gasque GM, Azcárate AV, et al. Has platelet-rich plasma any role in anterior cruciate ligament allograft healing? *Arthroscopy.* 2009;25(11):1206–1213.

149. Silva A, Sampaio R. Anatomic ACL reconstruction: does the platelet-rich plasma accelerate tendon healing? *Knee Surg Sports Traumatol Arthrosc.* 2009;17(6):676–682.

150. Figueroa D, Melean P, Calvo R, et al. Magnetic resonance imaging evaluation of the integration and maturation of semitendinosus-gracilis graft in anterior cruciate ligament reconstruction using autologous platelet concentrate. *Arthroscopy.* 2010;26(10):1318–1325.

151. Rupreht M, Vogrin M, Hussein M. MRI evaluation of tibial tunnel wall cortical bone formation after platelet-rich plasma applied during anterior cruciate ligament reconstruction. *Radiol Oncol.* 2013;47(2):119–124.

152. Rupreht M, Jevtic V, Serša I, et al. Evaluation of the tibial tunnel after intraoperatively administered platelet-rich plasma gel during anterior cruciate ligament reconstruction using diffusion weighted and dynamic contrast-enhanced MRI. *J Magn Reson Imaging.* 2013;37(4):928–935.

153. Vogrin M, Rupreht M, Dineki D, et al. Effects of a platelet gel on early graft revascularization after anterior cruciate ligament reconstruction: a prospective, randomized, double-blind, clinical trial. *Eur Surg Res.* 2010;45(2):77–85.

154. Radice F, Yánez R, Gutiérrez V, et al. Comparison of magnetic resonance imaging findings in anterior cruciate ligament grafts with and without autologous platelet-derived growth factors. *Arthroscopy.* 2010;26(1):50–57.

155. Valentí Azcárate A, Lamo-Espinosa J, Aquerreta Beola JD, et al. Comparison between two different platelet-rich plasma preparations and control applied during anterior cruciate ligament reconstruction. Is there any evidence to support their use? *Injury.* 2014;45 Suppl 4:S36–S41.

156. Eirale C, Mauri E, Hamilton B. Use of platelet-rich plasma in an isolated complete medial collateral ligament lesion in a professional football (soccer) player: a case report. *Asian J Sports Med.* 2013;4(2):158–162.

157. Rowden A, Dominici P, D'Orazio J, et al. Double-blind, randomized, placebo-controlled study evaluating the use of platelet-rich plasma therapy (PRP) for acute ankle sprains in the emergency department. *J Emerg Med.* 2015;49(4):546–551.

158. Laver L, Carmont MR, McConkey MO, et al. Plasma rich in growth factors (PRGF) as a treatment for high ankle sprain in elite athletes: a randomized control trial. *Knee Surg Sports Traumatol Arthrosc.* 2015;23(11):3383–3392.

159. Podesta L, Crow SA, Volkmer D, et al. Treatment of partial ulnar collateral ligament tears in the elbow with platelet-rich plasma. *Am J Sports Med.* 2013;41(7):1689–1694.

160. Wetzel RJ, Patel RM, Terry MA. Platelet-rich plasma as an effective treatment for proximal hamstring injuries. *Orthopedics.* 2013;36(1):e64–e70.

161. Bubnov R, Yevseenko V, Semeniv I. Ultrasound guided injections of platelet-rich plasma for muscle injury in professional athletes. Comparative study. *Med Ultrason.* 2013;15(2):101–105.

162. Ekstrand J, Healy JC, Waldén M, et al. Hamstring muscle injuries in professional football: the

correlation of MRI findings with return to play. *Br J Sports Med*. 2012;46(2):112–117.

163. Orchard JW, Seward H, Orchard JJ. Results of 2 decades of injury surveillance and public release of data in the Australian Football League. *Am J Sports Med*. 2013;41(4):734–741.

164. Hamid AM, Mohamed Ali MR, Yusof A, et al. Platelet-rich plasma injections for the treatment of hamstring injuries: a randomized controlled trial. *Am J Sports Med* 2014;42(10):2410–2418.

165. Hamilton B, Tol JL, Almusa E, et al. Platelet-rich plasma does not enhance return to play in hamstring injuries: a randomised controlled trial. *Br J Sports Med*. 2015;49(14):943–950.

166. Reurink G, Goudswaard GJ, Moen MH, et al.; Dutch hamstring injection therapy (HIT) study investigators. Platelet-rich plasma injections in acute muscle injury. *N Engl J Med*. 2014;370(26): 2546–2547.

167. Reurink G, Goudswaard GJ, Moen MH, et al.; Dutch HIT-study Investigators. Rationale, secondary outcome scores and 1-year follow-up of a randomised trial of platelet-rich plasma injections in acute hamstring muscle injury: the Dutch hamstring injection therapy study. *Br J Sports Med*. 2015;49(18):1206–1212.

168. Martinez-Zapata MJ, Orozco L, Balius R, et al. Efficacy of autologous platelet-rich plasma for the treatment of muscle rupture with haematoma: a multicentre, randomised, double-blind, placebo-controlled clinical trial. *Blood Transfus*. 2016;14(2):245–254.

169. Filardo G, Kon E, Buda R, et al. Platelet-rich plasma intra-articular knee injections for the treatment of degenerative cartilage lesions and osteoarthritis. *Knee Surg Sports Traumatol Arthrosc*. 2011;19(4): 528–535.

170. Kon E, Buda R, Filardo G, et al. Platelet-rich plasma: intra-articular knee injections produced favorable results on degenerative cartilage lesions. *Knee Surg Sports Traumatol Arthrosc*. 2010;18(4): 472–479.

171. Napolitano M, Matera S, Bossio M, et al. Autologous platelet gel for tissue regeneration in degenerative disorders of the knee. *Blood Transfus*. 2012; 10(1): 72–77.

172. Wang-Saegusa A, Cugat R, Ares O, et al. Infiltration of plasma rich in growth factors for osteoarthritis of the knee: short-term effects on function and quality of life. *Arch Orthop Trauma Surg*. 2011;131(3):311–317.

173. Sánchez M, Anitua E, Azofra J, et al. Intra-articular injection of an autologous preparation rich in growth factors for the treatment of knee OA: a retrospective cohort study. *Clin Exp Rheumatol*. 2008;26(5):910–913.

174. Lai LP, Stitik TP, Foye PM, et al. Use of platelet-rich plasma in intra-articular knee injections for osteoarthritis: a systematic review. *PM R*. 2015;7(6):637–648.

175. Li M, Zhang C, Ai Z, et al. [Therapeutic effectiveness of intra-knee-articular injection of platelet-rich plasma on knee articular cartilage degeneration]. *Zhongguo Xiu Fu Chong Jian Wai Ke Za Zhi*. 2011;25(10):1192–1196.

176. Raeissadat SA, Rayegani SM, Babaee M, et al. The effect of platelet-rich plasma on pain, function, and quality of life of patients with knee osteoarthritis. *Pain Res Treat*. 2013;2013:165967. doi:10.1155/2013/165967

177. Gobbi A, Karnatzikos G, Mahajan V, et al. Platelet-rich plasma treatment in symptomatic patients with knee osteoarthritis: preliminary results in a group of active patients. *Sports Health*. 2012;4(2): 162–172.

178. Rayegani SM, Raeissadat SA, Taheri MS, et al. Does intra articular platelet-rich plasma injection improve function, pain and quality of life in patients with osteoarthritis of the knee? A randomized clinical trial. *Orthop Rev (Pavia)*. 2014;6(3). doi:10.4081/or.2014.5405

179. Sampson S, Reed M, Silvers H, et al. Injection of platelet-rich plasma in patients with primary and secondary knee osteoarthritis: a pilot study. *Am J Phys Med Rehabil*. 2010;89(12):961–969.

180. Vaquerizo V, Plasencia MÁ, Arribas I, et al. Comparison of intra-articular injections of plasma rich in growth factors (PRGF-Endoret) versus durolane hyaluronic acid in the treatment of patients with symptomatic osteoarthritis: a randomized controlled trial. *Arthroscopy*. 2013;29(10):1635–1643.

181. Spaková T, Rosocha J, Lacko M, et al. Treatment of knee joint osteoarthritis with autologous platelet-rich plasma in comparison with hyaluronic acid. *Am J Phys Med Rehabil*. 2012;91(5):411–417.

182. Raeissadat SA, Rayegani SM, Hassanabadi H, et al. Knee osteoarthritis injection choices: platelet-rich plasma (PRP) versus hyaluronic acid (A one-year randomized clinical trial). *Clin Med Insights Arthritis Musculoskelet Disord*. 2015;8:1–8.

183. Sánchez M, Fiz N, Azofra J, et al. A randomized clinical trial evaluating plasma rich in growth factors

(PRGF-Endoret) versus hyaluronic acid in the short-term treatment of symptomatic knee osteoarthritis. *Arthroscopy*. 2012;28(8):1070–1078.

184. Kon E, Mandelbaum B, Buda R, et al. Platelet-rich plasma intra-articular injection versus hyaluronic acid viscosupplementation as treatments for cartilage pathology: from early degeneration to osteoarthritis. *Arthroscopy*. 2011;27(11):1490–1501.

185. Görmeli G, Görmeli CA, Ataoglu B, et al. Multiple PRP injections are more effective than single injections and hyaluronic acid in knees with early osteoarthritis: a randomized, double-blind, placebo-controlled trial. *Knee Surg Sports Traumatol Arthrosc*. 2017;25(3):958–965.

186. Montañez-Heredia E, Irizar S, Huertas PJ, et al. Intra-articular injections of platelet-rich plasma versus hyaluronic acid in the treatment of osteoarthritic knee pain: a randomized clinical trial in the context of the Spanish national health care system. *Int J Mol Sci*. 2016;17(7):1064. doi:10.3390/ijms17071064

187. Cerza F, Carnì S, Carcangiu A, et al. Comparison between hyaluronic acid and platelet-rich plasma, intra-articular infiltration in the treatment of gonarthrosis. *Am J Sports Med*. 2012;40(12):2822–2827.

188. Filardo G, Kon E, Di Martino A, et al. Platelet-rich plasma vs. hyaluronic acid to treat knee degenerative pathology: study design and preliminary results of a randomized controlled trial. *BMC Musculoskelet Disord*. 2012;13:229. doi:10.1186/1471-2474-13-229

189. Filardo G, Di Matteo B, Di Martino A, et al. Platelet-rich plasma intra-articular knee injections show no superiority versus viscosupplementation: a randomized controlled trial. *Am J Sports Med*. 2015;43(7):1575–1582.

190. Patel S, Dhillon MS, Aggarwal S, et al. Treatment with platelet-rich plasma is more effective than placebo for knee osteoarthritis: a prospective, double-blind, randomized trial. *Am J Sports Med*. 2013;41(2):356–364.

191. Forogh B, Mianehsaz E, Shoaee S, et al. Effect of single injection of platelet-rich plasma in comparison with corticosteroid on knee osteoarthritis: a double-blind randomized clinical trial. *J Sports Med Phys Fitness*. 2016;56(7–8):901–908.

192. Sánchez M, Guadilla J, Fiz N, et al. Ultrasound-guided platelet-rich plasma injections for the treatment of osteoarthritis of the hip. *Rheumatology*. 2012;51(1):144–150.

193. Battaglia M, Guaraldi F, Vannini F, et al. Efficacy of ultrasound-guided intra-articular injections of platelet-rich plasma versus hyaluronic acid for hip osteoarthritis. *Orthopedics*. 2013;36(12):e1501–e1508.

194. Battaglia M, Guaraldi F, Vannini F, et al. Platelet-rich plasma (PRP) intra-articular ultrasound-guided injections as a possible treatment for hip osteoarthritis: a pilot study. *Clin Exp Rheumatol*. 2011;29(4):754.

195. Dallari D, Stagni C, Rani N, et al. Ultrasound-guided injection of platelet-rich plasma and hyaluronic acid, separately and in combination, for hip osteoarthritis: a randomized controlled study. *Am J Sports Med*. 2016;44(3):664–671.

196. Mei-Dan O, Carmont MR, Laver L, et al. Platelet-rich plasma or hyaluronate in the management of osteochondral lesions of the talus. *Am J Sports Med*. 2012;40(3):534–541.

197. Angthong C, Khadsongkram A, Angthong W. Outcomes and quality of life after platelet-rich plasma therapy in patients with recalcitrant hindfoot and ankle diseases: a preliminary report of 12 patients. *J Foot Ankle Surg*. 2013;52(4):475–480.

198. Guney A, Akar M, Karaman I, et al. Clinical outcomes of platelet-rich plasma (PRP) as an adjunct to microfracture surgery in osteochondral lesions of the talus. *Knee Surg Sports Traumatol Arthrosc*. 2015;23(8):2384–2389.

199. Blanke F, Vavken P, Haenle M, et al. Percutaneous injections of platelet-rich plasma for treatment of intrasubstance meniscal lesions. *Muscles Ligaments Tendons J*. 2015;5(3):162–166.

200. Griffin JW, Hadeed MM, Werner BC, et al. Platelet-rich plasma in meniscal repair: does augmentation improve surgical outcomes? *Clin Orthop Relat Res*. 2015;473(5):1665–1672.

201. Pujol N, Salle De Chou E, Boisrenoult P, et al. Platelet-rich plasma for open meniscal repair in young patients: any benefit? *Knee Surg Sports Traumatol Arthrosc*. 2015;23(1):51–58.

202. Levi D, Horn S, Tyszko S, et al. Intradiscal platelet-rich plasma injection for chronic discogenic low back pain: preliminary results from a prospective trial. *Pain Med*. 2016;17(6):1010–1022.

203. Tuakli-Wosornu YA, Terry A, Boachie-Adjei K, et al. Lumbar intradiskal platelet-rich plasma (PRP) injections: a prospective, double-blind, randomized controlled study. *PMR*. 2016;8(1):1–10; quiz 10.

CHAPTER 8

PLATELET-RICH PLASMA TO ENHANCE ORTHOPEDIC PROCEDURES

Fadi Hassan, William D. Murrell , Suad Trebinjac, and Zaid Hashim

WHAT IS PLATELET-RICH PLASMA?

Definition

Platelet-rich plasma (PRP) is an orthobiologic agent that can contain a high concentration of platelets (above baseline) with the aim of accelerating tissue healing, modulating inflammation, and providing symptomatic relief (1–8). PRP was first used in the United States in 1987 to accelerate postoperative wound healing and since then, it has gained popularity in a number of medical fields, such as sports medicine, dentistry, ophthalmology, urology, and cosmetic surgery (9–12).

PRP has been increasingly used as a treatment for various orthopedic conditions in recent years due to evolving literature demonstrating its potential benefit in a wide range of conditions, such as osteoarthritis, lateral epicondylitis, rotator cuff disease, Achilles and patella tendinopathy, hamstring injuries, and degenerative spine disease (13–18). Despite great interest, and a plethora of studies that have been published, the evidence basis varies due to significant variation in preparations and lack of agreement in classification systems, and appropriate application (2,10,19). There has been some interest in using PRP to enhance tissue healing following various surgical procedures involving tendons, ligament, and cartilage. This chapter reviews the application of PRP to enhance the outcomes of various orthopedic surgical procedures.

How Does PRP Work?

Theoretically, PRP is thought to work via the release of supra-physiologic levels (above circulating baseline) of growth factors and other bioactive molecules that can initiate, and accelerate the healing process as well as modulate the inflammatory response (20,21). The cytokines released from the alpha granules of platelets include transforming growth factor-β (TGF-β), platelet-derived growth factor (PDGF), insulin-like growth factors I and II, fibroblast growth factors, epidermal growth factors, vascular endothelial growth factor (VEGF), and endothelial growth factors, among others (12,22).

Furthermore, other nongrowth factor bioactive substances are released and those include serotonin, histamine, dopamine, calcium, and adenosine (23). Those substances are thought to attract mesenchymal stem cells (MSCs), macrophages, and fibroblasts, which all can promote the removal of necrotic tissue and enhance tissue regeneration (24,25). Overall, PRP can possibly modulate proliferation and remodelling of tissue as well as influence the process of inflammation.

ATTRIBUTES OF PRP PREPARATIONS

What Platelets Concentrations Are Considered Ideal?

The evidence varies on this point. Normal range for platelet count is 150,000 µ/L to 350,000 µ/L and anything above that baseline range is considered supra-physiologic (26,27). Literature suggests that platelet concentrations of 2.5× to 3× baseline are ideal, with higher concentrations potentially slowing tissue healing, but this is currently under debate (28–30). Recent evidence provides contrasting results as concentrations of 5× to 7× baseline were found to be beneficial with no evidence of slower healing, as long as the concentration does not exceed 10× baseline (31). However, the "ideal" concentration might differ depending on the tissue treated (bone vs. cartilage vs. tendon) and the stage of the disease (32). Today, the ideal platelet concentration for specific pathologies remains unknown and a prime area for future research.

Reporting Concentration

One problem arising from reporting the quantity of platelets as "3× baseline" is that we still do not know the exact concentration of platelets delivered, as 3× the lower end of the range differs significantly from 3× the upper end of the normal baseline range. Hence, it is preferred to report the exact quantity of platelets (concentration × volume) in order to be more precise concerning the actual injectate.

White Blood Cells

There has been a considerable debate in recent years about whether the presence of white blood cells (WBCs) can affect the healing process in a negative or positive manner. The proposed concern with WBCs is the potential pro-inflammatory effect, especially with neutrophils, which may exacerbate the underlying condition and slow the healing process due to the hydrolytic properties present (33). However, it is much more complex than that. Some properties of WBCs can have potential benefit in chronic tendinopathy but can result in tissue damage in the early inflammatory stages of tendinopathies (34–36). Braun et al. studied the effect of PRP formulation on human synoviocytes and concluded that leukocyte-rich PRP and red blood cells (RBCs) can lead to significant cell death via the production of harmful pro-inflammatory mediators (37). The study also showed that leukocyte-rich PRP causes a significant increase in all four major pro-inflammatory mediators (interleukin-1β [IL-1β], interleukin [IL]-6, interferon [IFN]-γ, and tumor necrosis factor [TNF]-α), which contributes to inflammation and further cartilage degeneration. Furthermore, leukocyte-poor PRP was shown to induce the production of anti-inflammatory mediators (IL-4 and IL-10) in significant amounts leading to a potential therapeutic effect (37). Hence, it is possible that specific WBCs subtypes, in certain concentrations, can be beneficial for certain conditions and this is a topic that future investigation could explore further.

Red Blood Cells

Similarly, RBCs have been reported to be harmful to tissue repair by altering the local environment through changes in the pH, release of catabolic mediators (IFN-γ and IL-1), and decreasing sensitivity to anti-inflammatory mediators, thus promoting local inflammation and apoptosis of chondrocytes (34,37–39). It was thought that RBCs induce damage both directly (via reactive oxygen species) and indirectly (via hemosiderin-induced activation of synovium) (39,40).

The negative effect of RBCs has been investigated previously in a number of in vivo and in vitro studies that suggested hemarthrosis, which often occurs in patients with hemophilia, can lead to early knee arthritis (41–45). Furthermore, significant cartilage damage has been demonstrated after a single exposure of cartilage cells to RBCs, either through traumatic sporting injuries or atraumatic events in hemophilia patients (46). Therefore, removing RBCs from PRP may be beneficial for chondrocyte viability.

Activators

Activation of platelets results in the degranulation of the platelet α-granules, and release of more than 400 different growth factors and other bioactive proteins. The main activators are thrombin, collagen, or calcium. All three activators have different properties and different clinical effects. In terms of speed of activation, thrombin acts faster than calcium, which in turn acts faster than collagen (21). Synthetic activators, such as recombinant thrombin, can help augment this mechanism and offer more sustained release of growth factors (47). However, opposing opinion suggests that natural activation from interaction with the individual's own collagen is a better alternative, as it allows slower release of growth factors, which goes in tune with the body's natural physiologic healing response (48). Again, this is an area of considerable debate and limited evidence evaluating the efficacy of activated versus inactivated PRP and more basic science investigations as well as clinical trials are needed to clarify any substantive difference.

CLASSIFICATION SYSTEMS

In order to draw valid and meaningful conclusions from clinical trials, PRP attributes need to be reported in a way that allows for useful comparison of different preparations. Classification

systems have been proposed and there are several reported in the literature. However, some published classifications do not account for all attributes of the PRP preparation and miss key elements that might influence efficacy, such as, the actual platelet concentration (number/ μL), the volume delivered (mL), the presence of RBCs and WBCs and whether exogenous activation was performed (21). Furthermore, the lack of a consensus on a classification system and reporting of PRP preparations may be the critical limitation in the evidence available and could hamper the broad interpretation of such results. It is recommended that future investigations report the crucial aspects and attributes of the PRP protocols used, as all the elements discussed earlier can have an impact on the efficacy of the preparation in different pathologies. It is a challenging area but having a consensus on classification system will allow different preparations to be compared, hence, allowing researchers to make valid conclusions and comparisons.

Mishra's Classification

This classification system is based on two methods of processing and handling platelets and WBCs; the buffy coat system and the single-spin suspension system (Table 8.1) (49).

1. The buffy coat system: In this system, platelets are highly concentrated (more than 5×) and WBCs are increased, while RBCs are reduced.

2. The single-spin suspension system: This system produces relatively low platelet concentrations (1×–3×) and a very little amount of WBCs and RBCs.

The main problem with this classification is that science has moved forward in terms of our knowledge of PRP and other important attributes that can influence efficacy as well as the development of new PRP systems that can produce specific products in specific amounts (i.e., producing high platelet concentrations without having high amounts of neutrophils). In addition,

TABLE 8.1 The Mishra et al. Platelet-Rich Plasma Classification System

Type	White Blood Cells	Activated?
1	Increased over baseline	No
2	Increased over baseline	Yes
3	Minimal or no WBC	No
4	Minimal or no WBC A: >5× platelets B: <5× platelets	Yes

WBC, white blood cells.
Source: From Ref. (19). Mishra A, Woodall J Jr, Vieira A. Treatment of tendon and muscle using platelet-rich plasma. *Clin Sports Med*. 2009;28(1):113–125.

this classification system fails to require the reporting of the *actual* platelet count provided.

Dohan Ehrenfest et al. (2009)

This system classifies PRP according to platelet concentration, leukocyte concentration, and the presence of fibrin. PRP systems were divided into four categories; pure PRP (P-PRP), leukocyte and PRP (L-PRP), pure platelet-rich fibrin (P-PRF), and, leukocyte and platelet-rich fibrin (L-PRF) (50). However, this system does not account for RBCs or other WBC subtypes, such as neutrophils and again fails to require the reporting of the actual platelet count provided. Furthermore, this system is based mainly on surgical procedures and has limited nonoperative uses.

PAW Classification (See Figure 10.1)

PRP is defined in this system based on platelet concentration (P), activation (A), and the amount of WBCs and neutrophils (W) (51).

1. Platelet concentration is further categorised as P1 (less than or equal to baseline)

to P4 (greater than 1.2 million platelets/μL)

2. Activation is reported as either exogenous (×) or not.

3. WBCs and neutrophils are reported as either above or below baseline.

Similarly, RBC concentrations are not accounted for in this classification system and we know that RBCs can have a negative impact on the local chondrocytes. Additionally, classifying WBCs as above or below baseline can be misleading (see Figure 10.1).

PRLA Classification (See Figure 10.2)

This system is based on platelet count (P), RBC presence (R), leukocyte presence (L), and use of activation (A). This system aims to more clearly define the PRP subtypes to better determine the efficacy of a *defined* PRP product in the treatment of various clinical conditions and it is the preferred system by researchers currently (21). The elements of this system are:

1. Platelet count: calculated from the volume injected and reported as cells/μL

2. Leukocyte presence:
   a. More than 1% considered positive
   b. Less than 1% considered negative
3. RBC presence:
   a. More than 1% considered positive
   b. Less than 1% considered negative
4. The use of activation (Yes/No)

CLINICAL APPLICATIONS PRP TO ENHANCE ORTHOPEDIC PROCEDURES

The literature has a number of studies on the use of PRP in musculoskeletal medicine with mixed results of both positive (6,52–57) and negative (1,58,59) conclusions. One can argue that PRP does and does not work. However, many studies use different preparations that produce different products as a result of different centrifuge spin rates, platelet concentration, leukocyte concentration and different WBC or RBC counts. Therefore, comparing the results directly may be inequitable and may lead to biased conclusions. This highlights the need for standardizing PRP nomenclature and development of consensus on a classification system, which will allow for better comparison of assessing efficacy for different PRP preparations and impact of modulating various PRP attributes.

In this section, we look into the controversies of the clinical application of PRP to enhance orthopedic surgical conditions and assess published efficacy of different preparations.

ROTATOR CUFF DISEASE

Shoulder soft tissue injury is common with a prevalence of 7% to 66%; 50% resolve in 6 months and 60% resolve in 1 year in primary care (60,61); rotator cuff injury constitutes up to 70% of these injuries (62). However, the management of these conditions remains an area of controversy as the literature is limited with limited levels 1 and 2 evidence to support one management over another. It is clear, however, that the majority of these conditions can be managed nonsurgically (63).

In theory, repetitive stress due to high demand activity of the shoulder can lead to a myriad of rotator cuff syndromes that are again quite controversial in pathogenesis, resulting in various types of tendinopathy. These changes can eventually result in collagen fatigue and later partial or full thickness rotator cuff tears (64).

Conservative management has been shown to be beneficial (even in complete tears) and surgical management is usually indicated when conservative measures fail to treat persisting pain and functional symptoms (65–67). This is due to a combination of different risk factors, such as defect size, tissue quality, poor compliance, and finally poor vascularisation (68). It was hypothesised that the biology of healing needs to be addressed to augment the healing process of tendon-to-bone and PRP was suggested as a potential therapy (69).

Murrell et al. incorporated PRP into the arthroscopic repair of rotator cuff by using platelet-rich fibrin matrix (PRFM) (69). This was initially chosen due to the processing technique, which allowed for creation of the PRFM clot that can be held in place by running sutures through the material and placing it between the tendon and the bone. However, this technique never evolved over time and there are still questions over parameters, such as the number of clots and size of clots per torn area. Of the available literature (five studies) relating to PRFM repair, 80% showed no benefit to healing of rotator cuff tears (70–73). However, one study showed lower rate of re-tear when PRFM was added to arthroscopic repair (74). Antuna et al. prospectively evaluated the application of PRFM in massive rotator cuff tears with a follow-up period of 24 months and found that there was no significant difference in re-tear rate or subjective outcome measures among study groups (75).

Evidence regarding the use of PRP in rotator cuff disease suggests that leukocyte-poor PRP promotes a normal collagen matrix synthesis and decreases cytokines associated with matrix degradation and inflammation to a greater extent when compared with leukocyte-rich PRP in moderately degenerative tendons. However, in severely degenerative tendons, neither preparation enhanced matrix synthesis (76). Furthermore, initial case series studies examined the safety profile of PRP use intra-operatively and suggested that it was safe to use and can lead to good patient outcomes at 2 years (77,78).

There is also evidence that supports the use of PRP in refractory cases of rotator cuff tendinopathy. Scarpone et al. concluded that single ultrasound-guided, intralesional injection of PRP resulted in safe, significant, and sustained improvement of pain, function, and MRI outcomes in comparison to patients who received steroids injections and physical activity. However, the study has limitations, such as the lack of blinding that could have produced observer bias (79). These findings were replicated by Rha et al. in a level 1 study that compared the use of PRP with dry needling. The study found that ultrasound-guided injections of PRP can lead to progressive reduction in pain and disability and that the benefit was present even at 6 months (80).

There is little evidence focusing on exogenous activation and whether this can influence outcomes. One study used thrombin-activated PRP in augmentation of rotator cuff arthroscopic repair in a randomized controlled trial (RCT) and found no significant difference in clinical outcomes or re-tear rate between the two groups (81). The results contrast with a recently performed RCT in 102 patients with medium to large rotator cuff tears that were treated with either L-PRP or saline. At a 24-month follow-up the re-tear rate was significantly lower than in the control group (82). Additionally, another study recruited 60 patients with rotator cuff tendinopathy who had undergone arthroscopic decompression (78). Participants were randomly allocated to PRP and non-PRP-receiving groups and outcomes, such as the Oxford scores and histological analysis, were assessed at 2 years postoperatively. Results show no significant difference between the two groups in terms of pain and function and histology samples showed increased apoptosis in PRP-receiving groups. Hence, the authors did not recommend

co-application of PRP with surgical interventions. However, another double-blind RCT used LR-PRP in conjunction with arthroscopic rotator cuff repair in 53 patients and results showed that autologous PRP reduces pain in the first postoperative months; strength of external rotation was greater at all time intervals; and in the final follow-up at 24 months the rate of re-tear was significantly lower in the intervention group as compared with controls (83). The long-term results of subgroups of grade 1 and 2 tears suggest that PRP positively affected rotator cuff healing.

When considering rehabilitation, Beck et al. suggested that PRP can have negative impact on healing at 7 days; hence, a cautious rehabilitation process for the 3 weeks after surgery is warranted to maximize any benefit from PRP (84).

We have attempted to present a balanced view of the most robust studies conducted on PRP to date. Table 8.2 provides additional studies that further this discussion.

PLATELET-RICH PLASMA AUGMENTATION OF ACHILLES TENDON REPAIR

The rupture of the Achilles tendon is a common condition and is being seen with increasing frequency in recent decades (85). Although increases in incidence in sports-related trauma has been observed, the greatest increase in recent years has been demonstrated in non-sports-related ruptures (86). Systematic review and meta-analysis comparing nonoperative means versus surgical repair for Achilles rupture have concluded that surgical intervention results in decreased rerupture rates, but at the cost of incision problems and infection (87–89). However, a recent multicenter RCT demonstrated that both treatments are equally effective in outcome, with surgical treatment having a greater risk for infection (90).

It is reasonable to hypothesize that PRP could possibly assist with the healing of a ruptured tendon independently; however, on search,

(text continues on page 137)

TABLE 8.2 Summary of Additional Evidence

Study (y)	Design	Sample	Outcome Measures	Intervention	Results
Knee OA					
Cerza, 2012 (91)	RCT	120 participants M (53) and F (67) Mean age: 66.4 years	WOMAC Follow-up at 0, 4, 12, and 24 weeks	PRP group: 4 weekly intra-articular injections of 5.5 mL PRP (autologous conditioned plasma) ($n = 60$) Control: 4 weekly intra-articular injections of HA (20 mg/2 mL) (n = 60)	PRP treatment led to significant improvement in WOMAC score, which was sustained up to 24 weeks, compared to control group (36.5 vs. 65.1, p <.001).
Filardo, 2012 (92)	RCT	109 participants M (68) and F (41) Age >18 (mean 56.5) Chronic OA (symptoms >4 months) Imaging: Kellgren-Lawrence Score up to 3	IKDC EQ-VAS Tegner KOOS scores ROM and Knee circumference 2, 6, and 12 months follow-up	PRP group: 3-weekly intra-articular 8 mL PRP injections ($n = 54$) Control group: 3 weekly intra-articular injections of HA (>150 Kda) ($n = 55$)	Both groups showed clinical improvement but there was statistically significant difference in all scores. Trend favoring PRP was observed only in patients with low articular degeneration (Kellgren–Lawrence score up to 2). There was only one minor adverse event in PRP group (higher postinjection pain).
Patel, 2013 (93)	RCT	78 participants M (22) and F (53) Mean age: 52.8 years	WOMAC VAS 3 and 6 months follow-up	PRP groups: 26 patients received single injection of 8 mL of PRP and 25 patients received two injections of PRP 3 weeks apart Control group: 23 patients receiving single injection of normal saline (8 mL)	Statistically significant improvement in all WOMAC parameters was noted in patients receiving PRP (both groups), within 2–3 weeks and lasting until the final follow-up at 6 months. WOMAC scores deteriorated in control group. There was no improvement in control group compared to PRP group (p <.001). There was no difference between patients receiving one or two injections.

(continued)

TABLE 8.2 Summary of Additional Evidence *(continued)*

Study (y)	Design	Sample	Outcome Measures	Intervention	Results
Sanchez, 2012 (94)	RCT	178 participants M (85) and F (91) Mean age: (59.8) years	50% decrease in pain WOMAC Lequesne Follow-up at 1, 2, and 6 months	PRP group: 3 weekly intra-articular 8 mL PRGF Endoret ($n = 87$) Control group: 3 weekly intra-articular HA	PRGF showed superior short-term results when compared with HA. The rate of response to PRGF-Endoret was 14.1 percentage points higher (95% CI: 0.5–27.6, $p = .044$).
Vaquerizo, 2013 (95)	RCT	96 participants M (38) and F (58) Mean age: 63.6 years	WOMAC Lequesne OMERACT-ORASI Follow-up at 48 weeks	PRP group: 3 biweekly intra-articular injections of 8 mL PRGF endoret ($n = 48$) Control group: 1 intra-articular Durolane HA (n=48).	PRGF-Endoret was significantly more efficient than treatment with Durolane HA in reducing knee pain and stiffness and improving physical function in patients with knee OA. The rate of response to PRGF-Endoret was significantly higher than the rate of response to HA for all the scores.
Raeissadat, 2014 (96)	RCT	160 participants M (23) and F (116) Mean age: 58.8 years Imaging: Grade 1–4 Kellgren-Lawrence Scale	WOMAC SF-36 Follow-up at 52 weeks	PRP group: 2 intra-articular injections of 4–6 mL PRP, 4 weeks apart ($n = 87$). Control group: 3-weekly intra-articular HA injections ($n = 73$)	At 12 months, WOMAC pain scores significantly improved in both groups. Better results were achieved in PRP group compared to HA group ($p <.001$). Other WOMAC and SF-36 parameters improved only in the PRP group. More improvement (but not statistically significant) was seen in patients with grade 2 OA in both groups.
Smith, 2016 (97)	RCT	30 participants M (11) and F (19) Mean age: 50.1 years Imaging: Grade 2–3 Kellgren-Lawrence Scale	WOMAC Follow-up at 1, 2, 8, 12, 26, and 52 weeks	PRP group: three intra-articular injections of 3–8 mL LP-PRP, at 1-week intervals ($n = 15$) Control group: three intra-articular injections of 3–8 mL of phosphate buffered saline at 1-week intervals ($n = 15$)	PRP injections demonstrated a significant improvement in WOMAC score at all time points, and from controls from week 2 through 52 weeks. At 52 weeks the intervention group had 78% improvement in scores as compared with 7% in the control group.

(continued)

TABLE 8.2 Summary of Additional Evidence   (continued)

Study (y)	Design	Sample	Outcome Measures	Intervention	Results
Spakova, 2012 (98)	RCT	120 subjects M (63) and F (57) Mean age: 53 years Imaging: Grade 1–3 Kellgren-Lawrence Scale	WOMAC Numeric Rating Scale Follow-up at 3 and 6 months	PRP group: three intra-articular injections of LP-PRP, at 1-week intervals ($n = 60$) Control group: three intra-articular injections of 1.2% HA at 1-week intervals ($n = 60$)	PRP injections demonstrated a significant improvement in WOMAC and Numeric Rating Scales at both 3 and 6 months. No adverse events were reported.
Cole, 2016 (99)	RCT	99 subjects M (48) and F (51) Imaging: Grade 1–3 Kellgren-Lawrence Scale; one subject unknown	WOMAC Pain Score IKDC VAS Follow-up at 2, 3, 6, 12, 24, and 52 weeks	PRP group: three intra-articular injections of LP-PRP, at 1-week intervals (n = 49) Control group: three intra-articular injections of HA at 1-week intervals ($n = 50$)	PRP injections did not show any significant difference from HA group at any time frame in WOMAC pain score. K-L grade 1 IKDC score improved as compared with grade 3.
Kon, 2011 (100)	Prospective Cohort Study	150 subjects M (82) and F (68) Imaging: Grade 1–4 Kellgren Lawrence Scale	IKDC EQ VAS Follow-up at 2 and 6 months	LR-PRP group: three intra-articular injections at 2-week intervals LMW-HA Group: three intra-articular injections at 2-week intervals HMW-HA Group: three intra-articular injections at 2-week intervals	PRP injections demonstrated more and longer-lasting efficacy than HA injections. Results were better in younger and more active patients with low degree of cartilage degeneration. Worse outcomes were in more degenerated joints.
Say, 2012 (101)	Prospective Cohort Study	90 subjects M (11) and F (79) Imaging: Grade 1–3 Kellgren Lawrence Scale	KOOS VAS Follow-up at 3 and 6 months	LR-PRP Group: Single injection LMW-HA Group: three intra-articular injections at weekly intervals	There were no severe adverse events. KOOS and VAS significantly improved in PRP group as compared to HA at 3- and 6- month follow-up. PRP cost is lower than HA.

(continued)

TABLE 8.2 Summary of Additional Evidence   *(continued)*

Study (y)	Design	Sample	Outcome Measures	Intervention	Results
Filardo, 2012 (102)	RCT	144 subjects M (95) and F (49) Imaging: Grade 0–4 Kellgren Lawrence Scale	IKDC EQ-VAS Tegner Follow-up at 2, 6, and 12 months	Single-spin LP-PRGF three intra-articular injections given at 21-day intervals Double-spin LR-PRP three intra-articular injections given at 21-day intervals	Both PRGF and PRP showed significant improvement in all outcome measures at all time frames. Results were better in younger subjects with less disease. PRP had more adverse events as compared with PRGF.
Rotator cuff disease					
Antuna, 2013 (75)	Randomized Pilot Clinical Trial	28 adults; M and F participants with massive RC tears that failed conservative treatment Mean age: 65 years (53–77)	Constant score DASH VAS MRI	PRP group: 6 mL PRF applied over repair site ($n = 14$) Control group: No PRP Standard arthroscopic repair ($n = 14$)	Local application of autologous PRF to the repair site of massive rotator cuffs failed to improve the clinical outcome and the healing rate, compared with the control group.
Castricini, 2011 (71)	RCT	88 participants with repairable small- or medium- rotator cuff tears (supraspinatus) M and F Age: 37–72 years	Constant score MRI–integrity of RC repair and retear rate 16-month follow-up	PRP group: Single PRF matrix—9 mL of blood ($n = 43$) Control group: no PRP ($n = 45$)	There was no statistically significant difference in total constant score between the two groups (95% CIs [−3.43, 3.9]) ($p = .44$). There was no statistically significant difference in MRI results between two groups ($p = .07$).

(continued)

TABLE 8.2 Summary of Additional Evidence *(continued)*

Study (y)	Design	Sample	Outcome Measures	Intervention	Results
Gumina, 2012 (103)	RCT	80 participants undergoing arthroscopic RC repair Participants with large full-thickness RC tear M and F	Constant score Simple shoulder test MRI	All participants underwent arthroscopic RC repair PRP group: single, intra-operative platelet-leukocyte membrane inserted between the RC tendon and its footprint ($n = 40$) Control group: no PRP ($n = 40$)	Rotator cuff re-tears were observed only in the control group. The use of the platelet-leukocyte membrane was associated with significantly better repair integrity ($p = .04$). However, the improvement in repair integrity was not associated with greater clinical and functional improvement.
Malavolta, 2014 (81)	RCT	54 undergoing arthroscopic RC tear Skeletally mature Complete supraspinatus tear Pain and disability >3 months M and F	Constant score UCLA VAS Frequency of re-ruptures (MRI)	All participants underwent arthroscopic supraspinatus repair PRP: single intra-operative 30 mL of liquid PRP prepared by apheresis ($n = 27$) Control: no PRP ($n = 27$).	Both groups showed significant improvement ($p < .001$). There was no significant difference in UCLA scores, VAS and the mean constant score between the two groups. There were one complete re-tear and four partial re-tears in control group vs. two partial re-tears in PRP group ($p = .42$). PRP did not promote better clinical results at 24-month follow-up.
Randelli, 2011 (83)	RCT	53 participants undergoing arthroscopic RC repair M and F Complete RC tear Pre-op platelet count >150,000, hemoglobin >11.0 g/dL and have no infectious disease BMI <33	Constant score Simple shoulder test UCLA score VAS Strength of external rotation Rate of re-tear	PRP group: single, intra-operative injection of 6 mL of PRP + autologous thrombin through arthroscopic portals ($n = 26$) Control group: no PRP ($n = 27$)	The pain score in the treatment group was lower than the control group at 3, 7, 14, and 30 days postoperation ($p < .05$). The Simple Shoulder Test, UCLA, Constant scores, and external rotation strength were significantly higher in the treatment group than the control group at 3 months post-op ($p < .05$). Strength of external rotation was significantly higher in the PRP group, especially in grades 1 and 2 tears. There was no significant difference among groups after 6, 12, and 24 months. Hence, long-term effects are questionable but PRP offers short-term benefits.

(continued)

TABLE 8.2 Summary of Additional Evidence   *(continued)*

Study (y)	Design	Sample	Outcome Measures	Intervention	Results
Rodeo, 2012 (70)	RCT	79 undergoing arthroscopic RC repair Age ≥40 years Failed nonoperative management M and F	Ultrasound assessment ASES score L'Insalata score Shoulder strength	PRP group: single intraoperative PRF matrix produced from 9 mL of blood ($n = 40$) Control group: No PRP ($n = 39$)	There were differences in tendon-to-bone healing between the PRP and control groups (67% vs. 81%, $p = .20$). There was no significant differences in healing by ultrasound between 6 and 12 weeks. There was no significant difference between the two groups in ASES, shoulder strength, and L'Insalata outcomes.
Everts, 2008 (104)	RCT	40 participants with shoulder impingement syndrome M and F Mean age: PRP group (52 years) vs. Control (50 years)	ASES VAS ADL Shoulder ROM Use of pain medications	All participant underwent open subacromial decompression treatment group: Single intra-operative platelet-leukocyte gel application ($n = 20$) Control: No PRP ($n = 20$)	Treated patients demonstrated decreased VAS scores and used significantly less analgesia, and had improved ROM compared with control patients ($p <.001$). Treated patients performed more ADL ($p <.05$).
Carr, 2015 (78)	RCT	60 participants M (45%) and F (55%) Aged: 35–75	Oxford shoulder score Tendon biopsy specimens Follow-up up to 2 years	PRP group: Coapplication of subacromial PRP and arthroscopic acromioplasty Control group: arthroscopic acromioplasty alone	Significant increase in oxford shoulder scores was seen in both groups from 12 weeks onward. There was no significant difference in oxford shoulder score between the two groups at all follow-up points. There was no significant change in tissue structure with the co-application of PRP compared with control.

(continued)

TABLE 8.2 Summary of Additional Evidence   (*continued*)

Study (y)	Design	Sample	Outcome Measures	Intervention	Results
Rha, 2013 (80)	RCT	39 participants with supraspinatus tendon lesion	Shoulder pain and disability index Passive ROM Physician global rating scale Adverse events Ultrasound scan Follow-up at 6 months	PRP group: two ultrasound guided PRP injections at 4-week interval Control group: two ultrasound guided dry-needling procedures, 4 weeks apart	There was significant superior clinical outcomes in PRP group from 6 weeks to 6 months after initial injection, compared with control group ($p < .05$). Mean shoulder pain and disability index was 17.7 +/− 3.7 in PRP group vs. 29.5 +/− 3.8 in dry needling group ($p < .05$).
Knee cartilage repair					
Sanchez, 2003 (105)	Case Study	One subject articular cartilage avulsion without bone One 12-year-old subject	No outcome measures Postoperative MRI evaluation 2 and 6 weeks	PRGF 2 mL augmented surgery of reattachment of chondral lesion with absorbable pins	Subject was fully back to all activities 18 weeks after surgery. MRI at 2 and 6 weeks after surgery showed complete reattachment of avulsed lesion.
Dhollander, 2011 (106)	Prospective Case Series	Five subjects Symptomatic patellar cartilage defect	Pre- and post-MRI evaluation by MOCART score and modified MOCART Score 24-month follow-up	Microfracture and PRP gel and collagen-based scaffold	There was significant clinical improvement after 24-month follow-up. The formation of intralesional osteophytes was found in three of the five subjects recruited. All cases showed subchondral lamina and bone changes. Clinical outcome was not confirmed by MRI findings.
Siclari, 2014 (107)	Prospective Cohort Study	52 participants Aged: 19–31 M (20) and F (32)	KOOS MRI pre- and posttreatment ($n = 21$)—4 years MOCART score	Subchonral drilling with PGA-HA –PRP (3 mL) soaked implant	At 5-year follow-up, there was significant and clinically meaningful improvement in all categories of the KOOS score compared to baseline. Cartilage repair was complete in 20/21 patients who underwent MRI at 4 years postoperatively.

(*continued*)

TABLE 8.2 Summary of Additional Evidence *(continued)*

Study (y)	Design	Sample	Outcome Measures	Intervention	Results
Hip/labrum					
Dallari, 2016 (108)	RCT	111 participants Aged: 18–65 Hip OA Pain >20 on VAS	VAS WOMAC Follow-up 2, 6, 12 months	Group A: 3 weekly injections of PRP ($n = 44$) Group B: 3 weekly injections of PRP + HA ($n = 31$) Group C: 3 weekly injections of HA alone ($n = 36$)	Group A had the lowest VAS at all follow-up points, particularly at 6 months (21 vs 35 vs. 44). WOMAC score for group A was significantly better at 2 and 6 months but not 12 months.
Battaglia, 2013 (109)	RCT	100 participants Chronic unilateral hip OA	Harris Hip Score VAS Follow-up 1, 3, 6, and 12 months	Group A: Ultrasound guided PRP Group B: ultrasound-guided HA	There was improvement in both groups between 1 and 3 months. Despite some progressive worsening between 6- and 12-month follow-up, the final scores remained higher than baseline ($p < .0005$). There were no significant differences between PRP and HA.
Rafols, 2015 (110)	RCT	57 participants undergoing arthroscopic hip surgery	Modified Harris Hip Score (mHHS) VAS MRI Follow-up 3, 6, 24 months	Group A: intra-articular PRP at the end of arthroscopic surgery ($n = 30$) Control: no PRP ($n = 27$)	VAS was 3.04 in group A vs. 5.28 in control group ($p <.05$) 48 hours postoperation. At 3 months, the mHHS was 91.79 in group A vs. 90.97 in control ($p = .65$). At 24 months, it was 93.41 in group A ($p = .56$) vs. 92.32 in control ($p = .52$). At 6 months, MRI showed no effusion in 36.7% of patients in group A vs. 21.1% of patients in control group ($p = .013$). There was no significant difference in labral integration between two groups ($p = .76$).

(continued)

TABLE 8.2 Summary of Additional Evidence (*continued*)

Study (y)	Design	Sample	Outcome Measures	Intervention	Results
ACL reconstruction					
Almeida, 2012 (111)	RCT	27 participants undergoing ACLR Aged: <45 years M and F	VAS MRI Questionnaires (Lysholm, Kujala and Tegner) IKDC subjective score Isokinetic strength measurements	PRP group: single intraoperative 30–50 mL PRP + rehabilitation protocol ($n = 12$) Control group: no PRP + rehabilitation protocol ($n = 15$)	VAS score was lower in the PRP group immediately postoperatively (3.8 ± 1.0; 95% CI [3.18, 4.49]) than in the control group (5.1 ± 1.4; 95% CI [4.24, 5.90]; $p = .02$). There were no significant differences after 6 months in questionnaire and isokinetic testing. Patellar tendon gap area was significantly smaller in the PRP than in the control group.
Cervellin, 2012 (112)	RCT	40 participants undergoing arthroscopic ACLR. Aged: 18–29 years	VISA questionnaire VAS MRI	All patients had ACLR with bone-patellar-bone tendon graft PRP group: 54 mL of blood + 6 mL citrate anticoagulant centrifuged for 15 mins with participant's thrombin ($n = 40$) Control group: No PRP ($n = 40$)	VISA scores were significantly higher in PRP group compared with control (97.8 ± 2.5 and 84.5 ± 11.8, $p = .041$). There was no significant difference in postoperative VAS between the two groups. In 85% of PRP group patients, the tibial and patellar bone defect was satisfactorily filled by new bony tissue (>70% of gap filled), compared with 60% in control group (not statistically significant).
Orrego, 2008 (113)	RCT	108 participants undergoing ACLR Mature skeleton Total rupture of ACL Mean age: 30 years (15–57 years) M and F	MRI assessment IKDC	PRP group: single PRP treatment with 10 mL of PRP ($n = 26$) Control group: No PRP ($n = 27$) Bone plug group: 28 patients Combination of bone plug and PRP: 27 patients	The use of platelet concentrate had an enhancing effect on the graft maturation process evaluated only by MRI signal intensity, without showing any significant effect in the osteoligamentous interface or tunnel-widening evolution.

(continued)

TABLE 8.2 Summary of Additional Evidence   (*continued*)

Study (y)	Design	Sample	Outcome Measures	Intervention	Results
Vadalà, 2013 (114)	RCT	40 participants undergoing ACLR Chronic instability (>30 days of trauma) Mean age: 34.5 years (18–48 years) Gender: M	Tunnel enlargement Tegner activity score IKDC score Lysholm score	All participants underwent ACLR surgery PRP group: thick adhesive PRP gel obtained from 10 mL of blood and applied in the femoral and tibial tunnel ($n = 20$) Control group: No PRP ($n = 20$)	Femoral tunnel diameter increased from 9.0 ± 0.1 mm to 9.8 ± 0.3 mm in PRP group and from 9.0 ± 0.1 mm to 9.4 ± 0.5 mm in control group. Tibial tunnel diameter increased from 9.0 ± 0.2 mm to 10.9 ± 0.2 mm in PRP group and from 9.1 ± 0.1 mm to 10.1 ± 0.4 mm in control group. PRP was not effective in reducing tunnel enlargement.
Nín, 2009 (115)	RCT	100 participants undergoing ACLR Positive clinical tests for ACL instability and MRI findings Aged: 14–59 years M and F	VAS Anterior laxity (KT-1000) IKDC Protein-C MRI Radiographs	PRP group: 4 mL of PRP gel obtained from 40 mL of blood ($n = 50$) Control group: No PRP ($n = 50$)	There was no significant statistical differences between the groups in inflammatory parameters (CRP), MRI, VAS, IKDC, and KT-1000.
Vogrin, 2010 (116)	RCT	50 participants undergoing ACLR Aged: 18–50 years M and F	Knee stability (KT-2000) Tegner activity score Lysholm score IKDC	PRP group: single intra-operative application of 6 mL of PRP in bone tunnel activated with thrombin ($n = 25$) Control group: no PRP ($n = 25$)	Patients receiving platelet-rich gel showed significantly better anteroposterior knee stability than patients in the control group (3.1 +/– 2.5mm vs. 1.3 +/– 1.8 mm, $p = .011$).

This table provides brief summaries of additional studies not discussed in the body of the paper. This table lists by headings: Study, year published, bibliography citation number; Study design; Sample size; Outcome measures used; Intervention studied; Results.

ACL, anterior cruciate ligament; ACLR, anterior cruciate ligament reconstruction; ADL, activity of daily living; AOFAS, American Orthopaedic Foot and Ankle Score; ASES, American Shoulder and Elbow Surgeons scoring system; CI, confidence interval; DASH, disabilities of the arm, shoulder, and hand; EQ-VAS, European quality of life-visual analogue scale; ESWT, extracorporeal shockwave therapy; F, female; FRI, functional rating index; HA, hyaluronic acid; IKDC, International Knee Documentation Committee; KOOS, knee injury and osteoarthritis outcome score; M, male; MOCART, magnetic resonance observation of cartilage repair tissue; NASS, North American Spine Society; NRS, numerical rating scale; PRF, platelet-rich fibrin; PRGF, platelet-rich growth factor; PRTEE, patient-rated tennis elbow evaluation; RC, rotator cuff; RCT, randomized controlled trial; ROM, range of motion; SF, 36-item short-form; UCLA, The University of California at Los Angeles; VAS, Visual Analogue Scale; VISA, Victorian Institute of Sport Assessment; VISA-A, Victorian Institute of Sport Assessment-Achilles; VISA-P, Victorian Institute of Sport Assessment-Patella; WOMAC, Western Ontario and McMaster; y, year (s).

no studies using PRP to treat primary Achilles tendon rupture by injection alone were identified. The augmented surgical treatment of ruptured Achilles tendons was first published by Sánchez et al., an investigation using a platelet-rich plasma preparation rich in growth factors (PRGF), a platelet-rich concentrate product. The study was carried out in an athletic population of 12 patients, six undergoing augmented repair and six matched conventional surgical treatment followed by recording of functional outcomes, and ultrasound imaging at 32 and 50 months, respectively (117). Results demonstrated that the PRGF group regained motion earlier, and resumed training earlier, and the long-term cross-sectional area of the repaired tendon was significantly smaller as compared with controls. De Carli et al. again compared repair of Achilles tendon with and without PRP in 30 patients at the time of surgery, and 14 days postoperatively; there were no differences in clinical or functional results up to 24 months postoperation (118).

The first and only RCT investigating this area hypothesized that autologous PRP would stimulate healing of acute Achilles tendon ruptures. At the time of final closure for primary Achilles repair, tantalum beads were implanted, and before closure an injection of 10 cc of PRP 10× baseline concentration (double centrifugation—leukocyte rich) was injected in 16 of the 30 patients (119). At 7, 19, and 52 weeks postoperatively using three-dimensional (3D) radiographs, the bead distance was measured and estimated e-modulus determined resulting 13% higher, 2% lower, and no differences respectively in the PRP injection group as compared with controls. The Achilles Tendon Total Rupture Score (ATRS) demonstrated a lower score in the PRP indicating a possible detrimental effect.

ANTERIOR CRUCIATE LIGAMENT RECONSTRUCTION OR REPAIR

In essence, the sucesss of an anterior cruciate ligament reconstruction (ACLR) surgery depends on the biomechanics and biology as patients undergoing this surgery are young, active, and tend to have a short return to sports time. With respect to the biology of tissue, graft materials have been studied extensively but augmentation is a fairly recent science and is still being explored. An ideal augment should provide longevity represented by early sustainable bone- or soft-tissue graft integration and tensile strength to withstand patients' demands when getting back to high-level activity.

Imaging Studies

Previous imaging studies examined different stages and sites for healing and maturation. PRP was shown to promote graft site healing when patellar graft was used for ACLR radiographically and to reduce morbidity (111,112). As for graft tunnel sites, studies identified increased vascularization and new cortical bone formation at the site of osteo-ligamentous integration along with reduced bone edema at 1- to 6-month follow-ups, indicating that PRP is effective in early phases (120–122). These findings were not replicated in other trials at early stages (113,114,123). Further studies have been recommended to assess the impact of PRP on graft integration at long-term follow-up.

Few studies proved that PRP augmentation has faster and better graft maturation when compared with the control groups at 4 to 12 months when comparing graft homogeneity with intact posterior cruciate ligaments in the same patient (54,113,124). This was not the case in two other more recent studies that did not demonstrate better graft maturation following PRP augmentation (125,126).

Histology

Sánchez et al. conducted a study to investigate the effect of PRGF in tendon graft ligamentization and selected a group of volunteers to have a second-look arthroscopy (127). Results showed that the use of PRGF influenced histologic characteristics of grafts and led to more remodelling when compared with controls during the 6- to 24-month maturation period. Hence, PRP-augmented grafts appeared to have overall better tissue quality, which is consistent with imaging results.

Clinical Studies

Recent systematic review by Andriolo et al. (2015) showed the safety of intraoperative use of PRP as none of the clinical trials reviewed reported increased infection risk or other complications (128).

Seijas et al., in retrospect, reviewed the rate of return to play in 19 professional soccer players with partial ACL tears treated with arthroscopic 4 cc intra-ligament injection of $CaCl_2$-activated PRP in the remaining intact posterolateral bundle, and 6 cc intra-articular, that resulted in KT-1,000 normalization in all cases. Eighteen players were able to return to the previous level of play within 16.20 weeks (129).

Komzak et al. evaluated the use of PRP in a single-bundle ACLR in 20 of 40 patients, and at 3 and 12 months no difference was seen in bony ingrowth of the hamstring tendons (130). Radice et al., in a prospective study of 100 ACLRs, divided them into two groups, A—treated with platelet-rich plasma gel (PRPG) and B—control. MRI studies demonstrated that it took 179 days to complete graft homogeneity in group A as compared with 369 days in group B without PRPG (131). A double-blind RCT in 100 patients undergoing arthroscopic patellar tendon allograft ACL reconstruction (ACLR) where subjects were given activated PRP showed no significant difference in terms of subjective outcomes, biomechanical, or graft integration at 24-month follow-up compared to control group (115). A prospective study investigating hamstring ACLR with a graft soaked with $CaCl_2$-activated PRP in 36 subjects in intervention group and 27 controls was evaluated

by second-look arthroscopy and histology. It found that the gross appearance was no different; however, histologically newly formed connective tissue enveloping the graft was found in 77.3% of the intervention group versus 40% of the controls (127). An RCT of 50 patients of two equal groups, using hamstring ACLR was studied. The intervention group received thrombin-activated PRP-soaked graft. The authors noted improved anterior–posterior instrumented knee stability-KT 2000 at 6 months (116). Silva and Sampaio, prospectively evaluated graft-tunnel healing in anatomic ACLR in 40 patients sequentially divided into four groups: A—with PRP, B—with PRP femoral tunnel, C—with PRP femoral tunnels and intra-articular, D—thrombin-activated PRP femoral tunnel. An MRI at 3 months demonstrated no difference among groups in terms of bone-tunnel healing (132). A randomized, prospective study of the use of autologous platelet concentrate (APC) on 30 patients of group A versus control group of 20 patients of group B, was performed in subjects undergoing ACLR with hamstring grafts. At 6 months, an MRI evaluation was performed and demonstrated no differences in graft integration, bone-tunnel healing, or maturation (125). Ventura et al. demonstrated faster bony integration of hamstring tendons determined by CT scan at 6 months in 20 patients randomized to either PRP growth factor gel or control. Despite this difference, clinical outcomes were no different (132). Additional clinical studies are summarized in Table 8.2.

A systematic review of PRP augmentation is limited by a large variation in the type of graft construct used in hamstring tendons (gracilis and/or semitendinosus), bone-patellar tendon-bone graft (autologous vs. allograft), surgical technique, augment PRP preparations and administration techniques (simple intra-articular injection post operatively vs. applying it on graft pre- or postoperatively once it is fixed vs. graft substance injections vs. substrates incorporation vs. placing it inside the bone tunnels: tibia, femur, or both), devices used, patient comorbidity and length of follow-up, which makes it an area of controversy.

The majority of clinical outcomes of ACLR PRP augmentation showed no difference in results compared with control groups over early follow-up period. However, most of these studies considered clinical results as the secondary outcomes and were limited by a short follow-up (133,134).

In conclusion, early animal and in vitro studies on PRP have shown better healing outcomes on damaged ACLs, but this is yet to be proven clinically. More robust studies with large samples, unified preparations, administration techniques, short- and long-term follow-ups are needed to understand the PRP augment's role in ACLR and repair surgeries.

PLATELET-RICH PLASMA TO ENHANCE SURGICAL TREATMENT OF MENISCAL TEARS

The anatomy and vascular supply of the meniscus cartilage of the knee has been well studied and documented (135). Biomechanical and clinical data have demonstrated the importance of the meniscus and of meniscal preservation for protection of the articular cartilage, distribution of forces, and as a secondary stabilizer (136). Techniques for repair have evolved and include inside-out techniques, outside-in, and all-inside techniques. Although fixation methods have improved, there has been an increasing interest in biologic augmentation of these repairs to enhance healing given the limited blood supply. There are data demonstrating increased rates of meniscal healing following ACLR (vs. a repair in isolation) (137). This is thought to potentially be due to the release of marrow element during marrow stimulation techniques (138). Recent studies in a rabbit model have shown improvements in the quality and quantity of the reparative tissue bridging a meniscal repair using these marrow stimulation techniques (139). This is thought to potentially be due to the increased release of growth factors, including PDGF (140). These advances have resulted in a proliferation of research in the biologic realm of the augmentation of meniscal repair.

In a retrospective report of prospectively collected data of 35 isolated arthroscopic meniscal repairs, 15 were augmented with PRP, 20 without (141). At mean 4-year follow-up, more than 70% of patients were available for review. No differences in clinical outcomes were detected; however, with small numbers a moderate difference would be difficult to detect. Pujol and coworkers published a case–control study of 34 consecutive patients with grades 2 to 3 horizontal tears (142). One group had PRP injected in the area of the repair at the end of surgery, the other group had no PRP. MRI was repeated at 52 weeks postoperatively. The PRP group had a total of five MRIs that demonstrated resolution of any meniscal signal abnormalities with no improvement in MRI noted in the control group. Research in the area of meniscal repair or regeneration is in its infancy clinically; however, the results of many current trials is forthcoming. Summaries of the studies reviewed can be found in Table 8.2.

PLATELET-RICH PLASMA TO ENHANCE CARTILAGE REPAIR

Cartilage repair has long been an area of difficulty within orthopedics. Initial attempts at surgical treatment to address cartilage repair were described with the extensive debridement of osteoarthritic knee joints as described by Magnuson (143). The procedure involved removal of synovium, loose cartilage, and osteophytes thus prompting a "healing response," and this procedure was used for many years until supplanted by formal arthroplasty. Later, in the United Kingdom, Pridie expanded on the previous work of Magnuson and presented a technique of closely spaced multiple drilling of knee arthritic articular cartilage defects to promote a regenerative response (144). Microfracture is another healing response treatment, but was created to treat full-thickness cartilage injury in contrast to arthritis, as Pridie drilling was intended. The initial technique was described in 1994 (145). Around the same time, another method of cartilage repair called "autologous chondrocyte implantation" was published (146). It seems that the procedures to repair or regenerate knee articular cartilage were becoming more and more complex and expensive; however, the results are still not as good as we desire. The thought of using an easily accessible agent to aid in augmenting a commonly performed procedure would be ideal. This could include cell-augmented marrow stimulation procedures (microfracture and/or drilling) of both focal lesions as well as arthritis with an agent, such as PRP.

To date only a limited number of clinical investigations have been carried out in humans. The largest of the three published studies was completed by Siclari et al., who used Pridie drilling along with a PRP-soaked polyglycolic acid-hyaluronan (PGA-HA) scaffold in 52 patients and demonstrated good clinical outcomes at a 5-year follow-up and complete healing of cartilage defects in 21/52 patients who underwent MRI at 4-year follow-up (107). Dhollander et al., presented a case series of patellar osteochondral lesions that used microfracture and a collagen-based scaffold with PRP that resulted in improved MRI findings at 24-month follow-up (106). Sánchez et al. published the first case report using PRP to augment the repair of a pure chondral lesion in the knee, and at 18 weeks post surgery, the patient was able to return to the previous sporting activity (105). Summaries of studies reviewed can be found in Table 8.2.

In conclusion, PRP use for enhancing current cartilage repair procedures should be considered investigational at this stage, and further basic sciences as well as clinical investigations are warranted before widespread clinical application (147).

PLATELET-RICH PLASMA AND KNEE OSTEOARTHRITIS

Osteoarthritis (OA) is the leading cause of physical disability, often associated with pain, swelling, and significant impairment in the quality of life (148).

The impact of OA is expected to grow as the population continues to both increase and age in the coming years (149). OA can be treated effectively with conservative or interventional therapies.

PRP has demonstrated positive effects on chondrogenesis and MSC proliferation as well as the ability to modify the catabolic degenerative microenvironment. PRP can increase the synthetic capacity of chondrocytes via upregulation of genes that produce proteoglycans and also can enhance type II collagen deposition (150). Theoretically, this makes PRP a good therapy to alleviate the burdens of degenerative pathology. However, the published literature surrounding the use of PRP varies greatly. Current guidelines from the American Academy of Orthopaedic Surgeons indicate an inability to "recommend for or against" the use of PRP for the treatment of knee OA while citing that the literature had moderate applicability and strength of evidence; however, many of the studies themselves showed significant decreased levels of pain in the postinjection period (151).

There has been an increasing number of studies assessing the efficacy of PRP to treat knee OA. The results of individual and additional studies are summarized in Table 8.2.

In review of the available overall literature, Campbell et al. conducted a systematic review of overlapping meta-analyses, which demonstrated that intra-articular PRP is a viable treatment for knee OA and has the potential for symptomatic relief for up to 12 months, with patients in earlier stage OA benefiting relatively more (152). Furthermore, the authors stated that it was unclear from the currently available evidence if the use of multiple injections, double-spinning technology, or an activating agent lead to better outcomes as there was not sufficient evidence to draw conclusions regarding those attributes. The review did, however, demonstrate the potential for local adverse reactions after multiple PRP injections (152).

Meheux et al. showed similar results in a recent systematic review, concluding that a PRP injection results in significant clinical improvements up to 12 months postinjection and that clinical outcomes for PRP were significantly better compared to placebo and to hyaluronic acid (HA) injections at 3 to 12 months (131). Furthermore, the authors of this review recommended clinicians to use PRP in symptomatic knee OA with Ahlback grades of 1 to 3 or Kellgren-Lawrence grades of 1 to 3 and that injections can be administered in two to four sessions, 2 to 4 weeks apart. Furthermore, younger and more active patients were shown to achieve better results with a low degree of cartilage degeneration (153).

Filardo et al. found limited evidence comparing leukocyte-rich versus leukocyte-poor PRP for example. However, out of the six included studies, only one study used leukocyte-rich PRP (154). This study showed no significant improvement in any clinical outcomes and, in fact, it showed that patients were less satisfied. It could be argued that in osteoarthritic joints, leukocyte-poor PRP might be a better alternative. However, more evidence is needed in the form of level 1 evidence that compares leukocyte-rich and leukocyte-poor PRP directly (154).

In conclusion, it is difficult to confirm that a specific PRP preparation can maximize symptomatic relief and induce cartilage regeneration due to the paucity of appropriately powered clinical trials. However, based on an assessment of the limited number of investigations currently available, it appears that a leukocyte/RBC-poor PRP product may be better suited to treat degenerative synovial joints.

PLATELET-RICH PLASMA TO TREAT DEGENERATIVE HIP DISEASE

There is little evidence on the effectiveness of PRP in treating hip pathologies. Dallari et al. conducted an RCT to evaluate the effectiveness of PRP, HA, and a combination of PRP and HA in hip OA (108). The authors included 111 patients aged between 18 and 65 years and evaluated outcomes relating to pain and function. The results demonstrated that intra-articular PRP injections can offer significant improvement in pain and function with a good safety profile. PRP was superior to the HA product and the combination of PRP with HA was not found to be superior to PRP alone. Those benefits were maintained for up to 12 months compared with other treatments. These findings were replicated by other studies assessing ultrasound-guided PRP, therefore supporting the safety and efficacy of findings (109,155). However, there is a need for more level 1 trials to support the results of the findings of Dallari et al. (Table 8.2).

Hip arthroplasty is a very common orthopedic procedure and can be associated with significant complications including significant blood loss, infection, and a longer hospital stay, which in itself is associated with more risks. Safdar et al. investigated the use of PRP in hip replacement surgeries and whether or not it has any effect on bleeding complications, analgesic requirement, and ultimately the duration of hospital stay (156). They found no difference in the drop of hemoglobin, transfusion requirements, analgesic requirements, or length of hospital stay. Thus, PRP was not shown to have efficacy in reducing peri- and postoperation morbidity. However, in another study, Rafols et al. showed PRP to result in lower postarthroscopy pain scores at 48 hours and less joint effusions at 6 months (110). This suggests that PRP may have potential benefit in reducing inflammation in the postoperative period but the long-term outcome is still unclear. Therefore, additional and more robust studies are required to make any valid conclusions regarding the use of PRP in hip arthroplasty or arthroscopic surgeries.

CONCLUSION

In summary, although in vitro studies and early clinical outcomes are promising, there currently exists only a small number of high-quality clinical trials with appropriately powered protocols to support the augmentation of common orthopedic procedures, which include: surgical rotator cuff, ACL repair or reconstruction, meniscal repair, and cartilage repair. This is related primarily to the fact that many studies include a poorly defined PRP product resulting in outcomes with conflicting results and conclusions. Recent meta-analysis of the literature also highlights the lack of standardization in study methodology, PRP preparation, and outcome measures (102). This wide variation is likely to result in a comparison of heterogeneous data and to make any conclusions difficult to ascertain with any level of confidence. It is clear that further coordinated investigations with well-designed clinical protocols and consistently *defined* PRP *products are required in the future* to better define where PRP can enhance orthopedic surgical outcomes.

REFERENCES

1. de Vos RJ, Weir A, van Schie HT, et al. Platelet-rich plasma injection for chronic Achilles tendinopathy: a randomized controlled trial. *JAMA.* 2010;303(2):144–149.
2. Hall MP, Band PA, Meislin RJ, et al. Platelet-rich plasma: current concepts and application in sports medicine. *J Am Acad Orthop Surg.* 2009;17(10):602–608.
3. Filardo G, Kon E, Della Villa S, et al. Use of platelet-rich plasma for the treatment of refractory jumper's knee. *Int Orthop.* 2010;34(6):909–915.
4. Gaweda K, Tarczynska M, Krzyzanowski W. Treatment of Achilles tendinopathy with platelet-rich plasma. *Int J Sports Med.* 2010;31(8):577–583.
5. Kon E, Filardo G, Delcogliano M, et al. Platelet-rich plasma: new clinical application: a pilot study for treatment of jumper's knee. *Injury.* 2009;40(6):598–603.
6. Peerbooms JC, Sluimer J, Bruijn DJ, et al. Positive effect of an autologous platelet concentrate in lateral epicondylitis in a double-blind randomized controlled trial: platelet-rich plasma versus corticosteroid injection with a 1-year follow-up. *Am J Sports Med.* 2010;38(2):255–262.
7. Gosens T, Peerbooms JC, van Laar W, et al. Ongoing positive effect of platelet-rich plasma versus corticosteroid injection in lateral epicondylitis: a double-blind randomized controlled trial with 2-year follow-up. *Am J Sports Med.* 2011;39(6):1200–1208.
8. Nguyen RT, Borg-Stein J, McInnis K. Applications of platelet-rich plasma in musculoskeletal and sports medicine: an evidence-based approach. *PM R.* 2011;3(3):226–250.
9. Ferrari M, Zia S, Valbonesi M, et al. A new technique for hemodilution: preparation of autologous platelet-rich plasma and intraoperative blood salvage in cardiac surgery. *Int J Artif Organs.* 1987;10(1):47–50.
10. Alsousou J, Thompson M, Hulley P, et al. The biology of platelet-rich plasma and its application in trauma and orthopaedic surgery. *Bone Joint J* [Internet]. 2009 Aug 3;91-B(8):987–96. http://www.bjj.boneandjoint.org.uk/content/91-B/8/987.abstract
11. Mehta S, Watson JT. Platelet-rich concentrate: basic science and current clinical applications. *J Orthop Trauma.* 2008;22(6):432–438.
12. Foster TE, Puskas BL, Mandelbaum BR, et al. Platelet-rich plasma: from basic science to clinical applications. *Am J Sports Med* [Internet]. 2009 Nov 1;37(11):2259–2272. http://ajs.sagepub.com/cgi/content/short/37/11/2259
13. Sundman EA, Cole BJ, Karas V, et al. The anti-inflammatory and matrix restorative mechanisms of platelet-rich plasma in osteoarthritis. *Am J Sports Med.* 2014;42(1):35–41.
14. Sadoghi P, Rosso C, Valderrabano V, et al. The role of platelets in the treatment of Achilles tendon injuries. *J Orthop Res.* 2013;31(1):111–118.
15. Malavolta EA, Gracitelli ME, Ferreira Neto AA, et al. Platelet-rich plasma in rotator cuff repair: a prospective randomized study. *Am J Sports Med.* 2014;42(10):2446–2454.
16. Dragoo JL, Wasterlain AS, Braun HJ, et al. Platelet-rich plasma as a treatment for patellar tendinopathy: a double-blind, randomized controlled trial. *Am J Sports Med.* 2014;42(3):610–618.
17. Hamid AMS, Mohamed Ali MR, Yusof A, et al. Platelet-rich plasma injections for the treatment of hamstring injuries: a randomized controlled trial. *Am J Sport Med.* 2014;42:2410–2418.
18. Kim HJ, Yeom JS, Koh YG, et al. Anti-inflammatory effect of platelet-rich plasma on nucleus pulposus cells with response of TNF-a and IL-1. *J Orthop Res.* 2014;32(4):551–556.
19. Mishra A, Woodall J Jr, Vieira A. Treatment of tendon and muscle using platelet-rich plasma. *Clin Sports Med.* 2009;28(1):113–125.
20. Moraes VY, Lenza M, Tamaoki MJ, et al. Platelet-rich therapies for musculoskeletal soft tissue injuries. *Cochrane Database Syst Rev.* 2014;4:CD010071. doi:10.1002/14651858.CD010071.pub3

21. Mautner K, Malanga GA, Smith J, et al. A call for a standard classification system for future biologic research: the rationale for new PRP nomenclature. *PM R* [Internet]. *Am Acad Phys Med Rehabil.* 2015;7(4):S53–S59. doi:10.1016/j.pmrj.2015.02.005

22. Bennett NT, Schultz GS. Growth factors and wound healing: biochemical properties of growth factors and their receptors. *Am J Surg.* 1993;165(6):728–737.

23. Boswell SG, Cole BJ, Sundman EA, et al. Platelet-rich plasma: a milieu of bioactive factors. *Arthroscopy.* 2012;28(3):429–439.

24. Molloy T, Wang Y, Murrell G. The roles of growth factors in tendon and ligament healing. *Sports Med.* 2003;33(5):381–394.

25. de Mos M, van der Windt AE, Jahr H, et al. Can platelet-rich plasma enhance tendon repair? A cell culture study. *Am J Sports Med.* 2008;36(6):1171–1178.

26. Pietrzak WS, Eppley BL. Platelet-rich plasma: biology and new technology. *J Craniofac Surg.* 2005;16(6):1043–1054.

27. Marx RE. Platelet-rich plasma (PRP): what is PRP and what is not PRP? *Implant Dent.* 2001;10(4):225–228.

28. Sampson S, Gerhardt M, Mandelbaum B. Platelet-rich plasma injection grafts for musculoskeletal injuries: a review. *Curr Rev Musculoskelet Med.* 2008;1(3–4):165–174.

29. Weibrich G, Hansen T, Kleis W, et al. Effect of platelet concentration in platelet-rich plasma on peri-implant bone regeneration. *Bone.* 2004;34(4):665–671.

30. Graziani F, Ivanovski S, Cei S, et al. The *in vitro* effect of different PRP concentrations on osteoblasts and fibroblasts. *Clin Oral Implants Res.* 2006;17(2):212–219.

31. Giusti I, Rughetti A, D'Ascenzo S, et al. Identification of an optimal concentration of platelet gel for promoting angiogenesis in human endothelial cells. *Transfusion.* 2009;49(4):771–778.

32. Kevy S, Jacobson MMR. Defining the composition and healing effect of platelet-rich plasma. Presented at Platelet-Rich Plasma Symposium, New York, NY, August 5, 2010.

33. Tidball JG. Inflammatory processes in muscle injury and repair. *Am J Physiol Regul Integr Comp Physiol.* 2005;288(2):R345–R353.

34. Braun HJ, Kim HJ, Chu CR, et al. The effect of platelet-rich plasma formulations and blood products on human synoviocytes: implications for intra-articular injury and therapy. *Am J Sports Med.* 2014;42(5):1204–1210.

35. Pizza FX, Peterson JM, Baas JH, et al. Neutrophils contribute to muscle injury and impair its resolution after lengthening contractions in mice. *J Physiol (Lond).* 2005;562(Pt 3):899–913.

36. Browning SR, Weiser AM, Woolf N, et al. Platelet-rich plasma increases matrix metalloproteinases in cultures of human synovial fibroblasts. *J Bone Joint Surg Am.* 2012;94(23):e1721–e1727.

37. Braun HJ, Kim HJ, Chu CR, et al. The effect of platelet-rich plasma formulations and blood products on human synoviocytes: implications for intra-articular injury and therapy. *Am J Sports Med* [Internet]. 2014;42(5):1204–1210. http://www.ncbi.nlm.nih.gov/pubmed/24634448

38. Hooiveld M, Roosendaal G, Wenting M, et al. Short-term exposure of cartilage to blood results in chondrocyte apoptosis. *Am J Pathol.* 2003;162(3):943–951.

39. Roosendaal G, Vianen ME, Marx JJ, et al. Blood-induced joint damage: a human *in vitro* study. *Arthritis Rheum.* 1999;42(5):1025–1032.

40. Valentino LA, Hakobyan N, Kazarian T, et al. Experimental haemophilic synovitis: rationale and development of a murine model of human factor VIII deficiency. *Haemophilia.* 2004;10(3):280–287.

41. Roosendaal G, Vianen ME, Marx JJ, et al. Blood-induced joint damage: a human *in vitro* study. *Arthritis Rheum.* 1999;42(5):1025–1032.

42. Madhok R, Bennett D, Sturrock RD, et al. Mechanisms of joint damage in an experimental model of hemophilic arthritis. *Arthritis Rheum.* 1988;31(9):1148–1155.

43. Roosendaal G, Vianen ME, van den Berg HM, et al. Cartilage damage as a result of hemarthrosis in a human *in vitro* model. *J Rheumatol.* 1997;24(7):1350–1354.

44. Stein H, Duthie RB. The pathogenesis of chronic haemophilic arthropathy. *J Bone Joint Surg Br.* 1981;63B:601–609.

45. Jansen NW, Roosendaal G, Bijlsma JW, et al. Exposure of human cartilage tissue to low concentrations of blood for a short period of time leads to prolonged cartilage damage: an *in vitro* study. *Arthritis Rheum.* 2007;56(1):199–207.

46. Hooiveld M, Roosendaal G, Wenting M, et al. Short-term exposure of cartilage to blood results in chondrocyte apoptosis. *Am J Pathol.* 2003;162(3):943–951.

47. Tsay RC, Vo J, Burke A, et al. Differential growth factor retention by platelet-rich plasma composites. *J Oral Maxillofac Surg*. 2005;63(4):521–528.

48. Han B, Woodell-May J, Ponticiello M, et al. The effect of thrombin activation of platelet-rich plasma on demineralized bone matrix osteoinductivity. *J Bone Joint Surg Am*. 2009;91(6):1459–1470.

49. Mishra A, Harmon K, Woodall J, et al. Sports medicine applications of platelet-rich plasma. *Curr Pharm Biotechnol*. 2012;13(7):1185–1195.

50. Dohan Ehrenfest DM, Rasmusson L, et al. Classification of platelet concentrates: from pure platelet-rich plasma (P-PRP) to leucocyte- and platelet-rich fibrin (L-PRF). *Trends Biotechnol*. 2009;27(3):158–167.

51. DeLong JM, Russell RP, et al. Platelet-rich plasma: the PAW classification system. *Arthroscopy*. 2012;28(7):998–1009.

52. Kon E, Buda R, Filardo G, et al. Platelet-rich plasma: intra-articular knee injections produced favorable results on degenerative cartilage lesions. *Knee Surg Sports Traumatol Arthrosc*. 2010;18(4):472–479.

53. Filardo G, Kon E, Buda R, et al. Platelet-rich plasma intra-articular knee injections for the treatment of degenerative cartilage lesions and osteoarthritis. *Knee Surg Sports Traumatol Arthrosc*. 2011;19(4):528–535.

54. Radice F, Yánez R, Gutiérrez V, et al. Comparison of magnetic resonance imaging findings in anterior cruciate ligament grafts with and without autologous platelet-derived growth factors. *Arthroscopy*. 2010;26(1):50–57.

55. Thanasas C, Papadimitriou G, Charalambidis C, et al. Platelet-rich plasma versus autologous whole blood for the treatment of chronic lateral elbow epicondylitis: a randomized controlled clinical trial. *Am J Sports Med*. 2011;39(10):2130–2134.

56. Gosens T, Peerbooms JC, van Laar W, et al. Ongoing positive effect of platelet-rich plasma versus corticosteroid injection in lateral epicondylitis: a double-blind randomized controlled trial with 2-year follow-up. *Am J Sports Med*. 2011;39(6):1200–1208.

57. Wang-Saegusa A, Cugat R, Ares O, et al. Infiltration of plasma rich in growth factors for osteoarthritis of the knee: short-term effects on function and quality of life. *Arch Orthop Trauma Surg* [Internet]. 2011;131(3):311–317. doi:10.1007/s00402-010-1167-3

58. de Jonge S, de Vos RJ, Weir A, et al. One-year follow-up of platelet-rich plasma treatment in chronic Achilles tendinopathy: a double-blind randomized placebo-controlled trial. *Am J Sports Med*. 2011;39(8):1623–1629.

59. Vogrin M, Rupreht M, Dinevski D, et al. Effects of a platelet gel on early graft revascularization after anterior cruciate ligament reconstruction: a prospective, randomized, double-blind, clinical trial. *Eur Surg Res*. 2010;45(2):77–85.

60. Luime JJ, Koes BW, Hendriksen IJ, et al. Prevalence and incidence of shoulder pain in the general population; a systematic review. *Scand J Rheumatol*. 2004;33(2):73–81.

61. Kuijpers T, van der Windt DA, van der Heijden GJ, et al. Systematic review of prognostic cohort studies on shoulder disorders. *Pain*. 2004;109(3):420–431.

62. Mitchell C, Adebajo A, Hay E, et al. Shoulder pain: diagnosis and management in primary care. *BMJ*. 2005;331(7525):1124–1128.

63. van de Sande MAJ, de Groot JH, Rozing PM. Clinical implications of rotator cuff degeneration in the rheumatic shoulder. *Arthritis Rheum*. United States; 2008 Mar;59(3):317–324.

64. Robb G, Arroll B, Reid D, et al. Summary of an evidence-based guideline on soft tissue shoulder injuries and related disorders–Part 1: assessment. *J Prim Health Care*. 2009;1(1):36–41.

65. Motamedi AR, Urrea LH, Hancock RE, et al. Accuracy of magnetic resonance imaging in determining the presence and size of recurrent rotator cuff tears. *J Shoulder Elbow Surg*. 2002;11(1):6–10.

66. Kluger R, Bock P, Mittlböck M, et al. Long-term survivorship of rotator cuff repairs using ultrasound and magnetic resonance imaging analysis. *Am J Sports Med*. 2011;39(10):2071–2081.

67. Abdul-Wahab TA, Betancourt JP, Hassan F, et al. Initial treatment of complete rotator cuff tear and transition to surgical treatment: systematic review of the evidence. *Muscles Ligaments Tendons J*. 2016;6(1):35–47.

68. de Mos M, van der Windt AE, Jahr H, et al. Can platelet-rich plasma enhance tendon repair? A cell culture study. *Am J Sports Med*. 2008;36(6):1171–1178.

69. Murrell WD, Anz AW, Badsha H, et al. Regenerative treatments to enhance orthopedic surgical outcome. *PM R*. 2015;7(4 Suppl):S41–S52.

70. Rodeo SA, Delos D, Williams RJ, et al. The effect of platelet-rich fibrin matrix on rotator cuff tendon healing: a prospective, randomized clinical study. *Am J Sports Med*. 2012;40(6):1234–1241.

71. Castricini R, Longo UG, De Benedetto M, et al. Platelet-rich plasma augmentation for arthroscopic rotator cuff repair: a randomized controlled trial. *Am J Sports Med.* 2011;39(2):258–265.

72. Bergeson AG, Tashjian RZ, Greis PE, et al. Effects of platelet-rich fibrin matrix on repair integrity of at-risk rotator cuff tears. *Am J Sports Med.* 2012;40(2):286–293.

73. Weber SC, Kauffman JI, Parise C, et al. Platelet-rich fibrin matrix in the management of arthroscopic repair of the rotator cuff: a prospective, randomized, double-blinded study. *Am J Sports Med.* 2013;41(2):263–270.

74. Barber FA, Hrnack SA, Snyder SJ, et al. Rotator cuff repair healing influenced by platelet-rich plasma construct augmentation. *Arthroscopy.* 2011;27(8):1029–1035.

75. Antuña S, Barco R, Martínez Diez JM, et al. Platelet-rich fibrin in arthroscopic repair of massive rotator cuff tears: a prospective randomized pilot clinical trial. *Acta Orthop Belg.* 2013;79(1):25–30.

76. Cross JA, Cole BJ, Spatny KP, et al. Leukocyte-reduced platelet-rich plasma normalizes matrix metabolism in torn human rotator cuff tendons. *Am J Sports Med.* 2015;43(12):2898–2906.

77. Saito M, Takahashi KA, Arai Y, et al. Intraarticular administration of platelet-rich plasma with biodegradable gelatin hydrogel microspheres prevents osteoarthritis progression in the rabbit knee. *Clin Exp Rheumatol.* 2009;27(2):201–207.

78. Carr AJ, Murphy R, Dakin SG, et al. Platelet-rich plasma injection with arthroscopic acromioplasty for chronic rotator cuff tendinopathy: a randomized controlled trial. *Am J Sports Med.* 2015;43(12):2891–2897.

79. Scarpone M, Rabago D, Snell E, et al. Effectiveness of platelet-rich plasma injection for rotator cuff tendinopathy: a prospective open-label study. *Glob Adv Health Med.* 2013;2(2):26–31.

80. Rha DW, Park GY, Kim YK, et al. Comparison of the therapeutic effects of ultrasound-guided platelet-rich plasma injection and dry needling in rotator cuff disease: a randomized controlled trial. *Clin Rehabil.* 2013;27(2):113–122.

81. Malavolta EA, Gracitelli ME, Ferreira Neto AA, et al. Platelet-rich plasma in rotator cuff repair: a prospective randomized study. *Am J Sports Med.* 2014;42(10):2446–2454.

82. Pandey V, Bandi A, Madi S, et al. Does application of moderately concentrated platelet-rich plasma improve clinical and structural outcome after arthroscopic repair of medium-sized to large rotator cuff tear? A randomized controlled trial. *J Shoulder Elbow Surg.* 2016;25(8):1312–1322.

83. Randelli P, Arrigoni P, Ragone V, et al. Platelet rich plasma in arthroscopic rotator cuff repair: a prospective RCT study, 2-year follow-up. *J Shoulder Elbow Surg.* 2011;20(4):518–528.

84. Beck J, Evans D, Tonino PM, et al. The biomechanical and histologic effects of platelet-rich plasma on rat rotator cuff repairs. *Am J Sports Med.* 2012;40(9):2037–2044.

85. Järvinen TA, Kannus P, Maffulli N, et al. Achilles tendon disorders: etiology and epidemiology. *Foot Ankle Clin.* 2005;10(2):255–266.

86. Lantto I, Heikkinen J, Flinkkilä T, et al. Epidemiology of Achilles tendon ruptures: increasing incidence over a 33-year period. *Scand J Med Sci Sports.* 2015;25(1):e133–e138.

87. Bhandari M, Guyatt GH, Siddiqui F, et al. Treatment of acute Achilles tendon ruptures a systematic overview and meta-analysis. *Clinical Orthopaedics and Related Research.* 2002;400:190–200.

88. Wilkins R, Bisson LJ. Operative versus nonoperative management of acute achilles tendon ruptures a quantitative systematic review of randomized controlled trials. *Am J Sports Med.* 2012;40(9):2154–2160.

89. Khan RJ, Fick D, Keogh A, et al. Treatment of acute Achilles tendon ruptures. A meta-analysis of randomized, controlled trials. *J Bone Joint Surg Am.* 2005;87(10):2202–2210.

90. Willits K, Amendola A, Bryant D, et al. Operative versus nonoperative treatment of acute Achilles tendon ruptures: a multicenter randomized trial using accelerated functional rehabilitation. *J Bone Joint Surg Am.* 2010;92(17):2767–2775.

91. Cerza F, Carnì S, Carcangiu A, et al. Comparison between hyaluronic acid and platelet-rich plasma, intra-articular infiltration in the treatment of gonarthrosis. *Am J Sports Med.* 2012;40(12):2822–2827.

92. Filardo G, Kon E, Di Martino A, et al. Platelet-rich plasma vs hyaluronic acid to treat knee degenerative pathology: study design and preliminary results of a randomized controlled trial. *BMC Musculoskelet Disord.* 2012;13:229. doi:10.1186/1471-2474-13-229

93. Patel S, Dhillon MS, Aggarwal S, et al. Treatment with platelet-rich plasma is more effective than placebo for knee osteoarthritis: a prospective, double-blind, randomized trial. *Am J Sports Med.* 2013;41(2):356–364.

94. Sánchez M, Fiz N, Azofra J, et al. A randomized clinical trial evaluating plasma rich in growth factors (PRGF-Endoret) versus hyaluronic acid in the short-term treatment of symptomatic knee osteoarthritis. *Arthroscopy.* 2012;28(8):1070–1078.

95. Vaquerizo V, Plasencia MÁ, Arribas I, et al. Comparison of intra-articular injections of plasma rich in growth factors (PRGF-Endoret) versus durolane hyaluronic acid in the treatment of patients with symptomatic osteoarthritis: a randomized controlled trial. *Arthroscopy.* 2013;29(10):1635–1643.

96. Raeissadat SA, Rayegani SM, Hassanabadi H, et al. Knee osteoarthritis injection choices: platelet- rich plasma (PRP) versus hyaluronic acid (a 1-year randomized clinical trial). *Clin Med Insights Arthritis Musculoskelet Disord.* 2015;8:1–8.

97. Smith PA. Intra-articular autologous-conditioned plasma injections provide safe and efficacious treatment for knee osteoarthritis: an FDA-sanctioned, randomized, double-blind, placebo-controlled clinical trial. *American Journal of Sports Medicine.* 2016;44(4):884–891. doi:10.1177/0363546515624678

98. Spaková T, Rosocha J, Lacko M, et al. Treatment of knee joint osteoarthritis with autologous platelet-rich plasma in comparison with hyaluronic acid. *Am J Phys Med Rehabil.* 2012;91(5):411–417.

99. Cole BJ, Karas V, Hussey K, et al. Hyaluronic acid versus platelet-rich plasma: a prospective, double-blind randomized controlled trial comparing clinical outcomes and effects on intra-articular biology for the treatment of knee osteoarthritis. *Am J Sports Med.* 2017;45(2):339–346. doi:10.1177/0363546516665809

100. Kon E, Mandelbaum B, Buda R, et al. Platelet-rich plasma intra-articular injection versus hyaluronic acid viscosupplementation as treatments for cartilage pathology: from early degeneration to osteoarthritis. *Arthroscopy.* 2011;27(11):1490–1501.

101. Say F, Gürler D, Yener K, et al. Platelet-rich plasma injection is more effective than hyaluronic acid in the treatment of knee osteoarthritis. *Acta Chir Orthop Traumatol Cech.* 2013;80(4):278–283.

102. Filardo G, Kon E, Pereira Ruiz MT, et al. Platelet-rich plasma intra-articular injections for cartilage degeneration and osteoarthritis: single- versus double-spinning approach. *Knee Surg Sports Traumatol Arthrosc.* 2012;20(10):2082–2091.

103. Gumina S, Campagna V, Ferrazza G, et al. Use of platelet-leukocyte membrane in arthroscopic repair of large rotator cuff tears: a prospective randomized study. *J Bone Joint Surg Am.* 2012;94(15):1345–1352.

104. Everts PA, Devilee RJ, Brown Mahoney C, et al. Exogenous application of platelet-leukocyte gel during open subacromial decompression contributes to improved patient outcome. A prospective randomized double-blind study. *Eur Surg Res.* 2008;40(2):203–210.

105. Sánchez M, Azofra J, Anitua E, et al. Plasma rich in growth factors to treat an articular cartilage avulsion: a case report. *Med Sci Sports Exerc.* 2003;35(10):1648–1652.

106. Dhollander AA, De Neve F, Almqvist KF, et al. Autologous matrix-induced chondrogenesis combined with platelet-rich plasma gel: technical description and a five pilot patients report. *Knee Surg Sports Traumatol Arthrosc.* 2011;19(4):536–542.

107. Siclari A, Mascaro G, Kaps C, et al. A 5-year follow-up after cartilage repair in the knee using a platelet-rich plasma-immersed polymer-based implant. *Open Orthop J.* 2014;8:346–354.

108. Dallari D, Stagni C, Rani N, et al. Ultrasound-guided injection of platelet-rich plasma and hyaluronic acid, separately and in combination, for hip osteoarthritis: a randomized controlled study. *Am J Sports Med.* 2016;44(3):664–671.

109. Battaglia M, Guaraldi F, Vannini F, et al. Efficacy of ultrasound-guided intra-articular injections of platelet-rich plasma versus hyaluronic acid for hip osteoarthritis. *Orthopedics.* 2013;36(12):e1501–e1508.

110. Rafols C, Monckeberg JE, Numair J, et al. Platelet-rich plasma augmentation of arthroscopic hip surgery for femoroacetabular impingement: A prospective study with 24-month follow-up. *Arthroscopy.* 2015;31(10):1886–1892.

111. de Almeida AM, Demange MK, Sobrado MF, et al. Patellar tendon healing with platelet-rich plasma: a prospective randomized controlled trial. *Am J Sports Med.* 2012;40(6):1282–1288.

112. Cervellin M, de Girolamo L, Bait C, et al. Autologous platelet-rich plasma gel to reduce donor-site morbidity after patellar tendon graft harvesting for anterior cruciate ligament reconstruction: a randomized, controlled clinical study. *Knee Surg Sports Traumatol Arthrosc.* 2012;20(1):114–120.

113. Orrego M, Larrain C, Rosales J, et al. Effects of platelet concentrate and a bone plug on the healing of hamstring tendons in a bone tunnel. *Arthroscopy.* 2008;24(12):1373–1380.

114. Vadalà A, Iorio R, De Carli A, et al. Platelet-rich plasma: does it help reduce tunnel widening after ACL reconstruction? *Knee Surgery, Sport Traumatol Arthrosc* [Internet]. 2013;21(4):824–829. doi:10.1007/s00167-012-1980-z

115. Nin JR, Gasque GM, Azcárate AV, et al. Has platelet-rich plasma any role in anterior cruciate ligament allograft healing? *Arthroscopy.* 2009;25(11):1206–1213.

116. Vogrin M, Rupreht M, Crnjac A, et al. The effect of platelet-derived growth factors on knee stability after anterior cruciate ligament reconstruction: a prospective randomized clinical study. *Wien Klin Wochenschr.* 2010;122 Suppl 2:91–95.

117. Sánchez M, Anitua E, Azofra J, et al. Comparison of surgically repaired Achilles tendon tears using platelet-rich fibrin matrices. *Am J Sports Med.* 2007;35(2):245–251.

118. De Carli A, Lanzetti RM, Ciompi A, et al. Can platelet-rich plasma have a role in Achilles tendon surgical repair?. *Knee Surgery, Sports Traumatology, Arthroscopy.* 2015:1–7.

119. Schepull T, Kvist J, Norrman H, et al. Autologous platelets have no effect on the healing of human Achilles tendon ruptures: a randomized single-blind study. *Am J Sports Med.* 2011;39(1):38–47.

120. Rupreht M, Vogrin M, Hussein M. MRI evaluation of tibial tunnel wall cortical bone formation after platelet-rich plasma applied during anterior cruciate ligament reconstruction. *Radiol Oncol* [Internet]. Versita, Warsaw; 2013 Jun 21;47(2):119–124. http://www.ncbi.nlm.nih.gov/pmc/articles/PMC3691087

121. Rupreht M, Jevtic V, Serša I, et al. Evaluation of the tibial tunnel after intraoperatively administered platelet-rich plasma gel during anterior cruciate ligament reconstruction using diffusion weighted and dynamic contrast-enhanced MRI. *J Magn Reson Imaging.* 2013;37(4):928–935.

122. Vogrin M, Rupreht M, Dinevski D, et al. Effects of a platelet gel on early graft revascularization after anterior cruciate ligament reconstruction: a prospective, randomized, double-blind, clinical trial. *Eur Surg Res.* 2010;45(2):77–85.

123. Mirzatolooei F, Alamdari MT, Khalkhali HR. The impact of platelet-rich plasma on the prevention of tunnel widening in anterior cruciate ligament reconstruction using quadrupled autologous hamstring tendon: a randomised clinical trial. *Bone Joint J.* 2013;95-B(1):65–69.

124. Seijas R, Ares O, Catala J, et al. Magnetic resonance imaging evaluation of patellar tendon graft remodelling after anterior cruciate ligament reconstruction with or without platelet-rich plasma. *J Orthop Surg (Hong Kong).* 2013;21(1):10–14.

125. Figueroa D, Melean P, Calvo R, et al. Magnetic resonance imaging evaluation of the integration and maturation of semitendinosus-gracilis graft in anterior cruciate ligament reconstruction using autologous platelet concentrate. *Arthroscopy.* 2010;26(10):1318–1325.

126. Valentí Nin JR, Mora Gasque G, Valentí Azcárate A, et al. Has platelet-rich plasma any role in anterior cruciate ligament allograft healing? *Arthroscopy.* 2009;25(11):1206–1213.

127. Sánchez M, Anitua E, Azofra J, et al. Ligamentization of tendon grafts treated with an endogenous preparation rich in growth factors: gross morphology and histology. *Arthroscopy.* 2010;26(4):470–480.

128. Di Matteo B, Loibl M, Andriolo L, et al. Biologic agents for anterior cruciate ligament healing: A systematic review. *World J Orthop.* 2016;7(9): 592–603.

129. Seijas R, Ares O, Cuscó X, et al. Partial anterior cruciate ligament tears treated with intraligamentary plasma rich in growth factors. *World J Orthop.* 2014;5(3):373–378.

130. Komzák M, Hart R, Šmíd P, et al. [The effect of platelet-rich plasma on graft healing in reconstruction of the anterior cruciate ligament of the knee joint: prospective study]. *Acta Chir Orthop Traumatol Cech.* 2015;82(2):135–139.

131. Radice F, Yánez R, Gutiérrez V, et al. Comparison of magnetic resonance imaging findings in anterior cruciate ligament grafts with and without autologous platelet-derived growth factors. *Arthroscopy.* 2010;26(1):50–57.

132. Silva A, Sampaio R. Anatomic ACL reconstruction: does the platelet-rich plasma accelerate tendon healing? *Knee Surg Sports Traumatol Arthrosc.* 2009;17(6):676–682.

133. Ventura A, Terzaghi C, Borgo E, et al. Use of growth factors in ACL surgery: preliminary study. *Journal of Orthopaedics and Traumatology.* 2005;6(2):76–79.

134. Figueroa D, Figueroa F, Calvo R, et al. Platelet-rich plasma use in anterior cruciate ligament

surgery: systematic review of the literature. *Arthroscopy*. 2015;31(5):981–988.

135. Arnoczky SP, Warren RF. Microvasculature of the human meniscus. *Am J Sports Med*. 1982;10(2):90–95.

136. Baratz ME, Fu FH, Mengato R. Meniscal tears: the effect of meniscectomy and of repair on intra-articular contact areas and stress in the human knee. A preliminary report. *Am J Sports Med*. 1986;14(4):270–275.

137. Wasserstein D, Dwyer T, Gandhi R, et al. A matched-cohort population study of reoperation after meniscal repair with and without concomitant anterior cruciate ligament reconstruction. *Am J Sports Med*. 2012;41(2):349–355. doi:10.1177/0363546512471134

138. Freedman KB, Nho SJ, Cole BJ. Marrow-stimulating technique to augment meniscus repair. *Arthroscopy*. 2003;19(7):794–798.

139. Driscoll MD, Robin BN, Horie M, et al. Marrow stimulation improves meniscal healing at early endpoints in a rabbit meniscal injury model. *Arthroscopy*. 2013;29(1):113–121.

140. de Girolamo L, Galliera E, Volpi P, et al. Why menisci show higher healing rate when repaired during ACL reconstruction? Growth factors release can be the explanation. *Knee Surg Sports Traumatol Arthrosc*. 2015;23(1):90–96.

141. Griffin JW, Hadeed MM, Werner BC, et al. Platelet-rich plasma in meniscal repair: does augmentation improve surgical outcomes? *Clin Orthop Relat Res*. 2015;473(5):1665–1672.

142. Pujol N, Salle De Chou E, Boisrenoult P, et al. Platelet-rich plasma for open meniscal repair in young patients: any benefit? *Knee Surg Sports Traumatol Arthrosc*. 2015;23(1):51–58.

143. Magnuson PB. Technic of debridement of the knee joint for arthritis. *Surg Clin North Am*. 1946;26:249–266.

144. Pridie KH, Gordon G. A method of resurfacing osteoarthritic knee joints. *J Bone Joint Surg-British*. 1959;41(3):618–619.

145. Rodrigo JJ, Steadman JR, Silliman JF, et al. Improvement of full-thickness chondral defect healing in the human knee after debridement and microfracture using continuous passive motion. *Am J Knee Surg*. 1994;7(3):109–116.

146. Brittberg M, Lindahl A, Nilsson A, et al. Treatment of deep cartilage defects in the knee with autologous chondrocyte transplantation. *N Engl J Med*. 1994;331(14):889–895.

147. Anz AW, Bapat A, Murrell WD. Concepts in regenerative medicine: past, present, and future in articular cartilage treatment. *J Clin Orthop Trauma*. 2016;7(3):137–144.

148. Curl WW, Krome J, Gordon ES, et al. Cartilage injuries: a review of 31,516 knee arthroscopies. *Arthroscopy*. 1997;13(4):456–460.

149. Herndon JH, Davidson SM, Apazidis A. Recent socioeconomic trends in orthopaedic practice. *J Bone Joint Surg Am*. 2001;83-A(7):1097–1105.

150. Smyth NA, Murawski CD, Fortier LA, et al. Platelet-rich plasma in the pathologic processes of cartilage: review of basic science evidence. *Arthroscopy*. 2013;29(8):1399–1409.

151. Brown GA. AAOS clinical practice guidelines. Treatment of osteoarthritis of the knee: evidence-based guideline, 2nd ed. *J Am Acad Orthop Surg*. 2013; 21:577–579.

152. Campbell KA, Saltzman BM, Mascarenhas R, et al. Does intra-articular platelet-rich plasma injection provide clinically superior outcomes compared with other therapies in the treatment of knee osteoarthritis? A systematic review of overlapping meta-analyses. *Arthrosc—J Arthrosc Relat Surg* [Internet]. *AANA*. 2015;31(11):2213–2221. doi:10.1016/j.arthro.2015.03.041

153. Meheux CJ, McCulloch PC, et al. Efficacy of intra-articular platelet-rich plasma injections in knee osteoarthritis: A systematic review. *Arthrosc—J Arthrosc Relat Surg* [Internet]. *AANA*. 2016;32(3):495–505. doi:10.1016/j.arthro.2015.08.005

154. Filardo G, Kon E, Di Martino A, et al. Platelet-rich plasma vs hyaluronic acid to treat knee degenerative pathology: study design and preliminary results of a randomized controlled trial. *BMC Musculoskelet Disord*. 2012;13:229. doi:10.1186/1471-2474-13-229

155. Sánchez M, Guadilla J, Fiz N, et al. Ultrasound-guided platelet-rich plasma injections for the treatment of osteoarthritis of the hip. *Rheumatology (Oxford)*. 2012;51(1):144–150.

156. Safdar A, Shaaban H, Tibayan R, et al. The clinical efficacy of using autologous platelet-rich plasma in hip arthroplasty: A retrospective comparative study. *J Nat Sci Biol Med*. 2015;6(1):49–55.

CHAPTER 9

AMNIOTIC AND UMBILICAL CORD PRODUCTS, ALPHA-2 MACROGLOBULIN, AND INTERLEUKIN-1 RECEPTOR ANTAGONIST PROTEIN

Sean Colio, Marko Bodor, and Ryan Dregalla

In this chapter we review several emerging areas in regenerative medicine for orthopedic conditions: amniotic and umbilical cord products, interleukin-1 receptor antagonist protein (IRAP), and alpha-2 macro-globulin (A2M). Amniotic fluid and membranes contain numerous growth factors, cytokines, anti-inflammatory proteins, collagen, fibronectin, mesenchymal stromal cells, epithelial cells, and hyaluronic acid. These components are appealing for their utility in treating various acute and chronic musculoskeletal pathologies. IRAP is a naturally occurring analog and a competitor of interleukin-1 (IL-1) and binds to the interleukin-1 receptor (IL-1R) causing suppression of inflammation typically caused by IL-1. By suppressing the IL-1 inflammatory cascade, it may be possible to prevent the activation of macrophages, monocytes, and stimulation of osteoclasts that break down

bone and cartilage matrix in orthopedic injuries and degenerative processes. A2M is a plasma glycoprotein with a unique ability to inhibit metalloproteinases (MMP) involved in degrading cartilage and inflammatory cytokines production. Similar to IRAP, A2M may help reduce the catabolic process in degenerative and inflammatory orthopedic conditions. Throughout this chapter we also review the current clinical evidence regarding the use of these techniques.

AMNIOTIC FLUID AND TISSUE PRODUCTS

Amniotic products are derived from human amniotic fluid and amniotic membranes. The membrane forms the amniotic sac and the lining of the placenta while the fluid surrounds

149

the fetus during pregnancy providing protection and nourishment. Amniotic membranes contain numerous growth factors, cytokines, anti-inflammatory proteins, collagen, fibronectin, mesenchymal stromal cells, epithelial cells, and hyaluronic acid (HA) (1,2). These components convey anti-inflammatory, antimicrobial, and anti-fibroblastic properties. Amniotic fluid contains nutrients necessary for fetal development and also a chemical profile similar to that of synovial fluid with hyaluronan, lubrican, cholesterol, and cytokines (3). Amniotic tissues are also non-immunogenic, a potential source of pluripotent cells, and provide a tissue scaffold promoting wound healing and reduced scar formation (1). Stromal and epithelial cells extracted from amniotic membranes display characteristics of mesenchymal stem cells (MSC) capable of differentiating into myocytes, osteocytes, and chondrocytes (4–9). Miki et al. have described these stem cells as being non-tumerogenic on transplantation (4,6,10).

Numerous commercial forms of amniotic products are available, containing varying amounts of cryopreserved amniotic fluid, amniotic fluid-derived cells, and amniotic membrane. With respect to orthopedic applications, commercial amniotic products either employ the use of amniotic fluid allegedly containing a cell suspension or a micronized amniotic membrane that can be suspended in liquid and administered by injection. It is believed that some of the biological properties of amniotic tissues are retained when processed to be stored in either cryopreserved or dehydrated states. Koob et al. demonstrated that cytokine content varied significantly among amniotic membrane products, but they were able to elute the growth factors into saline and stimulate the migration of MSC both in vitro and in vivo (2).

Human amniotic fluid and tissue products are manufactured to be regulated under the U.S. Food and Drug Administration (FDA) regulation of human cells and tissues intended for implantation, transplantation, or infusion through the Center for Biologics Evaluation and Research, under Code of Federal Regulation (CFR) title

21, parts 1270 and 1271. Most manufacturers of amniotic products seek to be regulated solely under Section 361 of the Public Health Service (PHS) Act of 1944. Per the FDA, this classification allows for low-risk human cell and tissue products to enter the market and be sold without any safety or efficacy studies. To be solely regulated under this section, a product must satisfy the FDA's definitions of being: (a) minimally manipulated, and free of any process that alters the original relevant or biological characteristics; (b) intended for homologous use, where the tissue used is known by the FDA to have the same basic function(s) in the recipient as in the donor; and (c) free of viable cells in the case of an allograft, as the product may not rely on metabolic activity of the product. If a human cell or tissue product does not meet *all* of the criteria mentioned, then it will be regulated by the FDA as a medical device (class II or III), a drug, or under Section 351 of the PHS Act, which parallels the approval process for a drug but for products composed exclusively of human cells and tissues. In each of these instances, premarket approval of the product by the FDA is required, which becomes intensely more time-consuming and financially burdensome. In recent history, many amniotic products intended for orthopedic applications have been disqualified from the privilege of being solely regulated under Section 361 for three primary reasons: (a) the product description includes claims of viable (allogeneic) cells in the product that are ancillary to the product's function; (b) the morselization of a membrane (particulate form, Figures 9.1 and 9.2) alters the original relevant characteristics of the product from a mechanical and dimensional perspective and therefore is more than minimally manipulated; and (c) any homogenized or morselized form of amniotic membranes labeled for orthopedic use (injectable) are not for homologous use as it does not "replace or supplement damaged or inadequate *integumental* tissue." Hence, many amniotic products intended for orthopedic applications have been reassigned to a new classification; most have received notification that the product will be regulated under Section 351

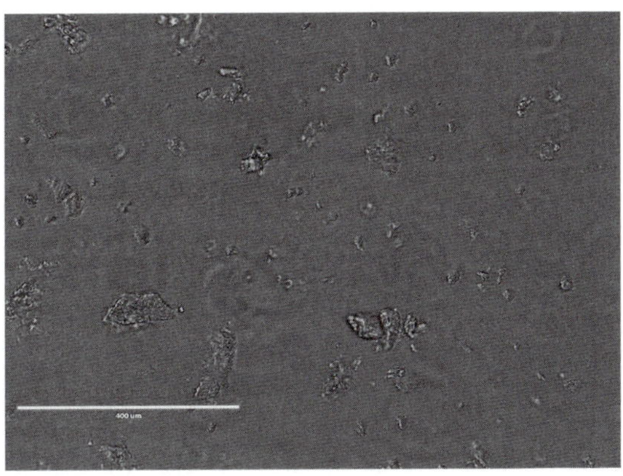

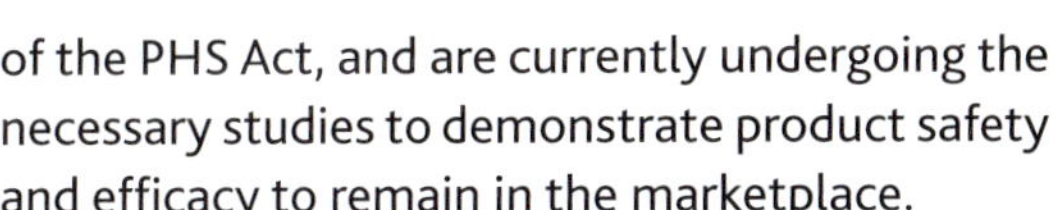

FIGURE 9.1

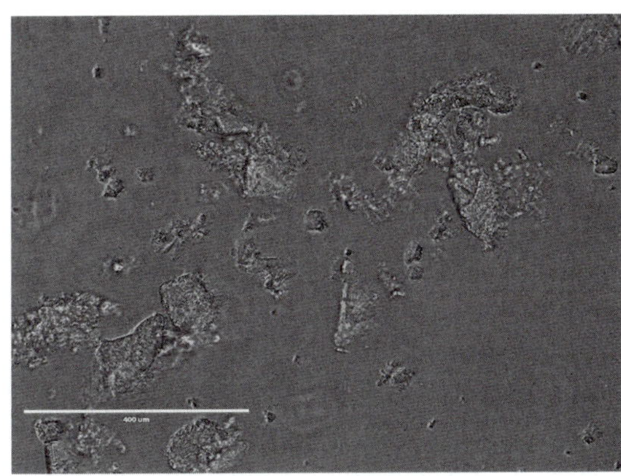

FIGURE 9.2

of the PHS Act, and are currently undergoing the necessary studies to demonstrate product safety and efficacy to remain in the marketplace.

Amnion-derived products have been utilized in the treatment of corneal injuries, skin wounds, burns, and leg ulcers (2,11–20). One of the earliest publications on their use for orthopedic conditions was in 1938 in which bovine amniotic fluid concentrate was used within the joints of 68 patients (21). In this study, Shimberg et al. recognized that the amniotic fluid mechanism of action was likely both mechanical and biological despite the limited understanding at the time of the composition of the amniotic concentrate.

The interpretation of their results was that there was a beneficial mechanical distention of the joint, a defense reaction in the intra-articular tissues due to fibrin formation, stimulation of a repair process, and improvement of intra-articular fluid viscosity by preventing adhesions (21).

Currently, there are numerous in vitro and in vivo studies evaluating the use of amniotic compounds in treating cartilage, tendon, ligament, and fascial injuries (22–31). The majority of these studies use animal models and at this time only three human studies have been published. Philip et al. and Kueckelhaus et al. demonstrated improved mechanical properties in Achilles tendons in rats after treatment with amniotic solutions (24,32). Coban et al. found no benefit in treating ruptured Achilles tendons

in rats with amniotic fluid and membrane (33). Other animal studies have looked at the effect of amniotic compounds on digital flexor tendon repair, demonstrating a decreased incidence of adhesion formation (34–36). There are no human studies evaluating the effects of amniotic compounds on human tendon and ligament healing; however, there are two studies on plantar fasciitis.

Zelen et al. published an industry-sponsored, prospective, randomized, single-center clinical trial of 45 patients with chronic refractory plantar fasciitis (37).They were randomized into three groups to receive an anesthetic injection of 2 mL 0.5% marcaine, followed by either 1.25 mL saline (controls), 0.5 mL micronized dehydrated amniotic membrane (MDAM), or 1.25 mL MDAM. Follow-up visits were scheduled weekly for 6 weeks, and a final study visit was scheduled at 8 weeks post injection. Three outcome measure scales were used during the evaluation: the American Orthopaedic Foot and Ankle Society (AOFAS) hindfoot scale, the Wong–Baker FACES Pain Rating Scale, and the SF-36v2 standard health survey. Baseline AOFAS scores were 54.4 ± 17.7, 41.3 ± 4.5, and 41.0 ± 7.7 in the control, 0.5 mL MDAM, and 1.25 mL MDAM groups, respectively. The scores rose in all groups throughout the study, with final scores at 8 weeks being 70.0 ± 9.6, 92.9 ± 8.7, 94.3 ± 5.6 in the control, 0.5 mL in the MDAM, and 1.25 mL in the MDAM groups respectively. Additionally, the SF36v2 mental and physical component scores rose and the FACES scores dropped for both MDAM groups more so than compared with the controls. Baseline scores on the SF36v2 physical component were 41.4 ± 6.1 for the control, 36.0 ± 5.9 for the 0.5 mL MDAM group, and 37.0 ± 3.8 for the 1.25 mL MDAM group and rose to 43.6 ± 5.6 for the control, 55.9 ± 3.5 for the 0.5 mL MDAM group, and 57.3 ± 2.6 for the 1.25 mL MDAM group. The authors reported no adverse events in either group. Due to the short 8-week follow-up, the editor of the journal termed this a feasibility study and noted that the authors were conducting a longer term follow-up study.

Hanselman et al. published an industry-sponsored–double-blind randomized, controlled, single-center pilot study of 24 patients with chronic plantar fasciitis (38). They randomized two groups: (a) a control group receiving corticosteroid (1 mL of 40 mg/mL Depo Medrol, 4 mL bupivacaine 0.5%) and (b) a study group receiving cryopreserved human amniotic membrane (1 mL cryopreserved human amniotic membrane [CHAM], 4 mL bupivacaine 0.5%). The groups were evaluated over three clinic visits: an initial visit at the time of the injection, a 6-week follow-up, and a 12-week follow-up. The primary outcome measure was the Foot Health Status Questionnaire (FHSQ) with higher scores implying reduced pain and improved function. The secondary outcome measure was the Visual Analog Scale (VAS) and the patient's verbal self-report of percent improvement. The average FHSQ scores at 6 weeks were: foot pain 24.6 in the corticosteroid group and 18.8 in the CHAM group, foot function 8.3 in the corticosteroid group and −2.1 in the CHAM group, and physical activity 14.8 in the corticosteroid group and 5.6 in the CHAM group. After the 6-week follow-up, when most of the FHSQ scores were higher in the corticosteroid group versus the CHAM group, the study groups were offered a second injection. Each group then underwent the same injection protocol with the same drug that corresponded to their initial injection, which was again blinded to both the investigator and the patient. They were then reevaluated twice more at 12-week and 18-week follow-up visits. At 18 weeks the FHSQ scores were as follows: foot pain 32.5 in the corticosteroid group and 66.3 in the CHAM group, foot function 33.3 in the corticosteroid group and 31.3 in the CHAM group, and physical activity 31.5 in the corticosteroid group and 33.3 in the CHAM group. Thus, at 18 weeks most of the FSHQ scores were higher in the CHAM group versus the corticosteroid group, a reversal of the findings seen at 6 weeks. The VAS scores decreased from baseline, with the single injection subset being −12.6 for the corticosteroid group and −17.8 for the CHAM group at 12 weeks, and the double injection subset being −25.7 for the corticosteroid group and −37.3 for the CHAM group at 18 weeks. The authors reported no adverse side effects from either injection. The editor of the journal opined that given the short follow-up period, the study showed that only CHAM was safe in the short term and about as equally effective as a corticosteroid injection but at a higher cost.

There are many cell culture and animal studies investigating the use of amniotic membranes for cartilage pathology (22,23,25,39–42). However, human studies are limited with only one published open-label, prospective feasibility study. In this study, Vines et al. selected six patients with Kellgren–Lawrence knee osteoarthritis grades of 3 and 4 (43). They administered a single intra-articular injection containing cryopreserved, particulate human amnion and amniotic fluid cells with follow-up of the patients at 1 and 2 weeks and at 3, 6, and 12 months posttreatment. Outcome measures included the Knee Injury and Osteoarthritis Outcome Score (KOOS), International Knee Documentation Committee scale (IKDC), and a single assessment numeric evaluation pain scale (SANE). The KOOS outcome score improved from a baseline of 43.35 to 70.23 by the 1-year time point. The IKDC assessment improved from an average score of 41.7 at baseline to 63.4 at 6 months and to 64.4 at 1 year. SANE scores improved from an average of 51.25 at baseline to 87.3 at 6 months and 85.8 at 1 year. The authors determined that statistical analysis was not appropriate for their data. The authors reported no adverse events other than a transient increase in knee pain that resolved at a 2-week follow-up (43).

In summary, although there are a number of animal and cell culture studies regarding the use of amniotic products for orthopedic conditions, the current clinical evidence for humans is limited to the one feasibility study for knee arthritis and the two small randomized controlled trials for plantar fasciitis. Additional clinical trials for more types of musculoskeletal pathologies along with larger sample sizes and longer follow-ups are needed. It is interesting to note that the published utilization of amniotic products in orthopedics dates as far back as 1938, preceding many other areas of regenerative medicine. Amniotic membranes are a potential source of viable pluripotent MSC in the fresh state and growth factors in the cryopreserved state, yet whether these products provide a benefit to MSC conditions remains unknown (1). With ongoing clinical research, the beneficial effects of amniotic products hypothesized by Shimberg et al. in 1938 may eventually be realized.

UMBILICAL CORD BLOOD

Umbilical cord blood (UCB) is blood left in the umbilical cord after childbirth. It consists of red and white blood cells, plasma, and platelets. It is also a rich source of hematopoietic and mesenchymal stromal cells. Collection of cord blood is typically done by cannulating the vein of the umbilical cord after it is severed. The amount of UBC from a donor differs but can range from 75 to 150 mL on an average (44). Processing then varies greatly depending on the tissue center or manufacturer. The UCB collected is then cryopreserved (45).

Clinical experience with UCB since its first use in the late 1980s is concerned mostly with hematopoietic reconstitution; however, increased understanding of the cell populations has expanded its potential in cellular immunotherapies for therapeutic use against malignancies (46).

UCB-derived MSC are in a more primitive state without antigen-producing cells, rendering them invisible to the host's immune system permitting allogenic cell therapy (47). Animal and human studies are currently underway in spinal cord and brain injury applications, cerebral palsy, lung disease, kidney injury, juvenile diabetes, and autoimmune applications (48).

Recently, a processing methodology (Progenokine®, Smart-Surgical Inc. dba Burst Biologics, Boise, Idaho) was developed to preserve the integrity of UCB cells and protecting cell viability. This processing method avoids using toxic media, including dimethyl sulfoxide (DMSO), to protect cell viability (49–51). As a result, these cells can self-renew after a freeze–thaw cycle and avoid apoptosis.

One of the first commercially available products using this method is an injectable/fluid allograft stem cell product derived from UCB (BioBurst Rejuv®, Burst Biologics, Boise, ID). It is regulated as a minimally manipulated tissue under CFR 1271 for homologous use only. Currently there are only unpublished anecdotal reports with clinical studies in process (52).

INTERLEUKIN-1 RECEPTOR ANTAGONIST PROTEIN

Inflammatory cytokines, such as tumor necrosis factor alpha (TNF-α) and IL-1 have been implicated in the pathogenesis of osteoarthritis due to their catabolic mechanisms on cartilage. These factors mediate the function of a variety of cells, including phenotype shifts in macrophages that are major players in the progression of osteoarthritis (53,54), express tissue-damaging metalloproteases (55) and contribute to disease progression through continued expression of proinflammatory cytokines (56,57). The discovery of competitive antagonists of these cytokines has greatly evolved the treatment of rheumatoid arthritis and is now offering insight into new techniques at halting the degenerative process of osteoarthritis. IRAP, also known as "IL-1 receptor antagonist (IL-1Ra)," is a naturally occurring analog and competitor of IL-1 and binds to the IL-1R receptor, with an affinity for type I and II receptors (58,59). When IL-1 binds to an IL-1R receptor, a cascade of inflammation is triggered, including activation of macrophages, monocytes, and stimulation of osteoclasts to break down bone and cartilage matrix (58–61). However, when IRAP binds to an IL-1R receptor, inflammation is suppressed. One hypothesis is that an appropriate balance of IRAP to IL-1 leads to a healthy equilibrium between anabolic and catabolic processes in joints and muscles (62–66). If that equilibrium is unbalanced toward excess IL-1 or insufficient IRAP, then a propensity toward the destruction of cartilage, muscles, and other joint structures ensues (62–66). Thus, there has been an interest in developing methods at isolating and producing IRAP.

In 1990, Seckinger et al. described natural and recombinant human IL-1 receptor antagonists blocking the effects of IL-1 on bone resorption and prostaglandin production (67). Since that time, recombinant versions of IRAP have been developed and tested with Jiang et al. publishing a multicenter, double-blind, dose-ranging, randomized, placebo-controlled study evaluating its utility for rheumatoid arthritis (RA) patients (68). They concluded that their systemic recombinant human IL-1 receptor antagonist reduced radiologic progression of RA. The recombinant version of IRAP was branded as anakinra and based on its effects on RA, Chevalier et al. investigated its use in osteoarthritis (OA). They published a safety study on the intra-articular injection of anakinra as an earlier use in RA was systemic administration (69). They reported that intra-articular injection of IRAP in patients with knee OA was well tolerated and did not induce any acute inflammatory reactions and also noted an improvement in Western Ontario and McMaster Universities Osteoarthritis Index (WOMAC) scores until month 3. Chevalier et al. followed up on this study with a multicenter, double-blind, placebo-controlled study and randomized 2:1:2 to receive a single intra-articular injection of placebo, anakinra 50 mg, or anakinra 150 mg in their symptomatic knee (70). The study groups were followed for 12 weeks with the primary end point being the change in the WOMAC score from baseline to week 4. Out of 160 (94%) patients who completed the study, the mean improvements from baseline to week 4 in WOMAC scores

were not statistically different among groups. They reported no adverse events.

Further studies on anakinra for intra-articular inflammatory processes have been more positive. Brown et al. retrospectively reviewed six patients (three female and three male), ranging in age from 17 to 50 years, who underwent injection of intra-articular anakinra, 200 mg, for persistent effusions of their postoperative knee (71). They reported that after intra-articular anakinra, 66% had improvement in knee arc of motion (15°–30°) and pain, five of six (83%) had improvement in swelling and all of these patients were able to return to sports. Kraus et al. evaluated 11 patients with acute anterior cruciate ligament (ACL) tear confirmed by MRI and randomized them to receive a single intra-articular injection of anakinra 150 mg or equal volume of saline placebo 2 weeks after injury and before surgical ACL reconstruction (72). They concluded that anakinra decreased pain and improved function (activities of daily living [ADL], sports function, and quality of life [QOL]) and exceeded the minimal perceptible clinical improvement in ADL for both the WOMAC and KOOS.

Arend et al. described IRAP production using surface-bound immunoglobulin G, lipopolysaccharide, phorbol myristate acetate, IL-1, and TNF-α to induce IRAP production by isolated human monocytes (73–77). Based on this understanding, Meijer et al. published a method to concentrate peripheral blood leukocytes from venous blood through centrifugation and then incubating them over glass beds to induce IRAP production de novo (78). This product was named as autologous-conditioned serum (ACS) and branded as Orthokine®. This process also produces a variety of likely beneficial growth factors and cytokines within ACS, including vascular endothelial growth factor (VEGF), platelet-derived growth factor (PDGF) AB, hepatocyte growth factor (HGF), insulin-like growth factor 1 (IGF-1), and transforming growth factor (TGF)-β (60,64).

There are several uncontrolled studies evaluating the use of multiple ACS injections for knee and hip OA all showing improvement in WOMAC scores (79–82). Two randomized placebo-controlled studies compared ACS with saline showed statistically significant improvements in KOOS and VAS scores (83,84). Yang et al. reported that ACS provided no greater improvement in WOMAC scores compared with saline and they concluded that because their primary efficacy objective was not met, they could not yet recommend the use of ACS for the treatment of OA (83). They also reported two adverse events, septic arthritis and an inflammatory reaction of the knee joint. Baltzer et al. included a HA group in their randomized controlled trial (RCT) and concluded that the effects of ACS were superior to those of HA and saline for all outcome measures and time points, and improvements were clinically relevant (84). They also reported that the frequency of adverse events was highest in the HA group.

Intra-articular application of ACS has been published as an adjunct to ACL reconstruction. Darabos et al. published level 1 therapeutic RCT study demonstrating that ACS reduced bone tunnel enlargement with four injections after ACL reconstruction (85). They reported that the enlargement in the ACS group at 6 months was 8%, 12 months being 13%; in the saline group at 6 months it was 31%, 12 months being 38%. They noted that WOMAC and IKDC scores were consistently better in patients treated with ACS than saline. Darabos followed up with a study comparing double-bundle anterior cruciate ligament reconstruction with and without ACS; however, the article was retracted at the request of the corresponding author due to inconsistencies in the described method and incorrect reporting of conflicts of interest (86).

ACS use for muscle injuries has been described by Wright-Carpenter et al.'s experimental study in which mice received blunt trauma to their gastrocnemius muscle (87). They divided the study group in half, with one group receiving saline and the other receiving ACS at 2, 24, and 48 hours after the injury. Histology results showed that satellite cell activation at 30 to 48 hours post injury was accelerated and the diameter of the regenerating myofibers was increased compared with the controls within the first week after injury (87). Based on these results

Wright-Carpenter et al. performed a pilot study of 18 athletes (soccer, basketball, ice hockey) with second-degree muscle strains diagnosed by MRI (hamstring, adductor, iliopsoas, gluteus, abdominal oblique, gastrocnemius, rectus femoris) (88). ACS injections started 2 days after the diagnosis and were administered every second day with the mean number of treatments per patient being 5.4. The control group in the study was a retrospective analysis of 11 patients treated with Actovegin®/Traumeel® therapy. The authors reported an average time to recovery of 16.6 ± 0.9 days with follow-up MRI scans taken at 14 to 16 days after injury showing near complete regression of the findings in the first scan concerning edema, bleeding into the muscle, and restitution of the muscle structure. In the control group they reported an average time to recovery of 22.3 ± 1.2 days with follow-up MRI scans taken at 14 to 16 days after injury showing only a mild regression of the findings in the first scan concerning edema and bleeding into the muscle. The authors reported no local or systemic side effects in either group.

Data regarding ACS use in tendon injuries is limited to two in vitro and in vivo studies. Both studies applied ACS to damaged rat Achilles tendons (89,90). Majewski et al. reported that ACS-treated tendons were thicker, with more type I collagen, and demonstrated an accelerated recovery of tendon stiffness and histologic maturity of the repair tissue (89). However, they reported that there were no differences in the maximum load to failure between the ACS and the untreated groups up to week 8. Heisterbach et al. noted that the expression of growth factors basic fibroblastic growth factor (bFGF), bone morphogenetic proteins (BMPs)-12 and TGF-β1 in the ACS-treated tendons was significantly greater than controls but VEGF was not affected (90). Both studies concluded that ACS has the potential to improve Achilles tendon healing.

ACS has been studied as a potential treatment for cervical and lumbar radiculopathy (91,92). Becker et al. published a single center, prospective, double-blind, reference-controlled, investigator-initiated study comparing 32 patients treated with epidural perineural ACS injections to 27 patients treated with 5 mg triamcinolone and 25 patients with 10 mg triamcinolone (91). ACS injections were performed once per week for 3 consecutive weeks and followed for 6 months. The primary outcome measure was the VAS and the Oswestry Disability Index (ODI) was the secondary end point of the study. The authors reported that from week 12 to the final evaluation at week 22, the ACS group had lower VAS scores compared with both triamcinolone groups, but statistical significance was observed only at week 22 in direct comparison with the triamcinolone 5 mg group. They noted that ODI scores were already reduced in all treatment groups at week 6 and, although the ACS group showed a greater reduction in ODI scores at week 10, at the final 6-month evaluation ODI scores were similar in all treatment groups.

Goni et al. published a prospective randomized pilot study on 40 patients with unilateral cervical radiculopathy equally divided into two groups: one receiving 2.5 to 3 mL of ACS and the other receiving 2.5 to 3 mL methylprednisolone both under fluoroscopic guidance into the neural foramen (92). They were followed for 6 months using the VAS for neck pain, neck disability index (NDI), and Short Form of Health Survey-12 (SF-12). They reported that the ACS group showed a 73.24% improvement in VAS scores over the mean baseline VAS at the end of 6 months. The methylprednisolone group showed a 58.54% improvement in VAS scores over baseline at the end of 6 months. They reported a decrease in the NDI in both groups with the percentage decrease in the ACS group being 74.47% compared with 52.80% in the methylprednisolone group. The SF-12 scores were divided into the Physical Health Component Score-12 (PCS-12) and Mental Health Component Score-12 (MCS-12). The mean PCS-12 score increased by 79.45% in the ACS group while the methylprednisolone group showed a 57.32% increase during the same duration of follow-up. In the ACS group, MCS-12 scores improved by 30.09% while the methylprednisolone group increased

by 16.16% at 6-month follow-up. In both groups they reported similar numbers of immediate (syncope, dizziness, sweating, tachycardia) and delayed complications (neck stiffness).

Based on early studies regarding the utility of IRAP in RA, further investigation regarding its ability to treat OA has been a logical outgrowth. However, the studies for both recombinant IRAP and ACS in knee OA are very limited compared with other areas of regenerative medicine. For other orthopedic conditions, both recombinant IRAP and ACS need larger, controlled studies with longer term follow-up. ACS and IRAP both appear safe with potential applications to many other inflammatory conditions.

ALPHA-2 MACROGLOBULIN

The Inflammatory cytokines TNF-α, IL-1b, and IL-6 are major contributors to both intra-articular and extra-articular joint pathologies and pain (93). These cytokines in turn enhance the inflammatory cascade by producing more pro-inflammatory agents, including enzymes of the MMP family. These MMPs target and degrade a wide array of extracellular matrices, which can result in the deterioration of cartilage, bone, tendon, and ligaments (94,95). Furthermore, MMP activity releases catabolic byproducts, which induce the production of more inflammatory cytokines (96–98). A2M is a plasma glycoprotein with a unique ability to inhibit all endoproteases and more specifically matrix MMP (99). Because of this effect, A2M may potentially slow cartilage damage by neutralizing cartilage catabolic enzymes. Wang et al. published their results on an ex vivo study showing that A2M decreased cartilage catabolism by inhibiting the protease activity of ADAMTS-5 and metalloproteinases (99).

The Autologous Protease Inhibitor Concentrate (APIC-CF) System is marketed as a method to concentrate A2M from 45 mL venous blood via centrifugation and ultrafiltration with a tangential flow filter (93). The APIC-CF system received the FDA approval for an Investigational New Drug (IND) Clinical Trial for the treatment of mild to moderate OA in July 2014. There are a few clinical studies investigating the use of A2M. In Wang et al.'s publication they used a rat model of anterior cruciate ligament transection-induced OA and found that supplemental intra-articular injection of A2M reduced the concentration of MMP-13 in synovial fluid, had a favorable effect on OA-related gene expression, and attenuated OA progression (99). Smith et al. published their findings of a specific cartilage degradation product, fibronectin-aggrecan complex (FAC), in the epidural space as a reliable predictor of response to the lumbar epidural steroid injection in patients with radiculopathy (100). Scuderi et al. reported in a poster presentation that patients who are FAC+ within the intervertebral disc are more likely to demonstrate clinical improvement in both VAS and ODI scores following intradiscal autologous A2M injection (101). They suggested that A2M may be an efficacious biologic treatment in discogenic pain and that the FAC may be an important biomarker in patient selection for this treatment. More clinical studies are needed to understand A2M's utility in degenerative and inflammatory orthopedic conditions.

CONCLUSION

The majority of studies investigating the use of amniotic products, IRAP, and A2M are limited to in vitro and animal studies with few human clinical trials. Additional randomized clinical trials including other musculoskeletal pathologies along with larger sample sizes and longer term follow-ups are needed to understand their future potential. Furthermore, most of the trials have compared their efficacy versus corticosteroids and saline rather than other orthobiologics. Corticosteroids have known dose-dependent side effects with risks, including osteoporosis, osteonecrosis, deterioration of articular cartilage and tendon or ligament weakening or rupture leading to minimizing their

chronic usage and in some cases avoiding them altogether. Intra-articular saline injections have been shown to yield a statistically and clinically meaningful improvement in knee OA symptoms for up to 6 months, which exceed a placebo effect (102). Therefore, a more logical comparison would be evaluating these products versus other regenerative medicine techniques, such as HA, platelet-rich plasma, or MSC. Nonetheless, improvements have been made in the production and isolation of these products allowing this research to advance, a great stride forward when compared with the early use of bovine amniotic fluid in the joints of patients described in 1938.

REFERENCES

1. Riboh JC, Saltzman BM, Yanke AB, et al. Human amniotic membrane-derived products in sports medicine: basic science, early results, and potential clinical applications. *Am J Sports Med.* 2016;44(9):2425–2434.

2. Koob TJ, Lim JJ, Zabek N, et al. Cytokines in single layer amnion allografts compared to multilayer amnion/chorion allografts for wound healing. *J Biomed Mater Res Part B Appl Biomater.* 2015;103(5):1133–1140.

3. Yu L. Human amniotic fluid-derived and amniotic membrane-derived stem cells. 2015. http://www.springer.com/978-94-017-7272-3

4. Miki T. Amnion-derived stem cells: in quest of clinical applications. *Stem Cell Res Ther.* 2011;2(3):25. doi:10.1186/scrt66

5. Kmiecik G, Niklinska W, Kuc P, et al. Fetal membranes as a source of stem cells. *Adv Med Sci.* 2013;58(2):185–195.

6. Miki T, Strom SC. Amnion-derived pluripotent/multipotent stem cells. *Stem Cell Rev.* 2006;2(2):133–142.

7. Insausti CL, Blanquer M, García-Hernández AM, et al. Amniotic membrane-derived stem cells: immunomodulatory properties and potential clinical application. *Stem Cells Cloning.* 2014;7: 53–63.

8. Wei JP, Nawata M, Wakitani S, et al. Human amniotic mesenchymal cells differentiate into chondrocytes. *Cloning Stem Cells.* 2009;11(1):19–26.

9. Ilancheran S, Michalska A, Peh G, et al. Stem cells derived from human fetal membranes display multilineage differentiation potential. *Biol Reprod.* 2007;77(3):577–588.

10. Miki T, Lehmann T, Cai H, et al. Stem cell characteristics of amniotic epithelial cells. *Stem Cells.* 2005;23(10):1549–1559.

11. Warner M, Lasyone L. An open-label, single-center, retrospective study of cryopreserved amniotic membrane and umbilical cord tissue as an adjunct for foot and ankle surgery. *Surg Technol Int.* 2014; 25:251–255.

12. Gaafar TM, El Hawary R, Osman A, et al. Comparative characteristics of amniotic membrane, endometrium and ovarian derived mesenchymal stem cells: a role for amniotic membrane in stem cell therapy. *Middle East Fertility Society J.* 2014;19(3): 156–170.

13. Fairbairn NG, Randolph MA, Redmond RW. The clinical applications of human amnion in plastic surgery. *J Plast Reconstr Aesthet Surg.* 2014;67(5): 662–675.

14. Perepelkin NM, Hayward K, Mokoena T, et al. Cryopreserved amniotic membrane as transplant allograft: viability and post-transplant outcome. *Cell Tissue Bank.* 2016;17(1):39–50.

15. Werber B, Martin E. A prospective study of 20 foot and ankle wounds treated with cryopreserved amniotic membrane and fluid allograft. *J Foot Ankle Surg.* 2013;52(5):615–621.

16. Zelen CM, Snyder RJ, Serena TE, et al. The use of human amnion/chorion membrane in the clinical setting for lower extremity repair: a review. *Clin Podiatr Med Surg.* 2015;32(1):135–146.

17. Koob TJ, Rennert R, Zabek N, et al. Biological properties of dehydrated human amnion/chorion composite graft: implications for chronic wound healing. *Int Wound J.* 2013;10(5):493–500.

18. Malhotra C, Jain AK. Human amniotic membrane transplantation: different modalities of its use in ophthalmology. *World J Transplant.* 2014;4(2): 111–121.

19. Wu KH, Zhou B, Mo XM, et al. Therapeutic potential of human umbilical cord-derived stem cells in ischemic diseases. *Transplant Proc.* 2007;39(5): 1620–1622.

20. Zelen CM, Serena TE, Snyder RJ. A prospective, randomised comparative study of weekly versus biweekly application of dehydrated human amnion/chorion membrane allograft in the management of diabetic foot ulcers. *Int Wound J.* 2014;11(2): 122–128.

21. Shimberg M. The use of amniotic-fluid concentrate in orthopaedic conditions. *Journal of Bone and Joint Surgery.* 1938;20(1):167–177.

22. Díaz-Prado S, Rendal-Vázquez ME, Muiños-López E, et al. Potential use of the human amniotic membrane as a scaffold in human articular cartilage repair. *Cell Tissue Bank.* 2010;11(2):183–195.

23. Garcia D, Longo UG, Vaquero J, et al. Amniotic membrane transplant for articular cartilage repair: an experimental study in sheep. *Curr Stem Cell Res Ther.* 2015;10(1):77–83.

24. Kueckelhaus M, Philip J, Kamel RA, et al. Sustained release of amnion-derived cellular cytokine solution facilitates Achilles tendon healing in rats. *Eplasty.* 2014;14:e29. https://www.ncbi.nlm.nih .gov/pmc/articles/PMC4124919

25. Lindenmair A, Nürnberger S, Stadler G, et al. Intact human amniotic membrane differentiated towards the chondrogenic lineage. *Cell Tissue Bank.* 2014;15(2):213–225.

26. Massee M, Chinn K, Lei J, et al. Dehydrated human amnion/chorion membrane regulates stem cell activity *in vitro. J Biomed Mater Res Part B Appl Biomater.* 2016;104(7):1495–1503.

27. Parolini O, Soncini M, Evangelista M, et al. Amniotic membrane and amniotic fluid-derived cells: potential tools for regenerative medicine? *Regen Med.* 2009;4(2):275–291.

28. Jin CZ, Park SR, Choi BH, et al. Human amniotic membrane as a delivery matrix for articular cartilage repair. *Tissue Eng.* 2007;13(4):693–702.

29. Lange-Consiglio A, Rossi D, Tassan S, et al. Conditioned medium from horse amniotic membrane-derived multipotent progenitor cells: immunomodulatory activity *in vitro* and first clinical application in tendon and ligament injuries in vivo. *Stem Cells Dev.* 2013;22(22): 3015–3024.

30. Lange-Consiglio A, Tassan S, Corradetti B, et al. Investigating the efficacy of amnion-derived compared with bone marrow-derived mesenchymal stromal cells in equine tendon and ligament injuries. *Cytotherapy.* 2013;15(8): 1011–1020.

31. Meller D, Pires RT, Tseng SC. Ex vivo preservation and expansion of human limbal epithelial stem cells on amniotic membrane cultures. *Br J Ophthalmol.* 2002;86(4):463–471.

32. Philip J, Hackl F, Canseco JA, et al. Amnion-derived multipotent progenitor cells improve Achilles tendon repair in rats. *Eplasty.* 2013;13:e31. http://www.eplasty.com/index.php?option=com_content&view=article&id=961&catid=186:volume-13-eplasty-2013

33. Coban I, Satoğlu IS, Gültekin A, et al. Effects of human amniotic fluid and membrane in the treatment of Achilles tendon ruptures in locally corticosteroid-induced Achilles tendinosis: An experimental study on rats. *FAS Foot and Ankle Surgery.* 2009;15(1):22–27.

34. Ozbölük S, Ozkan Y, Oztürk A, et al. The effects of human amniotic membrane and periosteal autograft on tendon healing: experimental study in rabbits. *The Journal of Hand Surgery (European Volume).* 2010;35(4):262–268.

35. Demirkan F, Colakoglu N, Herek O, et al. The use of amniotic membrane in flexor tendon repair: an experimental model. *Arch Orthop Trauma Surg.* 2002;122(7):396–399.

36. Ozgenel GY. The effects of a combination of hyaluronic and amniotic membrane on the formation of peritendinous adhesions after flexor tendon surgery in chickens. *J Bone Joint Surg Br.* 2004;86(2):301–307.

37. Zelen CM, Poka A, Andrews J. Prospective, randomized, blinded, comparative study of injectable micronized dehydrated amniotic/chorionic membrane allograft for plantar fasciitis: a feasibility study. *Foot Ankle Int.* 2013;34(10):1332–1339.

38. Hanselman AE, Tidwell JE, Santrock RD. Cryopreserved human amniotic membrane injection for plantar fasciitis: a randomized, controlled, double-blind pilot study. *Foot Ankle Int.* 2015;36(2):151–158.

39. Liu PF, Guo L, Zhao DW, et al. Study of human acellular amniotic membrane loading bone marrow mesenchymal stem cells in repair of articular cartilage defect in rabbits. *Genet Mol Res.* 2014;13(3):7992–8001.

40. Krishnamurithy G, Shilpa PN, Ahmad RE, et al. Human amniotic membrane as a chondrocyte carrier vehicle/substrate: *in vitro* study. *J Biomed Mater Res A.* 2011;99(3):500–506.

41. Nogami M, Tsuno H, Koike C, et al. Isolation and characterization of human amniotic mesenchymal stem cells and their chondrogenic differentiation. *Transplantation.* 2012;93(12):1221–1228.

42. Tan SL, Sulaiman S, Pingguan-Murphy B, et al. Human amnion as a novel cell delivery vehicle for chondrogenic mesenchymal stem cells. *Cell Tissue Bank.* 2011;12(1):59–70.

43. Vines JB, Aliprantis AO, Gomoll AH, et al. Cryopreserved amniotic suspension for the treatment of knee osteoarthritis. *J Knee Surg.* 2016;29(6):443–450.

44. Hillyer CD, Strauss RG, Luban NLC. *Handbook of pediatric transfusion medicine.* San Diego, CA: Elsevier Academic Press; 2004.

45. Roura S, Pujal JM, Gálvez-Montón C, et al. The role and potential of umbilical cord blood in an era of new therapies: a review. *Stem Cell Res Ther.* 2015;6:123. doi:10.1186/s13287-015-0113-2

46. Cany J, Dolstra H, Shah N. Umbilical cord blood-derived cellular products for cancer immunotherapy. *Cytotherapy.* 2015;17(6):739–748.

47. Lee M, Jeong SY, Ha J, et al. Low immunogenicity of allogeneic human umbilical cord blood-derived mesenchymal stem cells *in vitro* and in vivo. *Biochem Biophys Res Commun.* 2014;446(4):983–989.

48. Malgieri A, Kantzari E, Patrizi MP, et al. Bone marrow and umbilical cord blood human mesenchymal stem cells: state of the art. *Int J Clin Exp Med.* 2010;3(4):248–269.

49. Otrock ZK, Beydoun A, Barada WM, et al. Transient global amnesia associated with the infusion of DMSO-cryopreserved autologous peripheral blood stem cells. *Haematologica.* 2008;93(3):e36–e37.

50. Yuan C, Gao J, Guo J, et al. Dimethyl sulfoxide damages mitochondrial integrity and membrane potential in cultured astrocytes. *PLOS ONE.* 2014;9(9):e107447. doi:10.1371/journal.pone.0107447

51. Zambelli A, Poggi G, Da Prada G, et al. Clinical toxicity of cryopreserved circulating progenitor cells infusion. *Anticancer Res.* 1998;18(6B):4705–4708.

52. Ratajczak MZ, Jadczyk T, Pedziwiatr D, et al. New advances in stem cell research: practical implications for regenerative medicine. *Pol Arch Med Wewn.* 2014;124(7-8):417–426.

53. Gordon S, Taylor PR. Monocyte and macrophage heterogeneity. *Nat Rev Immunol.* 2005;5(12):953–964.

54. Utomo L, Bastiaansen-Jenniskens YM, Verhaar JA, et al. Cartilage inflammation and degeneration is enhanced by pro-inflammatory (M1) macrophages *in vitro*, but not inhibited directly by

anti-inflammatory (M2) macrophages. *Osteoarthr Cartil.* 2016;24(12):2162–2170.

55. Huang WC, Sala-Newby GB, Susana A, et al. Classical macrophage activation up-regulates several matrix metalloproteinases through mitogen activated protein kinases and nuclear factor-κB. *PLOS ONE.* 2012;7(8):e42507. doi:10.1371/journal.pone.0042507

56. Laskin DL. Macrophages and inflammatory mediators in chemical toxicity: a battle of forces. *Chem Res Toxicol.* 2009;22(8):1376–1385.

57. Daghestani HN, Pieper CF, Kraus VB. Soluble macrophage biomarkers indicate inflammatory phenotypes in patients with knee osteoarthritis. *Arthritis Rheumatol.* 2015;67(4):956–965.

58. Dinarello CA, Thompson RC. Blocking IL-1: interleukin-1 receptor antagonist *in vivo* and *in vitro*. *Immunol Today.* 1991;12(11):404–410.

59. Zumsteg U, Reimers JI, Pociot F, et al. Differential interleukin-1 receptor antagonism on pancreatic beta and alpha cells. Studies in rodent and human islets and in normal rats. *Diabetologia.* 1993;36(8):759–766.

60. Evans CH, Chevalier X, Wehling P. Autologous-conditioned serum. *Phys Med Rehabil Clin N Am.* 2016;27(4):893–908.

61. Evans CH, Kraus VB, Setton LA. Progress in intra-articular therapy. *Nat Rev Rheumatol.* 2014;10(1):11–22.

62. Fox BA, Stephens MM. Treatment of knee osteoarthritis with orthokine-derived autologous-conditioned serum. *Expert Rev Clin Immunol.* 2010;6(3):335–345.

63. O'Shaughnessey K, Matuska A, Hoeppner J, et al. Autologous protein solution prepared from the blood of osteoarthritic patients contains an enhanced profile of anti-inflammatory cytokines and anabolic growth factors. *J Orthop Res.* 2014;32(10):1349–1355.

64. Wehling P, Moser C, Frisbie D, et al. Autologous-conditioned serum in the treatment of orthopedic diseases: the orthokine therapy. *BioDrugs.* 2007;21(5):323–332.

65. Alvarez-Camino JC, Vázquez-Delgado E, Gay-Escoda C. Use of autologous-conditioned serum (orthokine) for the treatment of the degenerative osteoarthritis of the temporomandibular joint. Review of the literature. *Med Oral Patol Oral Cir Bucal.* 2013;18(3):e433–e438.

66. Frizziero A, Giannotti E, Oliva F, et al. Autologous-conditioned serum for the treatment of osteoarthritis and other possible applications in musculoskeletal disorders. *Br Med Bull.* 2013;105:169–184.

67. Seckinger P, Klein-Nulend J, Alander C, et al. Natural and recombinant human IL-1 receptor antagonists block the effects of IL-1 on bone resorption and prostaglandin production. *J Immunol.* 1990;145(12):4181–4184.

68. Jiang Y, Genant HK, Watt I, et al. A multicenter, double-blind, dose-ranging, randomized, placebo-controlled study of recombinant human interleukin-1 receptor antagonist in patients with rheumatoid arthritis: radiologic progression and correlation of Genant and Larsen scores. *Arthritis Rheum.* 2000;43(5):1001–1009.

69. Chevalier X, Giraudeau B, Conrozier T, et al. Safety study of intra-articular injection of interleukin-1 receptor antagonist in patients with painful knee osteoarthritis: a multicenter study. *J Rheumatol.* 2005;32(7):1317–1323.

70. Chevalier X, Goupille P, Beaulieu AD, et al. Intra-articular injection of anakinra in osteoarthritis of the knee: a multicenter, randomized, double-blind, placebo-controlled study. *Arthritis Rheum.* 2009;61(3):344–352.

71. Brown C, Toth A, Magnussen R. Clinical benefits of intra-articular anakinra for persistent knee effusion. *J Knee Surg.* 2011;24(1):61–65.

72. Kraus VB, Birmingham J, Stabler TV, et al. Effects of intra-articular IL1-Ra for acute anterior cruciate ligament knee injury: a randomized controlled pilot trial (NCT00332254). *Osteoarthr Cartil.* 2012;20(4):271–278.

73. Arend WP. Interleukin-1 receptor antagonist: a new member of the interleukin-1 family. *J Clin Invest.* 1991;88(5):1445–1451.

74. Arend WP, Guthridge CJ. Biological role of interleukin-1 receptor antagonist isoforms. *Ann Rheum Dis.* 2000;59(Suppl 1):i60–i64.

75. Arend WP, Dayer JM. Inhibition of the production and effects of interleukin-1 and tumor necrosis factor alpha in rheumatoid arthritis. *Arthritis Rheum.* 1995;38(2):151–160.

76. Arend WP, Welgus HG, Thompson RC, et al. Biological properties of recombinant human monocyte-derived interleukin-1 receptor antagonist. *J Clin Invest.* 1990;85(5):1694–1697.

77. Gabay C, Smith MF, Eidlen D, et al. Interleukin-1 receptor antagonist (IL-1Ra) is an acute-phase protein. *J Clin Invest.* 1997;99(12):2930–2940.

78. Meijer H, Reinecke J, Becker C, et al. The production of anti-inflammatory cytokines in whole

blood by physico-chemical induction. *Inflamm Res.* 2003;52(10):404–407.

79. Baltzer AW, Ostapczuk MS, Stosch D, et al. A new treatment for hip osteoarthritis: clinical evidence for the efficacy of autologous-conditioned serum. *Orthop Rev (Pavia).* 2013;5(2):59–64.

80. Baltzer AWA, Drever R, Granrath M, et al. Intra-articular treatment of osteoarthritis using autologous interleukine-1 receptor antagonist (IL-1Ra) conditioned serum. *Deutsche Zeitschrift fur Sportmedizin.* 2003;54(6):209–211.

81. Baselga García-Escudero J, Miguel Hernández Trillos P. Treatment of osteoarthritis of the knee with a combination of autologous-conditioned serum and physiotherapy: a two-year observational study. *PLOS ONE.* 2015;10(12):e0145551. doi:10.1371/journal.pone.0145551

82. Fathalla M, Abd-El Motaal F, Abdulkareem O, et al. Low-dose intra-articular autologous conditioned serum in treatment of primary knee osteoarthritis. *Egypt Rheumatol Rehabil Egyptian Rheumatology and Rehabilitation.* 2014;41(3):98–102.

83. Auw Yang KG, Raijmakers NJ, van Arkel ER, et al. Autologous interleukin-1 receptor antagonist improves function and symptoms in osteoarthritis when compared to placebo in a prospective randomized controlled trial. *Osteoarthr Cartil.* 2008;16(4):498–505.

84. Baltzer AW, Moser C, Jansen SA, et al. Autologous-conditioned serum (Orthokine) is an effective treatment for knee osteoarthritis. *Osteoarthr Cartil.* 2009;17(2):152–160.

85. Darabos N, Haspl M, Moser C, et al. Intra-articular application of autologous-conditioned serum (ACS) reduces bone tunnel widening after ACL reconstruction surgery in a randomized controlled trial. *Knee Surg Sports Traumatol Arthrosc.* 2011;19 Suppl 1:S36–S46.

86. Darabos N, Trsek D, Miklic D, et al. RETRACTED ARTICLE: comparison of double-bundle anterior cruciate ligament reconstruction with and without autologous-conditioned serum application. *Knee Surg Sports Traumatol Arthrosc.* 2016;24(10):3377. doi:10.1007/s00167-014-3457-8

87. Wright-Carpenter T, Opolon P, Appell HJ, et al. Treatment of muscle injuries by local administration of autologous-conditioned serum: animal experiments using a muscle contusion model. *Int J Sports Med.* 2004;25(8):582–587.

88. Wright-Carpenter T, Klein P, Schäferhoff P, et al. Treatment of muscle injuries by local administration of autologous-conditioned serum: a pilot study on sportsmen with muscle strains. *Int J Sports Med.* 2004;25(8):588–593.

89. Majewski M, Ochsner PE, Liu F, et al. Accelerated healing of the rat Achilles tendon in response to autologous-conditioned serum. *Am J Sports Med.* 2009;37(11):2117–2125.

90. Heisterbach PE, Todorov A, Flückiger R, et al. Effect of BMP-12, TGF-ß1 and autologous-conditioned serum on growth factor expression in Achilles tendon healing. *Knee Surg Sports Traumatol Arthrosc.* 2012;20(10):1907–1914.

91. Becker C, Heidersdorf S, Drewlo S, et al. Efficacy of epidural perineural injections with autologous-conditioned serum for lumbar radicular compression: an investigator-initiated, prospective, double-blind, reference-controlled study. *Spine.* 2007;32(17):1803–1808.

92. Goni VG, Singh Jhala S, Gopinathan NR, et al. Efficacy of epidural perineural injection of autologous-conditioned serum in unilateral cervical radiculopathy: a pilot study. *Spine.* 2015;40(16):E915–E921.

93. Cuéllar JM, Cuéllar VG, Scuderi GJ. a2-Macroglobulin: autologous protease inhibition technology. *Phys Med Rehabil Clin N Am.* 2016;27(4):909–918.

94. Murphy G, Lee MH. What are the roles of metalloproteinases in cartilage and bone damage? *Ann Rheum Dis.* 2005;64(Suppl 4):iv44–47.

95. Del Buono A, Oliva F, Osti L, et al. Metalloproteases and tendinopathy. *Muscles Ligaments Tendons J.* 2013;3(1):51–57.

96. Miller RE, Lu Y, Tortorella MD, et al. Genetically engineered mouse models reveal the importance of proteases as osteoarthritis drug targets. *Curr Rheumatol Rep.* 2013;15(8):350. https://www.ncbi.nlm.nih.gov/pmc/articles/PMC4062186

97. Homandberg GA, Wen C, Hui F. Cartilage damaging activities of fibronectin fragments derived from cartilage and synovial fluid. *Osteoarthr Cartil.* 1998;6(4):231–244.

98. Tetlow LC, Adlam DJ, Woolley DE. Matrix metalloproteinase and proinflammatory cytokine production by chondrocytes of human osteoarthritic cartilage: associations with degenerative changes. *Arthritis Rheum.* 2001;44(3):585–594.

99. Wang S, Wei X, Zhou J, et al. Identification of a2-macroglobulin as a master inhibitor of cartilage-degrading factors that attenuates the progression of posttraumatic osteoarthritis. *Arthritis Rheumatol.* 2014;66(7):1843–1853.

100. Smith MW, Ith A, Carragee EJ, et al. Does the presence of the fibronectin-aggrecan complex predict outcomes from lumbar discectomy for disc herniation? *The Spine Journal.* doi:10.1016/j.spinee.2013.06.064 [Epub ahead of print].

101. Scuderi GJ, Montesano PX, Cuellar J. Improving response to treatment for patients with ddd with the use of the fibronectin-aggrecan complex. *Medicine & Science in Sports & Exercise.* 2016;48(5S):511–512.

102. Saltzman BM, Leroux T, Meyer MA, et al. The therapeutic effect of intra-articular normal saline injections for knee osteoarthritis. *Am J Sports Med.* 2016. doi:10.1177/363546516680607

CHAPTER 10

SETUP AND PROCEDURES FOR PERFORMING PLATELET-RICH PLASMA INJECTIONS

Robert W. Engelen and José A. Ramírez-Del Toro

Autologous cell therapies such as platelet-rich plasma (PRP) are being increasingly used to treat soft tissue and joint-related conditions. Its use has spanned across various fields of medicine, including dermatology, sports medicine, wound management, oral maxillofacial surgery, and plastic surgery (1). Marx et al. initially demonstrated the use of PRP in the 1990s. They showed improved density of mandibular defects with PRP-enhanced autografts versus autografts alone (2). The use of biologic agents in sports and musculoskeletal medicine has grown dramatically over the past decade (3). Mishra and Pavelko recognized the value of PRP in sports medicine injuries in 2006 with the treatment of chronic lateral elbow tendinosis. In patients with persistent pain for a mean of 15 months despite standardized physical therapy, they noted a 60% improvement in their visual analog pain scores at 8 weeks after PRP injection versus 16% in the control group (4).

PRP is proposed to modulate inflammation and promote repair of tendon, ligament, or joint injuries through the release of powerful growth factors to enhance the body's natural healing response (4). The current concept of tendinopathy as a degenerative process with failure of normal repair rather than an acute inflammatory condition has further supported the use and investigation of PRP as an aid to healing. Unfortunately, most clinical investigations have not used a standardized classification system to describe the various components of the PRP preparation. In this chapter, we discuss the various preparation methods, classification systems, the role of growth factors, and a step-by-step pictorial preparation guide with necessary equipment and personnel.

DEFINITION

PRP is derived by centrifuging autologous blood to separate out different cell types based on their densities to obtain supra-physiologic amount of platelets in a small volume of plasma (5). It results in the formulation of a concentrated plasma layer containing platelets at various concentrations above the baseline blood level. In reference, the normal adult human platelet count ranges from between 150,000 and 350,000/µL (4). The platelet concentration of PRP can vary from 500,000 to 1,500,000 platelets/uL depending on the preparation method (6). Presently, there is no universally defined "ideal" platelet concentration for use in the treatment of musculoskeletal conditions. In addition to the platelet concentration, the inclusion of leukocytes, erythrocytes, type of anticoagulant, and method of activation must be taken into account as these may alter the intended biologic actions (6).

BIOLOGIC HEALING RESPONSE

The normal biologic healing response involves three phases: (a) inflammatory phase, (b) proliferative phase, and (c) the maturation and/or remodeling phase (5,7) (Table 10.1). The inflammatory phase involves hemostasis with clot formation and recruitment of inflammatory mediators. This typically occurs in the initial couple of days after the inciting injury. The clot will contain cells and platelets that will begin to release growth factors. The growth factors will attract macrophages and neutrophils to clean up necrotic debris, such as disorganized collagen matrix via phagocytosis. The proliferative and reparative phase takes place between 2 and 14 days after initial injury. It begins with the formation of an extracellular matrix through collagen deposition and the development of granulation tissue. Lastly, the remodeling phase begins with decreased vascularity, increased type 1 collagen deposition, and reorganization of tissue fibers (5,7).

TABLE 10.1 **Summary of the Healing Process in Tendons and Ligaments**

Time (Days)	Phase	Description
0	Immediately post injury	Clot formation around the wound
0–1	Inflammatory	First battery of growth factors and inflammatory molecules produced by cells within the blood clot
1–2	Inflammatory	Invasion by extrinsic cells, phagocytosis
2–4	Proliferation	Further invasion by extrinsic cells, followed by a second battery of growth factors that stimulate fibroblast proliferation
4–7	Reparative	Collagen deposition; granulation tissue formation; revascularization
7–14	Reparative	Injury site becomes more organized; extracellular matrix is produced in large amounts
14–21	Remodeling	Decreases in cellular and vascular content; increases in collagen type I
21+		Collagen continues to become more organized and cross-linked with healthy matrix outside the injury area. Collagen ratios, water content, and cellularity begin to approach normal levels

Source: Modified from Ref. (7). Molloy T, Wang Y, Murrell G. The roles of growth factors in tendon and ligament healing. *Sports Med*. 2003;33(5):381–394, with permission of Springer.

ROLE OF GROWTH FACTORS

Platelets and the liquid plasma portion of the blood contain many factors that are required for healing. These factors are essential for cell recruitment, multiplication, and specialization. Platelets contain two basic types of granules: alpha granules and dense granules. The dense granules release serotonin, adenosine, dopamine, calcium, and histamine (5). The alpha granules contain many growth factors, including platelet-derived growth factor (PDGF), transforming growth factor-beta (TGF-β), vascular endothelial growth factor (VEGF), epithelial growth factor (EGF), insulin-like growth factor (IGF), and basic fibroblast growth factor (FGF) (8). The growth factors are small peptides that bind to membrane receptors and promote downstream biologic pathways (5). They are released after platelet activation at levels in an attempt to augment the body's natural regenerative process (4). They influence chemotaxis and can induce mitosis, extracellular matrix production, and angiogenesis (5). The anabolic growth factors include IGF-1, PDGF, TGF, VEGF, and FGF. They play an important role in cell proliferation or differentiation in the healing process. Interleukin-1 (IL-1) and metalloproteinases-9 (MMP-9) are catabolic cytokines that play a role in inflammation or matrix degradation (9). Based on in vivo mouse models, Menetrey et al. found that beta-FGF and IGF-1 played a role in myogenesis with improved healing and fast-twitch strength at 1 month in injured mice gastrocnemius muscles (5,10). With regard to cartilage regeneration, TGF, IGF, and PDGF appear to have chondro-inductive effects (5).

PLATELET CONCENTRATION

The "ideal" platelet concentration for various clinical situations remains unknown. Normal platelet counts vary on an individual's blood morphology and can range from 150,000/μL to 350,000/μL (4). Most reporting of platelet concentration is described as "x baseline." Initial clinical studies by Anitua and Sanchez demonstrate effectiveness of PRP at platelet concentrations of 2X to 3X the baseline, with higher concentrations potentially inhibiting tissue healing (11,12). In 2010, Kevy et al. reported an ideal platelet concentration of 1.5 million/μL (5X–7X baseline) with no negative effects up to 3 million/μL (10X baseline) (12,13). However, a recent study by Giusti et al. noted that platelet counts higher than 2 million/uL were inhibitory to tenocyte behavior (14).Thus, the "ideal" platelet concentration may depend on the tissue being treated and the stage of disease process. To better determine the "ideal" concentration, future scientific studies should report on the actual quantity of platelets and specific growth factors being delivered to a specified tissue type.

ROLE OF LEUKOCYTES AND RED BLOOD CELLS

There remains considerable debate as to whether the inclusion of white blood cells (WBCs) in PRP formulations is detrimental to the healing process. WBCs are proposed to be pro-inflammatory resulting in a higher number of neutrophils and a greater release of matrix MMPs, ILs, and other pro-inflammatory mediators. The inclusion of WBCs may be beneficial in certain soft tissue conditions, such as tendinopathy, with neutrophils or macrophages being active in the removal of degenerative tissue or debris through the phagocytosis and the release of hydrolytic enzymes. This may be of value in tendinopathy but detrimental when applied to acute muscle injuries. Both platelets and leukocytes are important in the prevention of infection through an enhanced immune response (6). Braun et al. performed a controlled laboratory study to evaluate the effects of leukocyte-rich PRP (LR-PRP) versus leukocyte-poor PRP (LP-PRP) on human synoviocytes. LR-PRP and erthrocytes were found to be particularly cytotoxic to synviocytes by release of pro-inflammatory cytokines, such as IL-1 and IL-6 (15). Previous studies have indicated that red blood cells (RBCs) have a negative effect on chondrocytes. Hemarthrosis secondary to hemophilia or from a traumatic knee injury has resulted in a higher incidence of knee arthritis (12,16,17). PRP containing RBCs may have deleterious effect on the function of platelets and potentially promote chondrocyte death. Various types of PRP centrifuges and spinning methods are used to produce either LR or LP formulations. Slower and shorter spin regimens focus on intentionally excluding leukocytes. Alternatively, high spin rates and long spin regimens result in higher concentrations of WBCs and RBCs (9,12,15).

CLASSIFICATION SYSTEMS

As discussed previously, there is considerable variability in the blood products that are obtained from the many different PRP-concentrating systems. This variability could lead to altered clinical results. Therefore, two general classification systems have been proposed in an effort to standardize PRP preparations in order to improve clinical literature. The classification systems are the "PAW" and "PLRA" systems.

Delong et al. described the PAW system (Figure 10.1) in 2012 and recommended reporting PRP based on platelet concentration (P), exogenous or endogenous activation (A), and the amount of WBCs and neutrophils (W) relative to baseline (12).

The PLRA system proposed by Mautner et al. (Figure 10.2) in 2015 takes into account the aforementioned factors described in PAW but includes the RBC concentration. PLRA is defined as the absolute number of platelets/μL (P), leukocyte concentration, including neutrophils (L), red blood cell concentration (R), and activation by exogenous agents (A) (4).

PREPARATION METHODS

There is considerable variability in PRP preparation methods. Generally, after a blood sample is obtained from a patient, the specimen is put into a centrifuge to separate cells of varying densities, including platelet-rich plasma, platelet-poor plasma, erthrocytes, and leukocytes. The PRP portion is then collected the same day and

delivered to the injured area of bone or soft tissue, such as a tendon or ligament. PRP is given to patients through an injection preferably under ultrasound guidance to ensure precise placement. After the injection, a patient must avoid exercise for a short period of time before beginning a formal rehabilitation exercise program.

Some of the factors that can vary during PRP preparation include the number of centrifugation cycles, speed of centrifugation, and the duration of the spin. All of these may influence the final product in terms of different cellular types and amounts of bioactive proteins available (8). The two general preparation methods for PRP include plasma-based and buffy coat systems. Plasma-based methods use a slower and shorter spin regimen, which typically exclude more WBCs but generate lower platelet concentrations (300,000–500,000 platelets/μL) (12). Buffy coat systems isolate both a buffy coat and plasma layer. The buffy coat layer contains both leukocytes and erythrocytes. Inclusion of both layers yields higher platelet concentrations (500,000 to 1,500,000 platelets/uL) but also higher numbers of WBCs and RBCs. This method uses high spin rates and long spin regimens (1,12). The two general preparation methods for PRP include plasma-based and buffy coat systems, as detailed as follows.

Plasma-based method (1) (see Figure 10.3):

1. Obtain whole blood (WB) via venipuncture in centrifuge compatible tube containing anticoagulant.

2. Place WB tube in centrifuge (soft spin) with appropriate counterweight to separate out RBCs.

3. Transfer the suspension of plasma containing platelets into another sterile tube.

4. Centrifuge the tube containing the plasma suspension at higher speed to obtain a platelet concentrate.

5. Remove the supernatant containing platelet-poor plasma (PPP) and discard.

6. The remaining precipitate contains the platelet pellet that will be used for injection.

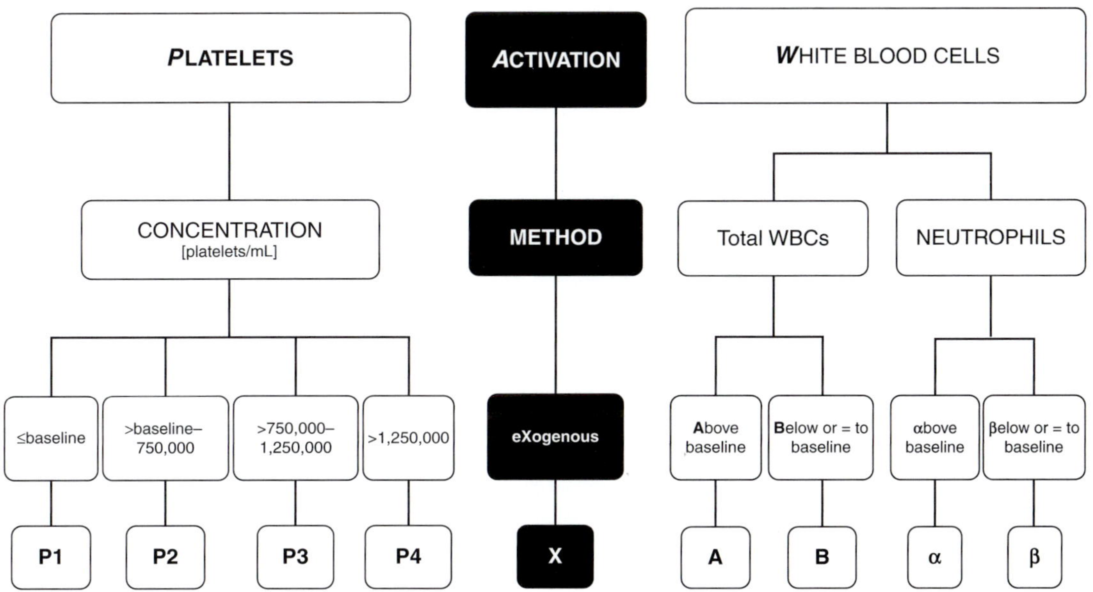

FIGURE 10.1: PAW Classification System developed by Delong et al. (12).

PRP, platelet-rich plasma; WBC, white blood cell.

Source: From Ref. (12). DeLong JM, Russell RP, Mazzocca AD. Platelet-rich plasma: the PAW classification system. *Arthroscopy*. 2012;28(7):998–1009.

PLRA Classification		Criteria	Final Score
P	Platelet count	_______P Volume injected	_______M Cells/µL
L	Leukocyte content*	>1% <1%	+ −
R	Red blood cell content	>1% <1%	+ −
A	Activation†	Yes No	+ −

Table created by Drs Patrick Nguyen and Walter Sussman.
* If white blood cells are present (+), the percentage of neutrophils should also be reported.
† The method of exogenous activation should be reported.

FIGURE 10.2: PLRA classification.

Source: From Ref. (4). Mautner K, Malanga GA, Smith J, et al. A call for a standard classification system for future biologic research: the rationale for new PRP nomenclature. *PM R*. 2015;7(4 Suppl):S53–S59.

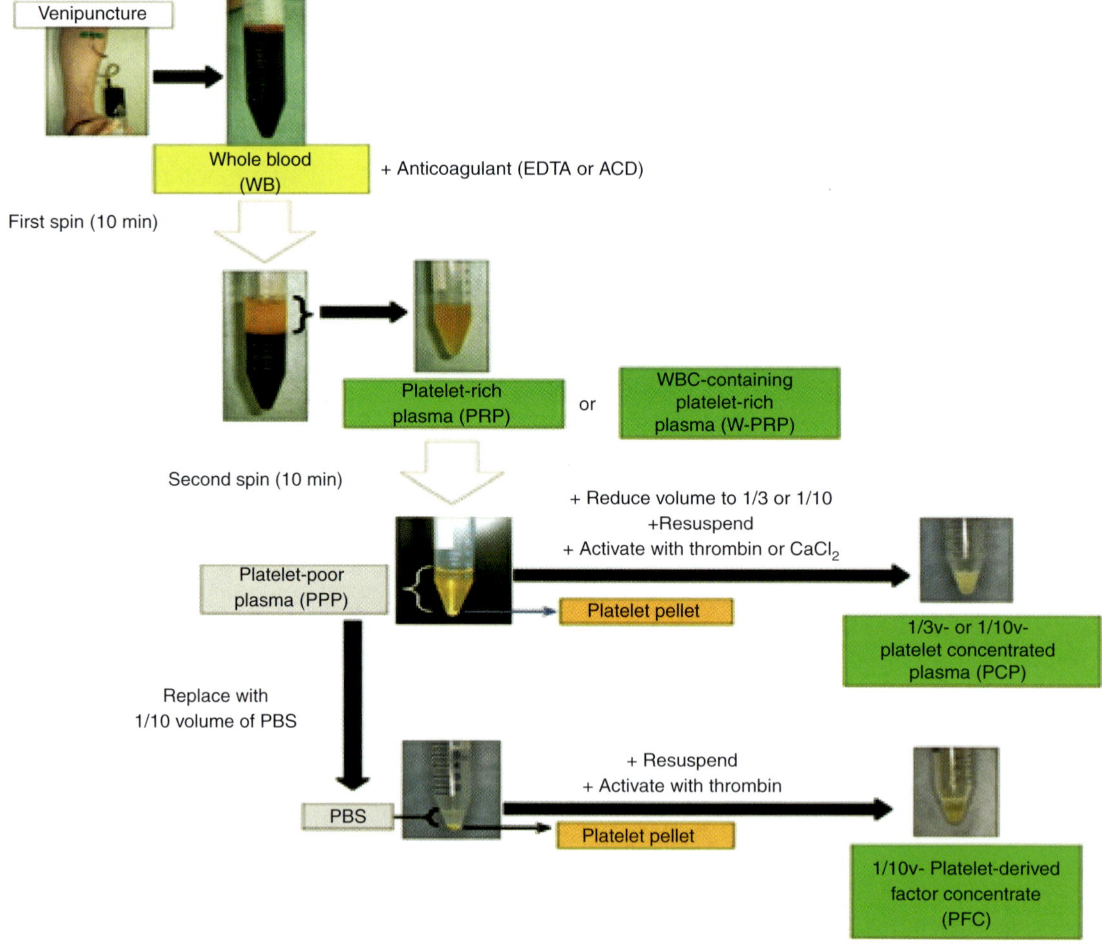

FIGURE 10.3: Flow chart for the preparation process of PRP using the plasma-based method.
PBS, phosphate-buffered saline; PCP, platelet concentrated plasma; PFC, platelet-derived factor concentrate;
PPP, platelet-poor plasma; W-PRP, WBC and plasma-rich plasma.

Source: Adapted from Ref. (18). Araki J , Jona M , Eto H , et al. Optimized preparation method of platelet-concentrated plasma and noncoagulating platelet-derived factor concentrates: maximization of platelet concentration and removal of fibrinogen. *Tissue Eng Part C Methods*. 2012;18(3):176–185.

Buffy coat method (1):

1. Obtain WB via venipuncture and place in a centrifuge compatible tube.

2. Place WB tube in centrifuge with appropriate counterweight for fast spin.

3. The resulting WB tube will contain three layers with the bottom layer consisting of RBCs, middle layer with platelets and WBCs (buffy coat), and the top suspension of PPP.

4. Remove the PPP suspension from the top of the tube and discard.

5. Transfer the buffy coat layer to another sterile tube and centrifuge to separate out the WBCs.

GROWTH FACTORS AND PREPARATION PROTOCOLS

The cell count alone cannot comprehensively identify the quantity and quality of growth factors due to the variability in centrifuge methods. A study by Oh et al. evaluated the differences in cellular composition and biomolecular characteristics of five PRP preparation methods. It included two manual protocols (single-spin [SS] at 900 g for 5 minutes; double-spin [DS] at 900 g for 5 minutes and then 1,500 g for 15 minutes) and three commercial methods (Arthrex ACP, Biomet GPS, and Prodizen Prosys; see Table 10.2 preparation protocols) (9).

Every PRP preparation demonstrated an increase in FGF, VEGF, TGF, and PDGF. The DS PRP had higher concentrations of platelets and leukocytes than SS PRP. PDGF and VEGF concentrations were higher in DS PRP, whereas TGF and FGF concentrations were higher in SS PRP. Arthrex ACP (SS method) had the highest FGF concentration but lowest PDGF concentration. Biomet had the highest VEGF concentration but also highest MMP-9. Prodizen Prosys had the highest IL-1 but also higher PDGF concentration than Arthrex ACP. As noted previously, IL-1 and MMP-9 are thought to play a role in inflammation or matrix degradation and identified as catabolic cytokines. The PDGF and VEGF concentrations correlated with a higher platelet count while the TGF and FGF correlated with a lower platelet count and an SS method (9). Furthermore, research in this area is needed to further specialize the use of PRP by identifying the type of growth factors needed for individual patient conditions.

ANTICOAGULATION

The use of autologous WB requires the addition of an anticoagulant to prevent premature clot formation. Many prefabricated PRP kits will include an anticoagulant solution, such as citrate dextrose (ACD), sodium citrate (SC), or ethylenediaminetetraacetic acid (EDTA). The choice of an anticoagulant solution may alter the normal physiologic tissue pH, platelet count, and growth factor content. A study by Amaral et al. compared the effect of ACD, SC, and EDTA on platelet numbers and growth factor release (19). Blood samples collected with EDTA yielded higher numbers of platelets, followed by SC

TABLE 10.2 **Preparation Protocols and Cellular Compositions of Five Platelet-Rich Plasma Preparations**

Centrifugation				
Preparation	**First Spin**	**Second Spin**	**Isolation**	**Final Vol/WB vol**
SS preparation	900 g, 5 min		Plasma layer	3 mL/30 mL
DS preparation	900 g, 5 min	1,500 g, 15 min	Plasma layer	3 mL/30 mL
Arthrex ACP			Plasma layer	3 mL/15 mL
Bioment GPS			Buffy coat layer	6 mL/54 mL
Prodizen Prosys[a]			Plasma layer	3 mL/30 mL

[a] The first-spin protocol of the Prodizen Prosys samples was subdivided into male and female subjects.

DS, double-spin method; SS, single-spin method; WB, whole blood.

Source: From Ref. (9). Oh JH, Kim W, Park KU, Roh YH. Comparison of the cellular composition and cytokine-release kinetics of various platelet-rich plasma preparations. *Am J Sports Med*. 2015;43(12):3062–3070.

and ACD. Although, SC samples produced the highest average platelet recovery at 81% in comparison to EDTA (76%) and ACD (45%). Interestingly, PRP prepared with ACD had the highest VEGF concentration. PRP prepared with SC had the highest TGF release and the preparations with EDTA had the lowest overall growth factor release. It is notable to mention that the only growth factors quantified were VEGF and TGF (18).

PLATELET ACTIVATION

Platelet activation may occur exogenously or endogenously. The issue of using exogenous activation is controversial and is not used by all clinicians. The types of exogenous activators include calcium chloride or thrombin. They are reported to result in a prompt release of 70% to 95% of the growth factors in 10 minutes (5,6,20). In addition, PRP combined with calcium or thrombin can produce gels or fibrin matrices that can serve as scaffolds (5). Endogenous activation may occur through mechanical trauma and subsequent release of collagen. Collagen is a natural activator of platelets (1,6). Employing un-activated PRP is thought to result in a physiologic manner with activation through exposure to the local biologic tissue (6).

PREPROCEDURE INSTRUCTIONS

A set of instructions should be provided to patients before the procedure day to ensure adequate preparation and understanding of the procedure. A standard consent form detailing the risks and potential complications should be reviewed and discussed with the patient before the procedure. As with all procedures, the patient's understanding of the procedure will assist with alleviating any undue anxiety pre- or postprocedure.

Nonsteroidal anti-inflammatory drugs (NSAIDs) should be discontinued 2 weeks before

the procedure and not used for 4 weeks after, as they may negatively influence platelet function. NSAIDs inhibit the prostaglandin pathway and may reduce the beneficial effects stimulated by the release of growth factors. In a single-center pilot study by Schippinger et al., the in vivo effect of NSAIDs on platelet function in autologous PRP was investigated. The NSAID study group demonstrated a massive inhibition of platelet aggregation in comparison to the control groups (21).

Patients who require anticoagulation for other medical issues can safely undergo PRP injections without the need for discontinuation of these medications. It is prudent to obtain an International Normalized Ratio (INR) to ensure the patient's levels are within therapeutic ranges and not supra-therapeutic. The smallest effective needle gauge should be used in these patients to prevent tissue damage and resultant bleeding.

EQUIPMENT AND PERSONNEL

There are many commercially marketed PRP systems that facilitate the application of platelet-rich suspensions. All operate on a small volume of drawn blood (20–60 mL) and various centrifuge spin protocols. As discussed previously, the systems differ in their ability to collect and concentrate platelets (1). The PRP kits are disposable units used for individual procedures and can include sterile centrifuge containers, blood draw kits, anticoagulant solution (sodium citrate), and a number of syringes. The cost of a PRP kit may range from $100 to $400 depending on the company, centrifuge system, and size of the kit. Presently, treatment with PRP is not covered by insurance plans (5).

In preparation for the procedure, the practitioner needs to ensure several items are available including (Figures 10.4 and 10.5):

1. Commercial PRP kit (as described earlier)

2. Sterile gloves

3. Anticoagulant, such as sodium citrate (Figure 10.6)

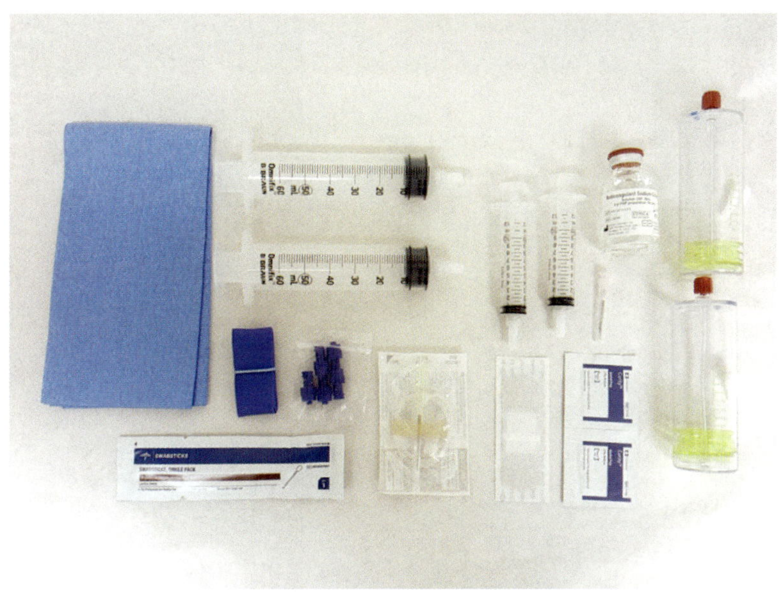

FIGURE 10.4: Necessary equipment and supplies for Exactech PRP system.

PRP, platelet-rich plasma.

Source: Image courtesy of Exactech, Inc.

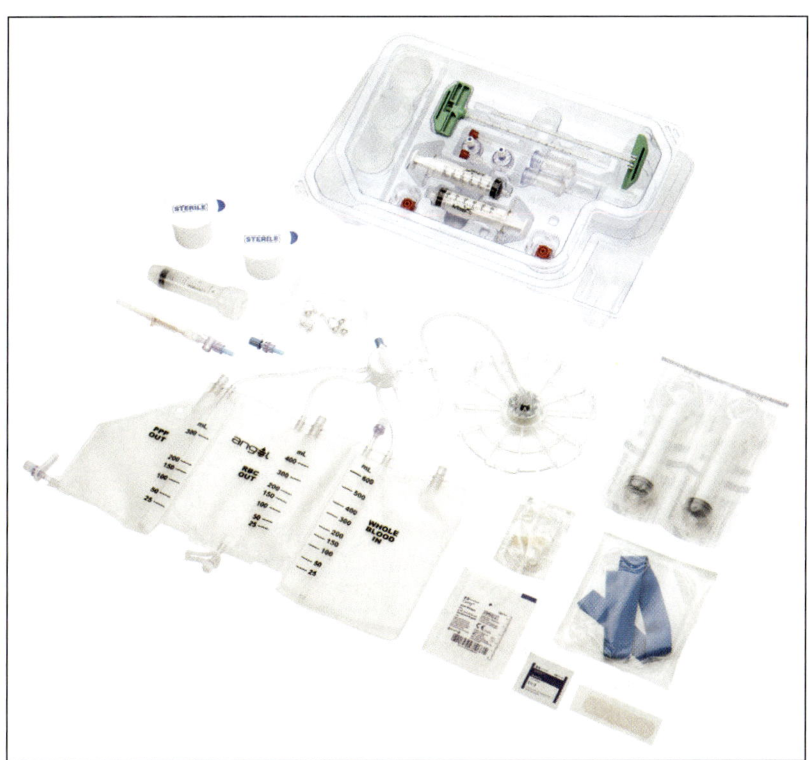

FIGURE 10.5: Supplies for Arthrex Angel PRP system.

PRP, platelet-rich plasma.

Source: Image courtesy of Arthrex, Inc.

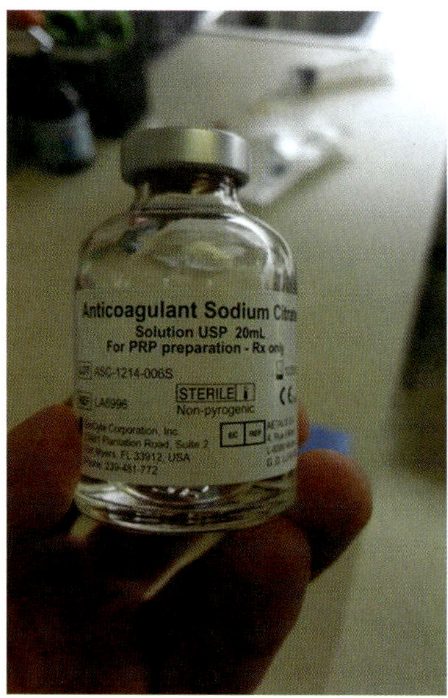

FIGURE 10.6: Anticoagulant—sodium citrate.

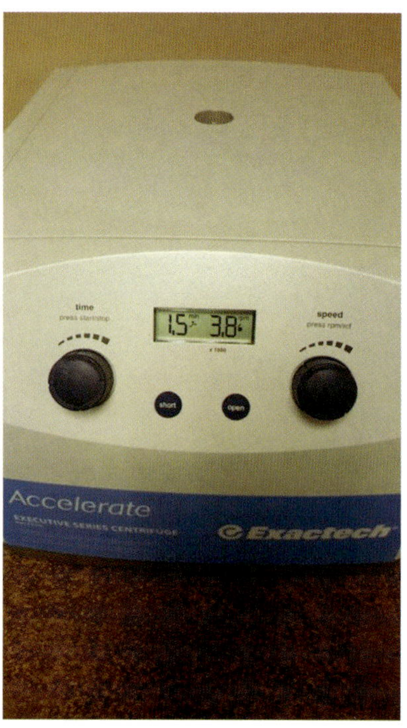

FIGURE 10.7: Centrifuge with controls for adjustment of duration (min) or speed (rpm).
Source: Image courtesy of Exactech, Inc.

4. Alcohol pad for venipuncture skin preparation

5. Tourniquet

6. Winged infusion set (butterfly needle with tubing)

7. 60 mL syringe for blood collection during venipuncture

8. Betadine or chlorhexadine for skin prep

9. Sterile drape

10. 18 to 22 gauge needles of 1 ½ to 3 ½ inches in length for PRP infusion (length dependent on tissue depth)

11. Centrifuge (Figures 10.7 and 10.8)

12. Blood pressure/pulse ox monitor (not pictured)

13. Ultrasound machine or C-arm (not pictured, procedure dependent)

In addition to the physician performing the procedure, other appropriate personnel should include nurse or medical assistant and radiology technician (if fluoroscopy is used). Ultrasound guidance has been recommended for the majority of tendon ligament and joint injections.

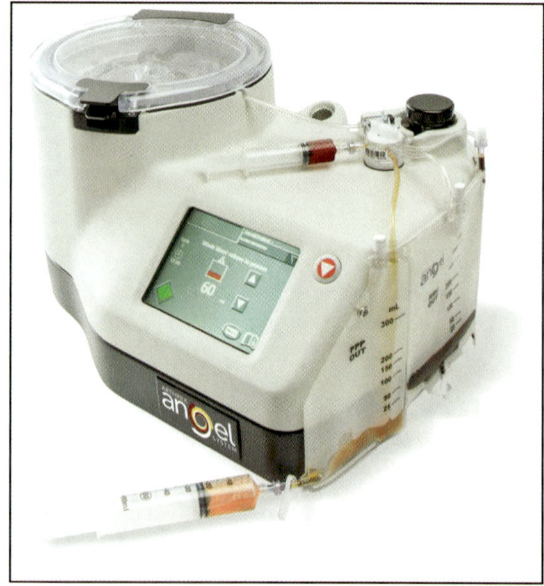

FIGURE 10.8: Arthrex Angel PRP centrifuge.

PRP, platelet-rich plasma.

Source: Image courtesy of Arthrex, Inc.

PROCEDURE DETAILS

Using standard exposure precautions, PRP is obtained from a sample of the patient's WB drawn at the time of treatment (Figure 10.9). A venous blood draw of 60 mL is performed and collected into a syringe filled with an anticoagulant solution, such as sodium citrate (Figure 10.6) to prevent clotting and platelet activation. Citrate may be used to inhibit the clotting cascade by binding ionized calcium. The preparation of PRP uses differential centrifugation relying on acceleration forces to separate out the previously described cellular constituents based on their individual specific gravities. Depending on the type of PRP kit, the collected WB will be transferred into a centrifuge-specific container (Figure 10.10). In some instances, the PRP kits may involve drawing the WB immediately into a centrifuge-specific container. Another centrifuge-specific container will then be filled with an equal amount of normal saline to be used as a counterweight (Figure 10.11). Place both containers in the centrifuge for a set spin time and speed depending on the chosen PRP system (Figure 10.12). After completion of the first spin, withdraw the suspension of plasma containing platelets into another sterile tube (Figure 10.13) and transfer it into another sterile centrifuge compatible tube (Figure 10.14). For a PRP system using a double spin method, centrifuge the tube containing the plasma suspension at a higher speed to obtain a platelet concentrate (Figure 10.15). After completion of the second spin, withdraw the supernatant containing PPP and discard (Figure 10.16). Finally, the remaining precipitate contains the platelet concentrate that will be withdrawn into another sterile syringe and used for injection (Figure 10.17).

INJECTION SETUP

After preparation of the PRP, the area of injection should be prepped and draped using a clean technique as to prevent contamination and reduce the potential for infection (Figure 10.18). The practitioner and any assistants should use universal contact precautions by wearing non-porous protective items, including gloves, face

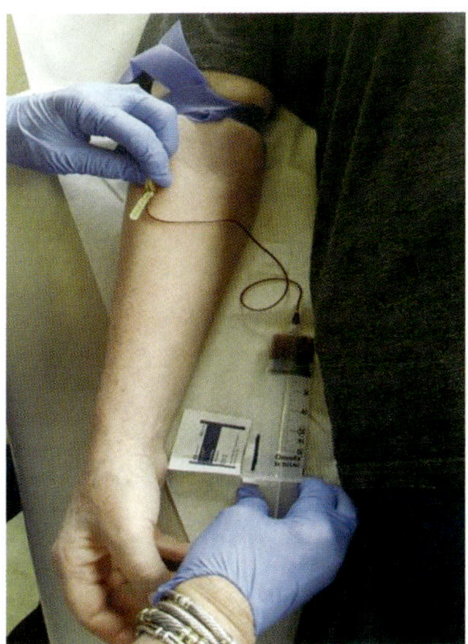

FIGURE 10.9: Obtain WB via venipuncture in a syringe containing anticoagulant.

WB, whole blood.

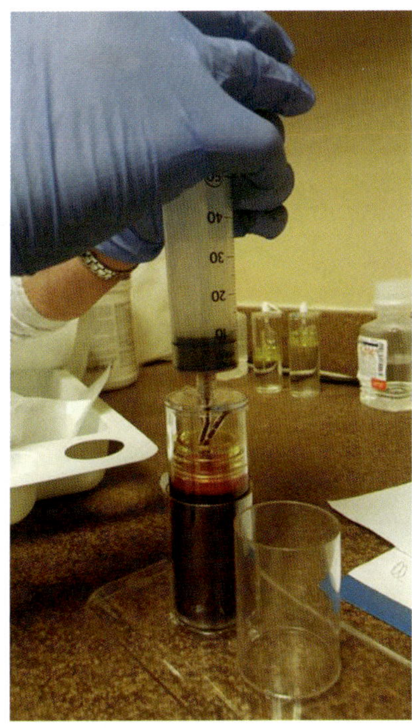

FIGURE 10.10: Transfer the WB into a sterile centrifuge compatible tube.

WB, whole blood.

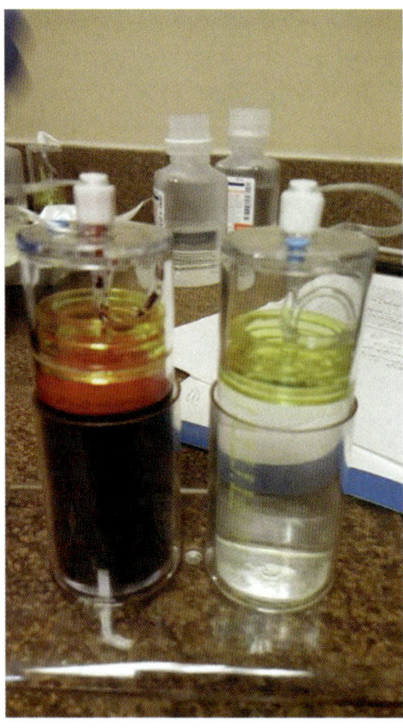

FIGURE 10.11: Fill another centrifuge compatible container with equivalent amount of sterile saline for use as a counterweight.

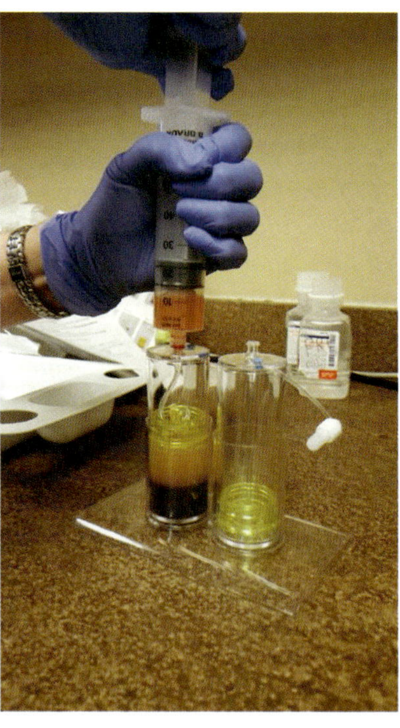

FIGURE 10.13: Withdraw the suspension of plasma containing platelets into another sterile tube.

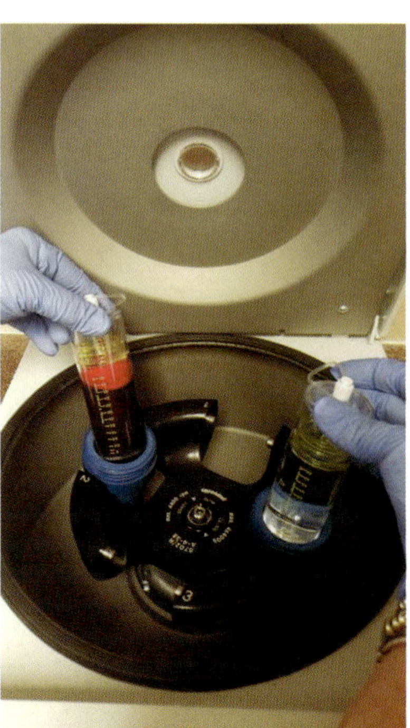

FIGURE 10.12: Place WB tube in centrifuge (soft spin) with appropriate counterweight to separate out RBCs.

RBCs, red blood cells; WB, whole blood.

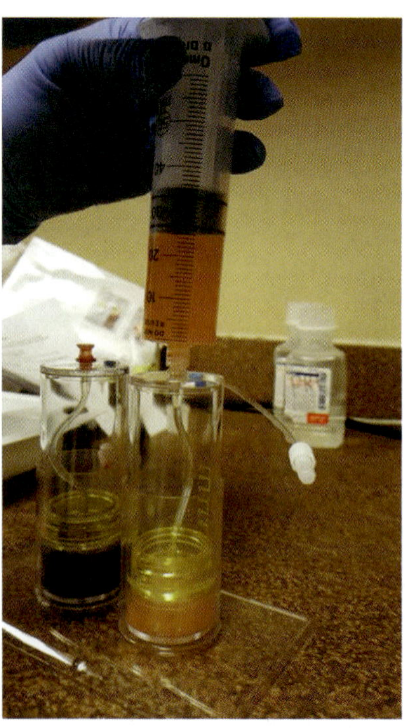

FIGURE 10.14: Transfer the suspension of plasma containing platelets into another sterile centrifuge compatible tube.

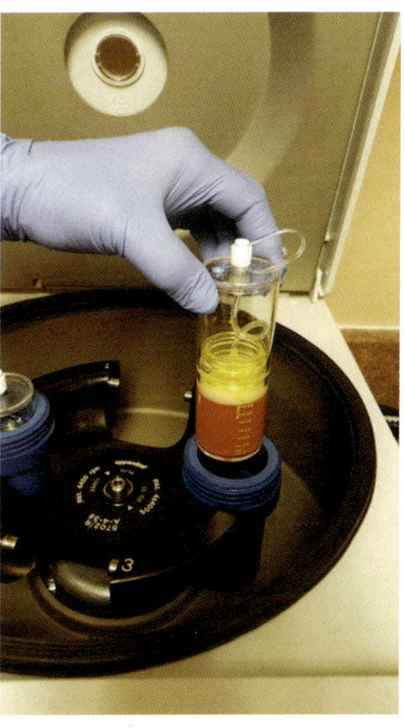

FIGURE 10.15: Centrifuge the tube containing the plasma suspension at a higher speed to obtain a platelet concentrate.

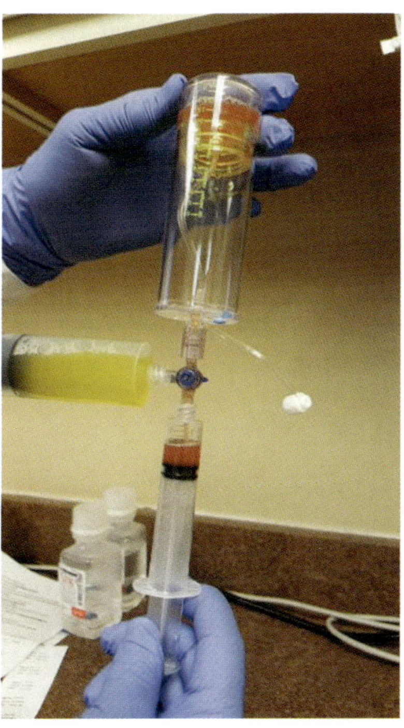

FIGURE 10.17: The remaining precipitate contains the platelet concentrate that will be used for injection.

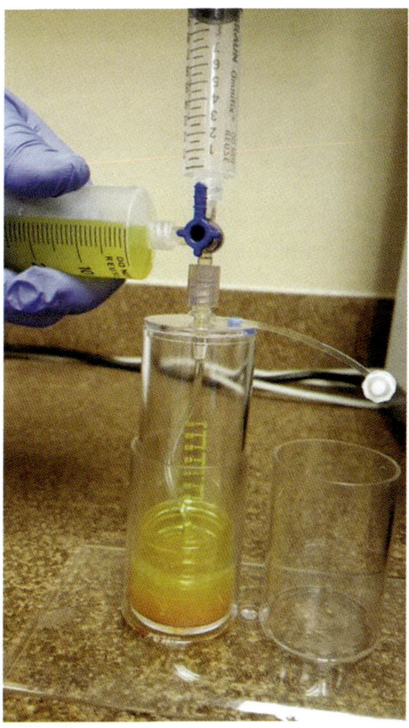

FIGURE 10.16: Withdraw the supernatant containing platelet-poor plasma (PPP) and discard.

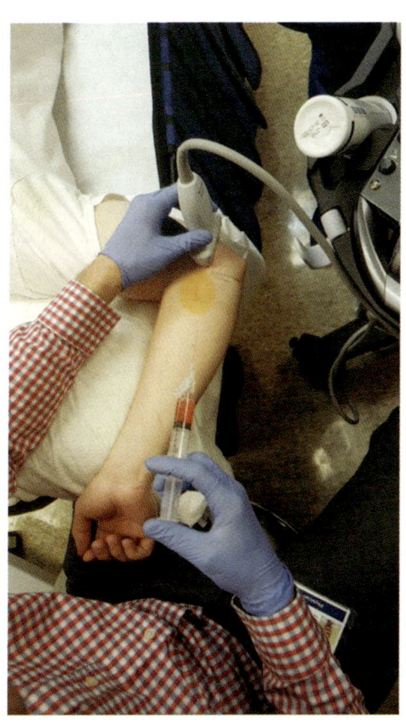

FIGURE 10.18: Injection setup.

mask, and goggles or face shield. Needle selection should be based on tissue depth to ensure adequate localization of the target tissue. If ultrasound guidance is used, it should be set up at the eye level and perpendicular to the practitioner as to avoid neck strain for the practitioner. If fluoroscopy is used, the practitioner and any assistants should wear leaded aprons, thyroid shields, and goggles to minimize radiation exposure.

IMAGING

A growing body of literature supports the use of ultrasound guidance. The therapeutic outcome is dependent on injection accuracy (22). The use of musculoskeletal ultrasound has enhanced the utility of PRP by allowing clinicians to effectively visualize the intended joint, tendon, or ligament. Eustace et al. showed that only 29% of palpation-guided injections for subacromial bursitis were actually placed in the intended bursa (23). Patel et al. compared the accuracy of palpation-guided versus ultrasound-guided glenohumeral injections using a posterior approach. The accuracy rate in 40 shoulders was 73% for palpation-guided injections and 93% for ultrasound-guided injections (24).

POSTINJECTION INSTRUCTIONS

There is no current evidence-based PRP postinjection protocol. Protocols are typically based on the injecting practitioner's preferences and the type of injury being treated. The University of Wisconsin Sports Medicine Department recently published online rehabilitation guidelines that seem to be comprehensive and well researched, but as stated earlier, no true evidence-based PRP postprocedure protocol currently exists (25).

Following is an example of general guidelines used in a private practice setting: Expect significant pain for 3 to 5 days. You may also experience redness and swelling in the treated area. Icing should consist of 10 to 15 minutes at a time,

approximately two to three times per day. Avoid excessive icing to prevent frostbite and allow for the intended inflammatory effect of PRP. Do not use any anti-inflammatory drugs (NSAIDs), such as Aleve, ibuprofen, Aspirin, Motrin, Excedrin for 2 weeks postinjection. You may then use acetaminophen or prescription pain medication as an acceptable alternative to NSAIDs. A more detailed postprocedure protocol is described in a separate chapter.

POST-PRP: REHABILITATION

Rehabilitation protocols after PRP procedures have not been well outlined in the literature. Verchenko and Aspenberg have shown that loading of a tendon after injection of PRP improves biomechanical properties in an acute injury model (26). The rehabilitation protocol should be customized to the athlete. Several factors should be considered, including severity of injury, location, sport, and competition phase. The different rehabilitation phases and sport-specific protocols are detailed later in the book, in the chapter on consideration for physical therapy in Chapter 13.

CONCLUSION

The use of biologic agents in sports and musculoskeletal medicine has grown dramatically over the past decade (2). Presently, there is no universally defined "ideal" platelet concentration for use in the treatment of musculoskeletal conditions. In addition to the platelet concentration, the inclusion of leukocytes, erythrocytes, type of anticoagulant, and method of activation must be taken into account as these may alter the intended biologic actions (6). Future studies on the application of PRP should include a description of the biomolecular characteristics including number and type of growth factors used (9). Unfortunately, most clinical investigations have not used a standardized classification system to describe the various components of the PRP preparation. Two general classification systems have been proposed in an effort to standardize PRP preparations in order to improve clinical literature. The classification systems are the "PAW" and "PLRA" systems (4,12). Concentration and content of bioactive factors present in PRP depend on the preparation and activation method and should be individually adapted to the respective application (8). These procedures should be performed by clinicians with a knowledge base of the various parameters that can affect the final PRP product. They should perform the actual injection using appropriate guidance to ensure proper placement to the targeted pathologic tissues. The post-PRP rehabilitation should be based on the knowledge of tissue healing time frames and rehabilitation principles. Finally, the clinician should consider measuring platelets before and after processing WB to determine the true concentration and the actual "dose," that is, platelet numbers that are being injected. There are many different types and brands of PRP systems on the market that are not depicted in this chapter. Each system uses their own unique method of PRP preparation; please follow brand-specific directions accordingly.

REFERENCES

1. Dhurat R, Sukesh M. Principles and methods of preparation of platelet-rich plasma: a review and author's perspective. *J Cutan Aesthet Surg*. 2014;7(4):189–197.
2. Marx RE, Carlson ER, Eichstaedt RM, et al. Platelet-rich plasma: Growth factor enhancement for bone grafts. *Oral Surg Oral Med Oral Pathol Oral Radiol Endod*. 1998;85(6):638–646.
3. Mishra A, Pavelko T. Treatment of chronic elbow tendinosis with buffered platelet-rich plasma. *Am J Sports Med*. 2006;34(11):1774–1778.
4. Mautner K, Malanga GA, Smith J, et al. A call for a standard classification system for future biologic research: the rationale for new PRP nomenclature. *PM R*. 2015;7(4 Suppl):S53–S59.
5. Nguyen RT, Borg-Stein J, McInnis K. Applications of platelet-rich plasma in musculoskeletal and sports medicine: an evidence-based approach. *PMR*. 2011;3(3):226–250.
6. Mishra A, Harmon K, Woodall J, et al. Sports medicine applications of platelet-rich plasma. *Curr Pharm Biotechnol*. 2012;13(7):1185–1195.
7. Molloy T, Wang Y, Murrell G. The roles of growth factors in tendon and ligament healing. *Sports Med*. 2003;33(5):381–394.
8. Krüger JP, Freymannx U, Vetterlein S, et al. Bioactive factors in platelet-rich plasma obtained by apheresis. *Transfus Med Hemother*. 2013;40(6):432–440.
9. Oh JH, Kim W, Park KU, et al. Comparison of the cellular composition and cytokine-release kinetics of various platelet-rich plasma preparations. *Am J Sports Med*. 2015;43(12):3062–3070.
10. Menetrey J, Kasemkijwattana C, Day CS, et al. Growth factors improve muscle healing in vivo. *J Bone Joint Surg Br*. 2000;82(1):131–137.
11. Sánchez M, Anitua E, Azofra J, et al. Comparison of surgically repaired Achilles tendon tears using platelet-rich fibrin matrices. *Am J Sports Med*. 2007;35(2):245–251.
12. DeLong JM, Russell RP, Mazzocca AD. Platelet-rich plasma: the PAW classification system. *Arthroscopy*. 2012;28(7):998–1009.
13. Kevy S, Jacobson M, Mandle R. Defining the composition and healing effect of platelet-rich plasma. Presented at the Platelet-Rich Plasma Symposium, New York, NY, August 5, 2010.
14. Giusti I, Rughetti A, D'Ascenzo S, et al. Identification of an optimal concentration of platelet gel for promoting angiogenesis in human endothelial cells. *Transfusion*. 2009;49(4):771–778.
15. Braun HJ, Kim HJ, Chu CR, et al. The effect of platelet-rich plasma formulations and blood products on human synoviocytes: implications for intra-articular injury and therapy. *Am J Sports Med*. 2014;42(5):1204–1210.
16. Hooiveld M, Roosendaal G, Wenting M, et al. Short-term exposure of cartilage to blood results in chondrocyte apoptosis. *Am J Pathol*. 2003;162(3):943–951.
17. Roosendaal G, Vianen ME, Marx JJ, et al. Blood-induced joint damage: a human *in vitro* study. *Arthritis Rheum*. 1999;42(5):1025–1032.
18. Araki J, Jona M, Eto H, et al. Optimized preparation method of platelet-concentrated plasma and noncoagulating platelet-derived factor concentrates: maximization of platelet concentration and removal of fibrinogen. *Tissue Eng Part C Methods*. 2012;18(3):176–185.
19. Amaral R, Silva N, Haddad N, et al. Platelet-rich plasma obtained with different anticoagulants

and their effect on platelet numbers and mesenchymal stromal cells behavior in vitro. *Stem Cells Int.* 2016; 1–11.

20. Liao H, Marra K, Rubin P. Application of platelet-rich plasma and platelet-rich fibrin in fat grafting: basic science and literature review. *Tissue Engineering.* 2014;20(4):267–276.

21. Schippinger G, Pruller F, Divjak M, et al. Autologous platelet-rich plasma preparation: influence of nonsteroidal anti-inflammatory drugs on platelet function. *Orthop J Sports Med.* 2015;3(6). doi:10.1177/2325967115588896

22. Curtiss HM, Finnoff JT, Peck E, et al. Accuracy of ultrasound-guided and palpation-guided knee injections by an experienced and less-experienced injector using a superolateral approach: a cadaveric study. *PM R.* 2011;3(6):507–515.

23. Eustace JA, Brophy DP, Gibney RP, et al. Comparison of the accuracy of steroid placement with clinical outcome in patients with shoulder symptoms. *Ann Rheum Dis.* 1997;56(1):59–63.

24. Patel DN, Nayyar S, Hasan S, et al. Comparison of ultrasound-guided versus blind glenohumeral injections: a cadaveric study. *J Shoulder Elbow Surg.* 2012;21(12):1664–1668.

25. Krogman K, Sherry M, Wilson J. "Platelet-Rich Plasma Rehabilitation Guidelines." University of Wisconsin Health Sports Rehabilitation. 2014. http://www.uwsportsmedicine.org

26. Virchenko O, Aspenberg P. How can one platelet injection after tendon injury lead to a stronger tendon after 4 weeks? Interplay between early regeneration and mechanical stimulation. *Acta Orthop.* 2006;77(5):806–812.

CHAPTER 11

BASIC SCIENCE AND RATIONALE FOR USING STEM CELLS FOR ORTHOPEDIC CONDITIONS

Christopher J. Williams, Walter I. Sussman, and Kenneth R. Mautner

DEFINING MESENCHYMAL STEM CELLS

Mesenchymal stem cells (MSCs) were first characterized in the literature in the 1950s and were later isolated by Friedenstein et al. in 1970 (1–3). In his pivotal study, Friedenstein originally described nonphagocytic, nonhematopoietic, fibroblastic-like cells isolated from the bone marrow of rats, which were plastic adherent and displayed multipotency. These cells were isolated in small numbers in culture and could differentiate in vitro into bone, cartilage, adipose tissue, tendon, muscle, and fibrous tissue. Since the initial identification of these cells, numerous names have been suggested for them. Caplan proposed the term "mesenchymal stem cells" for universal identification in 1991, and although there has been continued debate over the naming of these cells (4,5), the term MSC is still the most widely used and recognized nomenclature. Given the increasingly apparent roles these cells play in signaling, Caplan has recently proposed a new definition for MSC: medicinal signaling cell (6). The signaling properties include the secretion of immunomodulatory and trophic factors after an injury, which are explored in further detail later in this chapter.

MINIMAL CRITERIA AND SURFACE MARKERS

The Mesenchymal and Tissue Stem Cell Committee of the International Society for Cellular Therapy (ISCT) has proposed minimal criteria that cells must exhibit to be defined as MSCs (7). These criteria include: (a) polysterene (i.e., plastic) adherence with spindle-shaped morphology in laboratory culture; (b) the capacity to differentiate into at least osteoblasts, adipocytes, and chondroblasts in vitro; and (c) expression of a characteristic set of nonspecific surface markers CD73, CD90, and CD105, and a lack of expression of CD34, CD45, CD11b, CD14, CD19, CD79a, and HLA-DR (Table 11.1) (7–9).

TABLE 11.1 ISCT Minimal Criteria of MSCs

Positive Surface Markers	Differentiation Potential	Special Characteristics
CD73[+]	Osteogenic	Adherence to plastic
CD90[+]	Chondrogenic	Spindle-shaped morphology
CD105[+]	Adipogenic	
Negative surface markers		
CD34[−]		
CD45[−]		
CD11b[−]		
CD14[−]		
CD19[−]		
CD79a[−]		
HLA-DR[−]		

ISCT, International Society for Cellular Therapy; MSCs, mesenchymal stem cells.

Pericyte Origins

Additional functions of MSCs include supporting hematopoiesis and the secretion of immunomodulatory factors (10). It is widely accepted that MSCs exist in almost every tissue and share some properties distinct from their tissue of origin. Studies have shown that MSC-like precursor cells exist in all vascularized tissue, with two distinct perivascular populations: microvascular pericytes and adventitial cells (11–13). These cells have been termed "perivascular stem cells" (PSCs) and provide a rich supply of progenitor cells that respond swiftly to injury (10,14,15,171). Once released from the vessel wall, PSCs function as MSCs via immunomodulatory and trophic effects, hematopoiesis regulation, and tissue regeneration through multipotency and signaling (Figure 11.1) (10).

Differentiation and Basic Properties

MSCs display mesodermal trilineage differentiation into osteoblasts, chondrocytes, and adipocytes in vitro (16–20). However, more recent studies have also shown that under certain culture conditions, MSCs can differentiate into other mesodermal tissues (e.g., skeletal muscle, tendon, myocardium, smooth muscle, and endothelium) and also possess the ability to differentiate into other germinal lines of endodermic (e.g., epithelial cells) and ectodermic (e.g., neurons) origin (21–29). It should be noted that in vitro differentiation does not equate to in vivo function. In vivo studies supporting differentiation of MSCs are still lacking, and controversy exists whether the therapeutic effects are exerted through differentiation or trophic effects (i.e., the secretion of cytokines and growth factors) (30–32,180).

SOURCES OF MSCs

MSCs have been identified throughout the body (6), including adipose tissue, umbilical cord tissue (i.e., Wharton's jelly), tendons, epithelium, synovium, peripheral blood, muscle, and periosteum (Figure 11.2) (33–43). The optimal harvesting tissue for MSCs remains unclear, but the ideal source of MSCs would be autologous, easy to collect, have low associated morbidity, not require culturing, be readily available in therapeutic concentration, and meet ISCT minimal criteria for MSCs (Figure 11.3) (10,44–52).

In clinical practice, MSCs can be obtained from an autologous or allogenic source. Autologous cells are derived from and injected back into the same patient, while allogenic cells are collected from a donor(s) and injected into another person. Some of the drawbacks of autologous cells include the collection process and a decreasing differentiation potential with age (53,54). Allogenic cells have the advantage of being able to be mass produced, yielding a product ready to be used "off the shelf." However, allogenic cells may allow the transmission of pathologic genetic material and/or

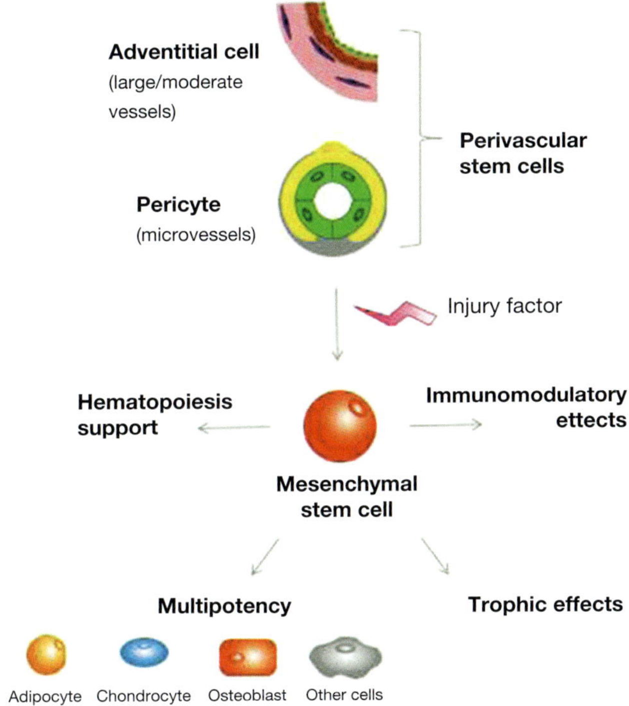

FIGURE 11.1: Diagram showing pericytes and adventitial cells in homeostasis, and in response to injury there is release of the PSCs from the peripheral vasculature. Migration and activation into MSCs occur in response to injury. MSCs are thought to contribute to healing primarily via immunomodulatory effects, trophic effects, and their multipotency.

MSCs, mesenchymal stem cells; PSCs, perivascular stem cells.

Source: Adapted from Refs. (7,10–14).

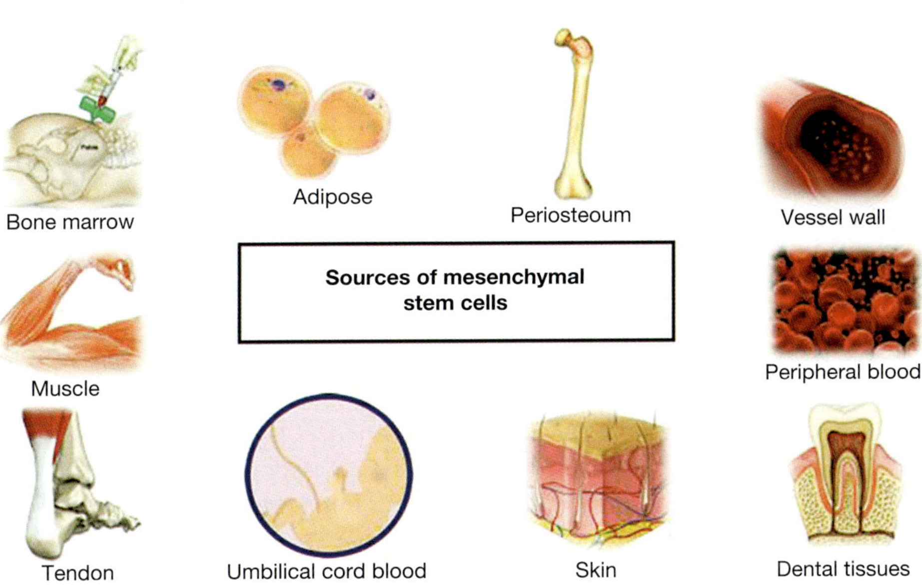

FIGURE 11.2: Common sources of mesenchymal stem cells.

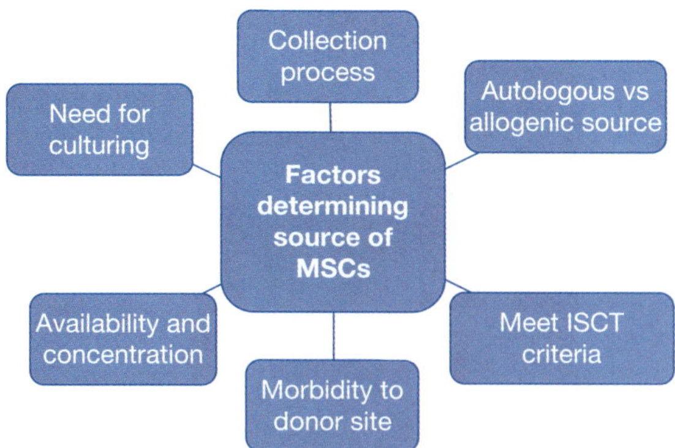

FIGURE 11.3: The ideal source of MSCs for therapeutic application would be autologous, easy to collect, have minimal procedure-associated morbidity, be readily available at a therapeutic concentration and not require culturing, and meet ISCT minimal criteria for MSCs.

ISCT, International Society for Cellular Therapy; MSCs, mesenchymal stem cells.

infectious diseases. Also, unlike autologous MSCs, they may lack their immunoprivilege properties and therefore have the potential to be recognized as a foreign tissue by the recipient immune system against the donor cells (55,56).

As bone marrow aspirate (BMA) was the first source of MSCs identified, it has been the most widely studied source for MSCs, especially in regard to orthopedic conditions. Several studies have shown that the nucleated cells collected from BMA yield only a small fraction of MSCs, approximately 0.001% to 0.02% (47,57). MSCs from BMA also exhibit a precipitous decline in yield as persons age (Figure 11.4) (50, 58–63). Although relatively safe, BMA has been perceived to have greater morbidity (i.e., donor site pain, bleeding, and infection) compared to adipose tissue (64,65). However, a large study completed in the United Kingdom with more than 19,000 patients found that the incidence of an adverse event with BMA was rare, occurring in only 0.08% of all reported BMA procedures (65). Hemorrhage was the most common adverse event, occurring in 70% of the 16 cases of adverse events. However, it should be noted that all of the patients in this study had hematologic diseases, including myeloid neoplasms (e.g., leukemia) and lymphoproliferative disorders (e.g., idiopathic thrombocytopenic purpura), which increase the risk of hemorrhage in general. Hemorrhage is unlikely to be observed in the general patient population seeking regenerative treatment for orthopedic conditions.

Adipose-derived stem cells (ASCs) are another common source of autologous stem cells in orthopedics. Human adipogenic stem cell precursors were first isolated by plastic adherence in 1976 and in human lipoaspirates in 2001 by Zuk et al. (66,67). Lipoaspiration is considered a minimally invasive, safe, and frequently performed procedure, with more than 400,000 liposuction surgeries performed in the United States each year (47,48,57,68,69). Historically, this has been performed by plastic surgeons for cosmetic purposes. ASCs are located in the stromal vascular fraction (SVF), which can only be accessed once separated from adipocytes by centrifugation after mechanical processing or enzymatic digestion (172). Crude SVF contains vascular endothelial cells, pericytes, smooth muscle cells, red blood cells, erythrocytes, and ASCs (70–72). Of the total nucleated portion, ASCs constitute approximately 1% to 7% of lipoaspirate cells and 30% to 40% of crude SVF cells (70,71,73). A schematic illustrating the basic processing steps and cellular content of MSCs from adipose tissue and BMA can be seen in Figure 11.5.

Older studies indicate that MSCs derived from BMA have superior differentiation into

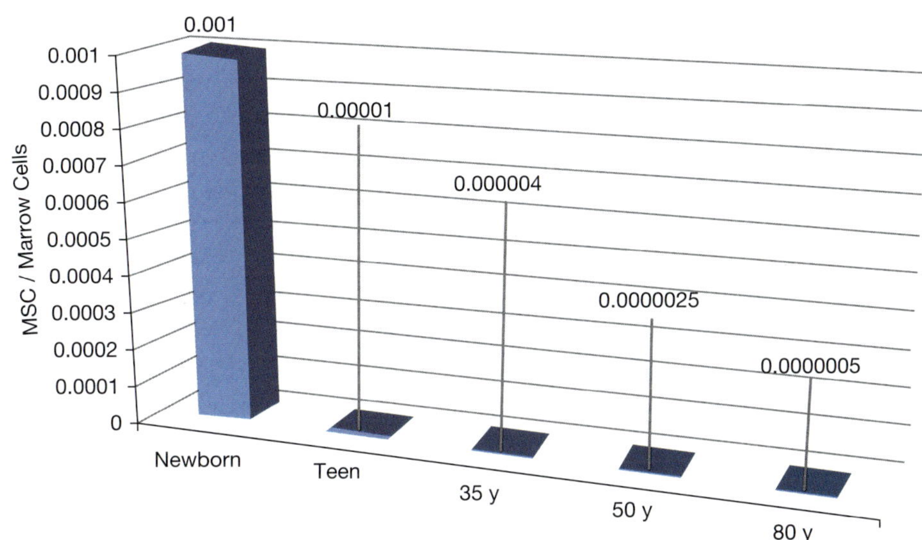

FIGURE 11.4: Human MSCs in bone marrow and their age-related decline.

MSCs, mesenchymal stem cells.

Source: Adapted from Refs. (50,58–63).

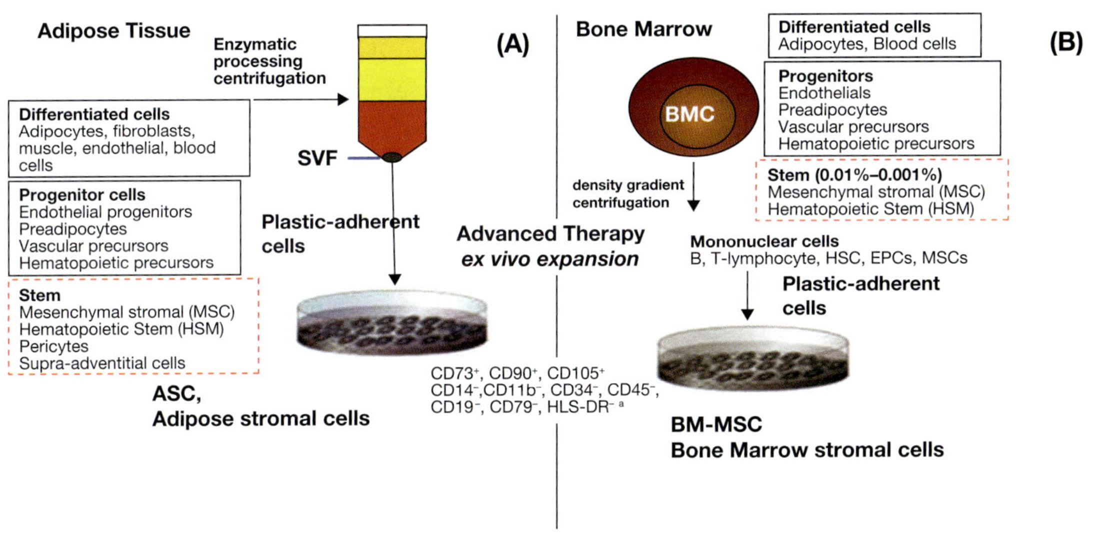

FIGURE 11.5: A schematic illustrating the processing and cellular content of MSCs derived from adipose tissue and bone marrow.

ASC, adipose stromal cells; BMC, bone marrow stromal cells; EPCs, endothelial progenitor cells; HSC, hematopoietic stem cells; MSCs, mesenchymal stem cells; SVF, stromal vascular fraction.

musculoskeletal tissues such as cartilage, bone, and muscle tissue capacity over adipose tissue; however, more recent publications demonstrate comparative osteogenic and chondrogenic potential of adipose-derived stem cells (48,66,74). Human ASCs have also been shown to be more genetically and morphologically stable, displaying a higher proliferative capacity, and some studies suggest that they retain a longer differentiation potential in culture when compared to BMA (75,173). In a recent study, Li et al. (2015) investigated the biological differences between cultured bone marrow and adipose-derived stem cells. Li et al. found negligible differences in cell morphology (e.g., cell surface markers); however, there were differences in differentiation potential (i.e., as previously mentioned) and protein secretion (e.g., growth factor secretion), and ASCs may exhibit superior immunogenic properties compared to bone marrow–derived cells (69). This is still a topic of great debate and further quality research is still needed.

Human umbilical cord (i.e., Wharton's jelly) is a rich source of MSCs, but many ethical concerns remain regarding its use (8,76,77). Other promising sources of MSCs, including amniotic fluid, tendons, and different germinal cell lines (i.e., of ectodermal and endodermal lineage), face current regulatory, safety, and ethical challenges (34–43).

MIGRATION TO SITES OF INJURY

Studies have also demonstrated that MSCs have the capacity to migrate to sites of inflammation after an injury, although the exact mechanisms remain unknown. One proposed mechanism for MSC migration is chemokine signaling, such as stromal cell-derived factor (SDF-1)/C-X-C chemokine receptor type 4 (CXCR4), vascular endothelial growth factor (VEGF)/VEGF receptor, platelet-derived growth factor (PDGF)/ PDGF receptor, and other cell adhesion molecules (78–83). Physiologic electric fields found in the extracellular microenvironment may also guide cell migration and influence differentiation of MSCs (84). Additional techniques are being explored to augment the natural MSC migration, including the use of viral vectors and exploring novel cell-culturing environments (e.g., inducing short-term hypoxia) (85).

TROPHIC PROPERTIES

MSCs release several trophic factors (e.g., exosomes) once being at the location of injury, which alter the local environment and affect local MSC differentiation, angiogenesis, and cytokine secretion (86–100,178) (Figure 11.6). Exosomes are released by most cells in the body and are thought to play a critical role in the

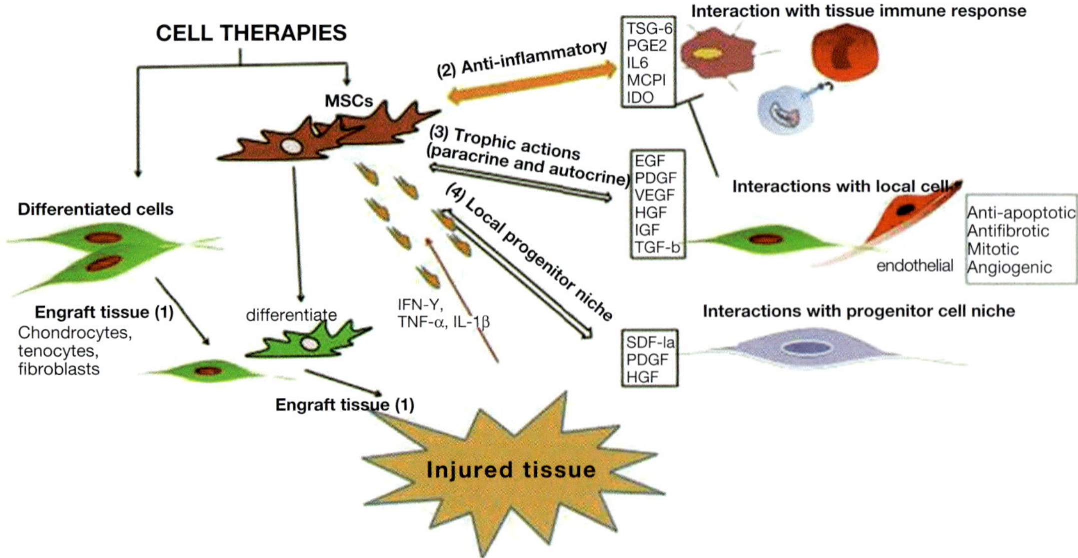

FIGURE 11.6: Trophic and inflammatory properties of MSCs in response to injured tissue.

EGF, endothelial growth factor; HGF, hepatocyte growth factor; IDO; IGF; IL-6, interleukin 6; MCP1; MSCs, mesenchymal stem cells; PGDF; PGE2; SDF-1a, stromal cell-derived factor 1a; TSG-6; VEGF, vascular endothelial growth factor.

local environment as well as cell signaling and immune regulation (101–113). As simply stated by Caplan et al., MSCs serve as "drugstores, to promote and support the natural regeneration of focal injuries" (15).

IMMUNOMODULATION

MSCs also participate in tissue repair through immunomodulation via potent immunosuppressive and anti-inflammatory interactions with the innate and adaptive immune systems (15,114–116). Under acute inflammatory conditions, MSCs suppress macrophage polarization to M1 and favor M2 polarization; inhibit natural killer and dendritic cell activation, differentiation, and effector functions; inhibit neutrophil apoptosis; and suppress mast cell degranulation. Cumulatively, these changes make the local environment less susceptible to autoimmune reactions (15,115–117). Under chronic inflammatory conditions, MSCs are polarized by M2 macrophages and are recruited into the fibrotic process (118–129).

Cells of the adaptive immune system include B cells and T cells primarily. A number of studies have shown that MSCs inhibit T-cell and B-cell proliferation, and arrest both cell types in the G0/G1 phase of the cell cycle (130). Inhibited T and B cells exhibit increased survival and less apoptosis (131). Furthermore, an immunosuppressive environment is induced by the generation of T-regulatory cells by MSCs through direct cell-to-cell contact and the production of soluble factors, including hepatocyte growth factor (HGF), nitric oxide (NO), transforming growth factor-B (TGF-β), and interleukin (IL)-10 (132,133).

Based on the microenvironment, which is directly related to the cytokine milieu (i.e., via tumor necrosis factor-α [TNF-α], interferons, matrix metalloproteinases [MMPs], HGF, NO, TGF-β, and toll-like receptor [TLR] stimulation), MSCs may be driven down a pro-inflammatory or anti-inflammatory pathway (134–136) (Figure 11.6).

CULTURING, SCAFFOLDS, AND REGULATORY ISSUES

In vitro studies frequently use culture-expanded MSCs to increase the cell yield before application. During the culturing process, centrifuged cellular aspirate from BMA or SVF cells are plated as a single layer into tissue culture polystyrene (i.e., TCPS) flasks, allowing the MSCs to adhere to the plastic surface (10,52,137–140). Plastic adherence allows for the isolation of the MSCs from the other plated nucleated cells, which do not attach to the TCPS flasks. While growing, the cells are fed nutrient broth (i.e., medium), which is changed after the initial 2 days to remove the non-MSC nucleated cells. The MSCs continue to grow until they come into contact with each other, which inhibits further growth. These cells are then trypsinized from the TCPS flask and replatted onto multiple new flasks with a fresh culture medium. This culturing step is termed "passaging." Through proliferation and expansion, MSCs become more abundant with each passage. However, the expression of different surface markers, multipotency, and the secretion of several chemokines have been shown to diminish with serial passaging of cultured human MSCs (141).

MSC culturing has several other drawbacks that must be taken into consideration. Culturing adds additional steps in the processing of MSCs, requires several weeks and has additional associated costs (10). Another significant concern has been the theoretical risk of tumorigenecity based on in vitro studies (65,142–147); however, clinical trials have not demonstrated any tumor growth associated with the long-term use of cultured MSCs in humans (144,147–150). Most importantly, no studies to date have suggested that culturing cells provides any clinical advantage to non-culture-based cell therapies.

Additionally, the most common medium supplement used for culturing (i.e., fetal bovine serum or FBS) may increase the risk of infection or autoimmune reaction (64,143,151,175). Although no cases of infection have been reported in the literature, there has been at least one case of an acute autoimmune disseminated encephalitis-like illness following the intrathecal infusion of cultured MSCs (143). It remains unclear whether the observed autoimmune reaction was related to the culturing process or was a consequence of the MSCs exerting their immunomodulatory effects.

Different culture media and scaffolds for MSCs have been explored in the literature (176,177). Platelet-rich plasma (PRP) and platelet lysate (PL) have shown promising results as a culture medium supplement or as a vehicle for injecting MSCs. As a culture medium supplement, platelet products have been shown to be an efficacious and comparable alternative to FBS, and may help diminish infection concerns (152–155,179). Platelets are one of the first responders to injury and contain greater than 1,500 protein-based growth factors (e.g., basic fibroblast growth factor; bFGF, vascular endothelial growth factor; VEGF, transforming growth factor-beta; TGF-B, platelet derived growth factor; PDGF, fibroblast growth factor 2; FGF2, insulin like growth factor 1 & 2; IGFI-II), chemokines, peptides, hormones, and proteins with antibacterial and fungicidal properties (50,156–160). When used as a scaffold adjunct, PRP has been shown to increase the osteogenic and chondrogenic differentiation potential of MSCs, while also imparting an anabolic effect on MSCs and the extracellular matrix (160).

Hyaluronic acid (HA) is also being investigated as an adjunct to MSCs. In older preclinical studies, HA has been shown to facilitate MSC migration, adherence, and integration when used as a culture medium supplement and/or scaffold (161–164). In one recent study by Succar et al., MSCs cultured with HA showed dose-dependent increased growth kinetics, adhesion, and growth factor secretion (165). Although more studies are needed, HA shows promise as a potential culture medium alternative and delivery method for MSCs.

Although there is a growing body of literature exploring the safety and efficacy of culture media and scaffolding adjuncts, regulatory issues limit the ability to implement this into clinical practice. The U.S. Food and Drug Administration (FDA) guidelines require that cells are processed in accordance with the current Good Manufacturing Practice Guidelines (166). Under current FDA regulation, cells that undergo "more than minimal manipulation" fall under these regulatory guidelines, which classify cultured cells as drugs. Culturing of cells, the use of enzymes for the digestion of adipose tissue, and/or the treatment of cellular products with growth factors do not meet minimal manipulation guidelines and require FDA approval (167,168). Regulatory issues are discussed more in depth in Chapter 3.

ADHERENCE, INTEGRATION, AND ENGRAFTMENT

Increasing the likelihood of cell integration and engraftment is paramount for successful treatment. Success involves taking into account several key components, including: (a) cellular integrity, (b) cellular administration and anchoring within the target lesion, (c) target-site remodeling, (d) cellular proliferation and differentiation, (e) appropriate space, and (f) adequate nutritional support (50,169). Recent literature has demonstrated that MSCs injected adhere after 3 hours and undergo fibroblastic differentiation after 8 hours (165). These findings can potentially affect postprocedure joint mobilization protocols, requiring longer immobilization to improve clinical outcomes (165). As mentioned previously, the use of other vehicle and/or scaffolding agents (e.g., HA or platelet products) may also aid in successful integration and engraftment.

FUTURE PERSPECTIVES

Although new research studies are being published regularly to further clarify the exact mechanisms of how MSCs function, there are several key issues that still need to be addressed, including: What are the optimal culturing conditions? What are the best delivery method(s) for MSCs? How many MSCs need to be injected for a desired therapeutic effect? How do we accurately track injected MSCs to better understand engraftment, adherence, and differentiation? Which MSC source is optimal (e.g., adipose tissue vs. bone marrow aspirate concentrate [BMAC]) and does the underlying pathology matter (i.e., is one source better for treating a specific disease process)?

Despite the paucity of level I and level II studies, regenerative treatments for various musculoskeletal conditions are currently offered by several medical specialists in the United States, largely driven by the lack of effective nonsurgical alternatives (49,50,52,160,170). The potential use of MSCs for tissue regeneration and orthopedic conditions is unlimited (174), but the clinical application of these cells should first be founded in basic science research.

KEY POINTS

- MSCs were first isolated in the 1970s and later named in the 1990s.

- The ISCT has minimal criteria for the classification of MSCs: (a) displaying a unique set of surface markers; (b) possessing trilineage differentiation potential into osteoblasts, chondrocytes, and adipocytes; (c) and spindle-shaped morphology with plastic adherence in a laboratory setting.

- PSCs (i.e., pericytes) are precursors to MSCs and reside around vascular tissue, activating after an injury.

- MSCs have been isolated from every tissue in the body. Most literature on MSCs for orthopedic conditions involves BMA, with more recent studies also using adipose tissue.

- The optimal source for MSCs has yet to be determined.

- Migration to sites of injury is believed to be influenced by chemokine and receptor interactions.

- Three key properties of MSCs include their trophic effects, immunomodulatory properties, and differentiation potential.

- Platelet products may offer an alternative to FBS as a culturing medium supplement and as a scaffolding adjunct.

- Current regulatory guidelines by the FDA allow only minimal manipulation of tissues and cells without approval.

- The basic science principles of regenerative treatments are still being explored, with new discoveries occurring at an exponential rate. The future of medicine and, in particular, the treatment of orthopedic conditions using MSCs is extremely promising.

REFERENCES

1. Berman L, Stulberg CS, Ruddle FH. Long-term tissue culture of human bone marrow. i. Report of isolation of a strain of cells resembling epithelial cells from bone marrow of a patient with carcinoma of the lung. *Blood.* 1955;10(9):896–911.

2. Mcculloch EA, Parker RC. Continuous cultivation of cells of hemic origin. *Proc Can Cancer Conf.* 1957;2:152–167.

3. Friedenstein AJ, Chailakhjan RK, Lalykina KS. The development of fibroblast colonies in monolayer cultures of guinea-pig bone marrow and spleen cells. *Cell Tissue Kinet.* 1970;3(4):393–403.

4. Caplan AI. Mesenchymal stem cells. *J Orthop Res.* 1991;9(5):641–650.

5. Horwitz EM, Le Blanc K, Dominici M, et al.; International Society for Cellular Therapy. Clarification of the nomenclature for MSC: the International Society for Cellular Therapy position statement. *Cytotherapy.* 2005;7(5):393–395.

6. Caplan AI. Adult mesenchymal stem cells: when, where, and how. *Stem Cells Int.* 2015;2015: 628767.

7. Dominici M, Le Blanc K, Mueller I, et al. Minimal criteria for defining multipotent mesenchymal stromal cells. The International Society for Cellular Therapy position statement. *Cytotherapy.* 2006;8:315–317.

8. Bieback K, Kern S, Klüter H, et al. Critical parameters for the isolation of mesenchymal stem cells from umbilical cord blood. *Stem Cells.* 2004;22(4):625–634.

9. Boxall SA, Jones E. Markers for characterization of bone marrow multipotential stromal cells. *Stem Cells Int.* 2012;2012:975871.

10. Murray IR, Corselli M, Petrigliano FA, et al. Recent insights into the identity of mesenchymal stem cells: implications for orthopaedic applications. *Bone Joint J.* 2014;96-B(3):291–298.

11. Caplan AI. All MSCs are pericytes? *Cell Stem Cell.* 2008;3(3):229–230.

12. da Silva Meirelles L, Caplan AI, Nardi NB. In search of the in vivo identity of mesenchymal stem cells. *Stem Cells.* 2008;26(9):2287–2299.

13. Corselli M, Chen CW, Sun B, et al. The tunica adventitia of human arteries and veins as a source of mesenchymal stem cells. *Stem Cells Dev.* 2012;21(8):1299–1308.

14. Sacchetti B, Funari A, Michienzi S, et al. Self-renewing osteoprogenitors in bone marrow sinusoids can organize a hematopoietic microenvironment. *Cell.* 2007;131(2):324–336.

15. Caplan AI, Correa D. The MSC: an injury drugstore. *Cell Stem Cell.* 2011;9(1):11–15.

16. Zhou S, Eid K, Glowacki J. Cooperation between TGF-beta and wnt pathways during chondrocyte and adipocyte differentiation of human marrow stromal cells. *J Bone Miner Res.* 2004;19(3):463–470.

17. Longobardi L, O'Rear L, Aakula S, et al. Effect of IGF-i in the chondrogenesis of bone marrow mesenchymal stem cells in the presence or absence of TGF-beta signaling. *J Bone Miner Res.* 2006;21(4):626–636.

18. Bosnakovski D, Mizuno M, Kim G, et al. Isolation and multilineage differentiation of bovine bone marrow mesenchymal stem cells. *Cell Tissue Res.* 2005;319(2):243–253.

19. Knippenberg M, Helder MN, Zandieh Doulabi B, et al. Osteogenesis versus chondrogenesis by BMP-2 and BMP-7 in adipose stem cells. *Biochem Biophys Res Commun.* 2006;342(3):902–908.

20. Bai Y, Li P, Yin G, et al. BMP-2, VEGF and BFGF synergistically promote the osteogenic differentiation of rat bone marrow-derived mesenchymal stem cells. *Biotechnol Lett.* 2013;35(3):301–308.

21. Dezawa M, Ishikawa H, Itokazu Y, et al. Bone marrow stromal cells generate muscle cells and repair muscle degeneration. *Science.* 2005;309 (5732):314–317.

22. Kuo CK, Tuan RS. Mechanoactive tenogenic differentiation of human mesenchymal stem cells. *Tissue Eng Part a.* 2008;14(10):1615–1627.

23. Shim WS, Jiang S, Wong P, et al. Ex vivo differentiation of human adult bone marrow stem cells into cardiomyocyte-like cells. *Biochem Biophys Res Commun.* 2004;324(2):481–488.

24. Jeon ES, Moon HJ, Lee MJ, et al. Sphingosylphosphorylcholine induces differentiation of human mesenchymal stem cells into smooth-muscle-like cells through a TGF-beta-dependent mechanism. *J Cell Sci.* 2006;119(Pt 23):4994–5005.

25. Oswald J, Boxberger S, Jørgensen B, et al. Mesenchymal stem cells can be differentiated into endothelial cells in vitro. *Stem Cells.* 2004;22(3):377–384.

26. Pittenger MF, Mackay AM, Beck SC, et al. Multilineage potential of adult human mesenchymal stem cells. *Science.* 1999;284(5411):143–147.

27. Schwartz RE, Reyes M, Koodie L, et al. Multipotent adult progenitor cells from bone marrow differentiate into functional hepatocyte-like cells. *J Clin Invest.* 2002;109(10):1291–1302.

28. Tropel P, Platet N, Platel JC, et al. Functional neuronal differentiation of bone marrow-derived mesenchymal stem cells. *Stem Cells.* 2006;24:2868–2876.

29. Cogle CR, Yachnis AT, Laywell ED, et al. Bone marrow transdifferentiation in brain after transplantation: a retrospective study. *Lancet.* 2004;363:1432–1437.

30. Rose RA, Keating A, Backx PH. Do mesenchymal stromal cells transdifferentiate into functional cardiomyocytes? *Circ Res.* 2008;103:e120. 17.

31. Lindner U, Kramer J, Rohwedel J, Schlenke P. Mesenchymal stem or stromal cells: toward a better understanding of their biology? *Transfus Med Hemother.* 2010;37(2):75–83.

32. Väänänen HK. Mesenchymal stem cells. *Ann Med.* 2005;37(7):469–479.

33. Zhang Y, Li C, Jiang X, et al. Human placenta-derived mesenchymal progenitor cells support culture expansion of long-term culture-initiating cells from cord blood CD34+ cells. *Exp Hematol.* 2004;32(7):657–664.

34. Petersen BE, Bowen WC, Patrene KD, et al. Bone marrow as a potential source of hepatic oval cells. *Science.* 1999;284(5417):1168–1170.

35. Bi Y, Ehirchiou D, Kilts TM, et al. Identification of tendon stem/progenitor cells and the role of the extracellular matrix in their niche. *Nat Med.* 2007;13(10):1219–1227.

36. Tan Q, Lui PP, Rui YF, et al. Comparison of potentials of stem cells isolated from tendon and bone marrow for musculoskeletal tissue engineering. *Tissue Eng Part a.* 2012;18(7–8):840–851.

37. Krampera M, Marconi S, Pasini A, et al. Induction of neural-like differentiation in human mesenchymal stem cells derived from bone marrow, fat, spleen and thymus. *Bone.* 2007;40(2):382–390.

38. Păunescu V, Deak E, Herman D, et al. In vitro differentiation of human mesenchymal stem cells to epithelial lineage. *J Cell Mol Med.* 2007;11:502–508.

39. Timper K, Seboek D, Eberhardt M, et al. Human adipose tissue-derived mesenchymal stem cells differentiate into insulin, somatostatin, and glucagon expressing cells. *Biochem Biophys Res Commun.* 2006;341(4):1135–1140.

40. Sato Y, Araki H, Kato J, et al. Human mesenchymal stem cells xenografted directly to rat liver are differentiated into human hepatocytes without fusion. *Blood.* 2005;106(2):756–763.

41. Aurich H, Sgodda M, Kaltwasser P, et al. Hepatocyte differentiation of mesenchymal stem cells from human adipose tissue in vitro promotes hepatic integration in vivo. *Gut.* 2009;58(4):570–581.

42. Khoo ML, Tao H, Meedeniya AC, et al. Transplantation of neuronal-primed human bone marrow mesenchymal stem cells in hemiparkinsonian rodents. *PLOS ONE.* 2011;6(5):e19025.

43. Hölig K, Kramer M, Kroschinsky F, et al. Safety and efficacy of hematopoietic stem cell collection from mobilized peripheral blood in unrelated volunteers: 12 years of single-center experience in 3928 donors. *Blood.* 2009;114(18):3757–3763.

44. Mafi R, Hindocha S, Mafi P, et al. Sources of adult mesenchymal stem cells applicable for musculoskeletal applications: a systematic review of the literature. *Open Orthop J.* 2011;5(Suppl 2):242–248.

45. Roubelakis MG, Pappa KI, Bitsika V, et al. Molecular and proteomic characterization of human mesenchymal stem cells derived from amniotic fluid: comparison to bone marrow mesenchymal stem cells. *Stem Cells Dev.* 2007;16(6):931–952.

46. Bochev I, Elmadjian G, Kyurkchiev D, et al. Mesenchymal stem cells from human bone marrow or adipose tissue differently modulate mitogen-stimulated B-cell immunoglobulin production in vitro. *Cell Biol Int.* 2008;32(4):384–393.

47. Alvarez-Viejo M, Menendez-Menendez Y, Blanco-Gelaz MA, et al. Quantifying mesenchymal stem cells in the mononuclear cell fraction of bone marrow samples obtained for cell therapy. *Transplant Proc.* 2013;45(1):434–439.

48. Kern S, Eichler H, Stoeve J, Klüter H, Bieback K. Comparative analysis of mesenchymal stem cells from bone marrow, umbilical cord blood, or adipose tissue. *Stem Cells.* 2006;24(5):1294–1301.

49. Bashir J, Sherman A, Lee H, et al. Mesenchymal stem cell therapies in the treatment of musculoskeletal diseases. *PM R.* 2014;6(1):61–69.

50. Mautner K, Blazuk J. Where do injectable stem cell treatments apply in treatment of muscle, tendon, and ligament injuries? *PM R.* 2015;7(4 Suppl):S33–S40.

51. Crisostomo PR, Wang M, Wairiuko GM, et al. High passage number of stem cells adversely affects stem cell activation and myocardial protection. *Shock.* 2006;26(6):575–580.

52. Murrell WD, et al. Regenerative treatments to enhance orthopedic surgical outcome. *PM R.* 2015:541–552.

53. Gibon E, Lu L, Goodman SB. Aging, inflammation, stem cells, and bone healing. *Stem Cell Res Ther.* 2016;7:44. doi:10.1186/s13287-016-0300-9

54. Marędziak M, Marycz K, Tomaszewski KA, et al. The influence of aging on the regenerative potential of human adipose derived mesenchymal stem cells. *Stem Cells Int.* 2016;2016, Article ID 2152435:15 pages. doi:10.1155/2016/2152435

55. Klyushnenkova E, Mosca JD, Zernetkina V, et al. T-cell responses to allogeneic human mesenchymal stem cells: immunogenicity, tolerance, and suppression. *J Biomed Sci.* 2005;12(1):47–57.

56. Ueda Y, Inaba M, Takada K, et al. Induction of senile osteoporosis in normal mice by intra-bone marrow-bone marrow transplantation from osteoporosis-prone mice. *Stem Cells.* 2007;25(6):1356–1363.

57. Peng L, Jia Z, Yin X, et al. Comparative analysis of mesenchymal stem cells from bone marrow, cartilage, and adipose tissue. *Stem Cells Dev.* 2008;17(4):761–773.

58. Zhu M, Kohan E, Bradley J, et al. The effect of age on osteogenic, adipogenic and proliferative potential of female adipose-derived stem cells. *J Tissue Eng Regen Med.* 2009;3(4):290–301.

59. Stolzing A, Jones E, McGonagle D, et al. Age-related changes in human bone marrow-derived mesenchymal stem cells: consequences for cell therapies. *Mech Ageing Dev.* 2008;129(3):163–173.

60. Majd H, Quinn TM, Wipff PJ, et al. Dynamic expansion culture for mesenchymal stem cells. *Methods Mol Biol.* 2011;698:175–188.

61. D'Ippolito G, Schiller PC, Ricordi C, et al. Age-related osteogenic potential of mesenchymal stromal stem cells from human vertebral bone marrow. *J Bone Miner Res.* 1999;14(7):1115–1122.

62. Muschler GF, Nitto H, Boehm CA, et al. Age- and gender-related changes in the cellularity of human bone marrow and the prevalence of osteoblastic progenitors. *J Orthop Res.* 2001;19(1):117–125.

63. Sorrell JM, Caplan AI. Topical delivery of mesenchymal stem cells and their function in wounds. *Stem Cell Res Ther.* 2010;1(4):30. doi:10.1186/scrt30

64. Prockop DJ, Brenner M, Fibbe WE, et al. Defining the risks of mesenchymal stromal cell therapy. *Cytotherapy.* 2010;12(5):576–578.

65. Bain BJ. Bone marrow biopsy morbidity: review of 2003. *Journal of Clinical Pathology.* 2005;58(4):406–408.

66. Zuk PA, Zhu M, Mizuno H, et al. Multilineage cells from human adipose tissue: implications for cell-based therapies. *Tissue Eng.* 2001;7(2):211–228.

67. Van RL, Bayliss CE, Roncari DA. Cytological and enzymological characterization of adult human adipocyte precursors in culture. *J Clin Invest.* 1976;58(3):699–704.

68. Chamberlain G, Fox J, Ashton B, et al. Concise review: mesenchymal stem cells: their phenotype, differentiation capacity, immunological features, and potential for homing. *Stem Cells.* 2007;25(11):2739–2749.

69. Li CY, Wu XY, Tong JB, et al. Comparative analysis of human mesenchymal stem cells from bone marrow and adipose tissue under xeno-free conditions for cell therapy. *Stem Cell Res Ther.* 2015;6:55. doi:10.1186/s13287-015-0066-5

70. Suga H, Matsumoto D, Inoue K, et al. Numerical measurement of viable and nonviable adipocytes and other cellular components in aspirated fat tissue. *Plast Reconstr Surg.* 2008;122(1):103–114.

71. Eto H, Suga H, Matsumoto D, et al. Characterization of structure and cellular components of aspirated and excised adipose tissue. *Plast Reconstr Surg.* 2009;124(4):1087–1097.

72. James AW, Zara JN, Corselli M, et al. An abundant perivascular source of stem cells for bone tissue engineering. *Stem Cells Transl Med.* 2012;1(9):673–684.

73. Bianchi F, Maioli M, Leonardi E, et al. A new nonenzymatic method and device to obtain a fat tissue derivative highly enriched in pericyte-like elements by mild mechanical forces from human lipoaspirates. *Cell Transplant.* 2013;22(11):2063–2077.

74. Zuk PA, Zhu M, Ashjian P, et al. Human adipose tissue is a source of multipotent stem cells. *Mol Biol Cell.* 2002;13(12):4279–4295.

75. Izadpanah R, Trygg C, Patel B, et al. Biologic properties of mesenchymal stem cells derived from bone marrow and adipose tissue. *J Cell Biochem.* 2006;99(5):1285–1297.

76. Baksh D, Yao R, Tuan RS. Comparison of proliferative and multilineage differentiation potential of human mesenchymal stem cells derived from umbilical cord and bone marrow. *Stem Cells.* 2007;25(6):1384–1392.

77. Subramanian A, Shu-Uin G, Kae-Siang N, et al. Human umbilical cord Wharton's jelly mesenchymal stem cells do not transform to tumor-associated fibroblasts in the presence of breast and ovarian cancer cells unlike bone marrow mesenchymal stem cells. *J Cell Biochem.* 2012;113(6):1886–1895.

78. Rui YF, Lui PP, Lee YW, et al. Higher BMP receptor expression and BMP-2-induced osteogenic differentiation in tendon-derived stem cells compared with bone-marrow-derived mesenchymal stem cells. *Int Orthop.* 2012;36(5):1099–1107.

79. Zhi L, Chen C, Pang X, et al. Synergistic effect of recombinant human bone morphogenic protein-7 and osteogenic differentiation medium on human bone-marrow-derived mesenchymal stem cells in vitro. *Int Orthop.* 2011;35(12):1889–1895.

80. Ode A, Kopf J, Kurtz A, et al. CD73 and CD29 concurrently mediate the mechanically induced decrease of migratory capacity of mesenchymal stromal cells. *Eur Cell Mater.* 2011;22:26–42.

81. Kitaori T, Ito H, Schwarz EM, et al. Stromal cell-derived factor 1/CXCR4 signaling is critical for the recruitment of mesenchymal stem cells to the fracture site during skeletal repair in a mouse model. *Arthritis Rheum.* 2009;60(3):813–823.

82. Shinohara K, Greenfield S, Pan H, et al. Stromal cell-derived factor-1 and monocyte chemotactic protein-3 improve recruitment of osteogenic cells into sites of musculoskeletal repair. *J Orthop Res.* 2011;29(7):1064–1069.

83. Mendelson A, Frank E, Allred C, et al. Chondrogenesis by chemotactic homing of synovium, bone marrow, and adipose stem cells in vitro. *FASEB J.* 2011;25(10):3496–3504.

84. Zhao Z, Watt C, Karystinou A, et al. Directed migration of human bone marrow mesenchymal stem cells in a physiological direct current electric field. *Eur Cell Mater.* 2011;22:344–358.

85. Sohni A, Verfaillie CM. Mesenchymal stem cells migration homing and tracking. *Stem Cells Int.* 2013;2013:130763. doi:10.1155/2013/130763

86. Caplan AI, Dennis JE. Mesenchymal stem cells as trophic mediators. *J Cell Biochem*. 2006;98(5):1076–1084.

87. Wu L, Leijten JC, Georgi N, et al. Trophic effects of mesenchymal stem cells increase chondrocyte proliferation and matrix formation. *Tissue Eng Part a*. 2011;17(9–10):1425–1436.

88. de Windt TS, Saris DB, Slaper-Cortenbach IC, et al. Direct cell-cell contact with chondrocytes is a key mechanism in multipotent mesenchymal stromal cell-mediated chondrogenesis. *Tissue Eng Part a*. 2015;21(19–20):2536–2547.

89. Nakamizo A, Marini F, Amano T, et al. Human bone marrow-derived mesenchymal stem cells in the treatment of gliomas. *Cancer Res*. 2005;65(8):3307–3318.

90. Son BR, Marquez-Curtis LA, Kucia M, et al. Migration of bone marrow and cord blood mesenchymal stem cells in vitro is regulated by stromal-derived factor-1-CXCR4 and hepatocyte growth factor-c-met axes and involves matrix metalloproteinases. *Stem Cells*. 2006;24(5):1254–1264.

91. Forte G, Minieri M, Cossa P, et al. Hepatocyte growth factor effects on mesenchymal stem cells: proliferation, migration, and differentiation. *Stem Cells*. 2006;24(1):23–33.

92. Ball SG, Shuttleworth CA, Kielty CM. Vascular endothelial growth factor can signal through platelet-derived growth factor receptors. *J Cell Biol*. 2007;177(3):489–500.

93. Fiedler J, Röderer G, Günther KP, et al. BMP-2, BMP-4, and PDGF-bb stimulate chemotactic migration of primary human mesenchymal progenitor cells. *J Cell Biochem*. 2002;87(3):305–312.

94. Shabbir A, Zisa D, Suzuki G, et al. Heart failure therapy mediated by the trophic activities of bone marrow mesenchymal stem cells: a noninvasive therapeutic regimen. *Am J Physiol Heart Circ Physiol*. 2009;296(6):H1888–H1897.

95. Nixon AJ, Watts AE, Schnabel LV. Cell- and gene-based approaches to tendon regeneration. *J Shoulder Elbow Surg*. 2012;21(2):278–294.

96. Doorn J, Moll G, Le Blanc K, et al. Therapeutic applications of mesenchymal stromal cells: paracrine effects and potential improvements. *Tissue Eng Part b Rev*. 2012;18(2):101–115.

97. Kinnaird T, Stabile E, Burnett MS, et al. Local delivery of marrow-derived stromal cells augments collateral perfusion through paracrine mechanisms. *Circulation*. 2004;109(12):1543–1549.

98. da Silva Meirelles L, Fontes AM, Covas DT, et al. Mechanisms involved in the therapeutic properties of mesenchymal stem cells. *Cytokine Growth Factor Rev*. 2009;20(5–6):419–427.

99. Mok PL, Leong CF, Cheong SK. Cellular mechanisms of emerging applications of mesenchymal stem cells. *Malays J Pathol*. 2013;35(1):17–32.

100. Ozaki K, Sato K, Oh I, et al. Mechanisms of immunomodulation by mesenchymal stem cells. *Int J Hematol*. 2007;86(1):5–7.

101. Valadi H, Ekström K, Bossios A, et al. Exosome-mediated transfer of MMAs and micro RNAs is a novel mechanism of genetic exchange between cells. *Nat Cell Biol*. 2007;9(6):654–659.

102. Lázaro-Ibáñez E, Sanz-Garcia A, Visakorpi T, et al. Different gDNAcontent in the subpopulations of prostate cancer extracellular vesicles: apoptotic bodies, microvesicles, and exosomes. *Prostate*. 2014;74(14):1379–1390.

103. Lotvall J, Valadi H. Cell to cell signalling via exosomes through esrna. *Cell Adh Migr*. 2007;1(3):156–158.

104. Huebner AR, Somparn P, Benjachat T, et al. Exosomes in urine biomarker discovery. *Adv Exp Med Biol*. 2015;845:43–58.

105. Keating A. How do mesenchymal stromal cells suppress T cells? *Cell Stem Cell*. 2008;2(2):106–108.

106. Ren G, Zhang L, Zhao X, et al. Mesenchymal stem cell-mediated immunosuppression occurs via concerted action of chemokines and nitric oxide. *Cell Stem Cell*. 2008;2(2):141–150.

107. Meisel R, Zibert A, Laryea M, et al. Human bone marrow stromal cells inhibit allogeneic T-cell responses by indoleamine 2,3-dioxygenase-mediated tryptophan degradation. *Blood*. 2004;103(12):4619–4621.

108. Joo SY, Cho KA, Jung YJ, et al. Mesenchymal stromal cells inhibit graft-versus-host disease of mice in a dose-dependent manner. *Cytotherapy*. 2010;12(3):361–370.

109. Zappia E, Casazza S, Pedemonte E, et al. Mesenchymal stem cells ameliorate experimental autoimmune encephalomyelitis inducing T-cell anergy. *Blood*. 2005;106(5):1755–1761.

110. González MA, Gonzalez-Rey E, Rico L, et al. Treatment of experimental arthritis by inducing immune tolerance with human adipose-derived mesenchymal stem cells. *Arthritis Rheum*. 2009;60(4):1006–1019.

111. Patel SA, Meyer JR, Greco SJ, et al. Mesenchymal stem cells protect breast cancer cells through regulatory T cells: role of mesenchymal stem cell-derived TGF-beta. *J Immunol*. 2010;184(10):5885–5894.

112. Nemeth K, Keane-Myers A, Brown JM, et al. Bone marrow stromal cells use TGF-beta to suppress allergic responses in a mouse model of ragweed-induced asthma. *Proc Natl Acad Sci USA.* 2010;107(12):5652–5657.

113. Madec AM, Mallone R, Afonso G, et al. Mesenchymal stem cells protect NOD mice from diabetes by inducing regulatory T cells. *Diabetologia.* 2009;52(7):1391–1399.

114. Shi Y, Hu G, Su J, et al. Mesenchymal stem cells: a new strategy for immunosuppression and tissue repair. *Cell Res.* 2010;20(5):510–518.

115. Fong EL, Chan CK, Goodman SB. Stem cell homing in musculoskeletal injury. *Biomaterials.* 2011;32(2):395–409.

116. Kumar S, Ponnazhagan S. Mobilization of bone marrow mesenchymal stem cells in vivo augments bone healing in a mouse model of segmental bone defect. *Bone.* 2012;50(4):1012–1018.

117. Jiang XX, Zhang Y, Liu B, et al. Human mesenchymal stem cells inhibit differentiation and function of monocyte-derived dendritic cells. *Blood.* 2005;105(10):4120–4126.

118. Glenn JD, Whartenby KA. Mesenchymal stem cells: emerging mechanisms of immunomodulation and therapy. *World J Stem Cells.* 2014;6(5):526–539.

119. Uccelli A, Moretta L, Pistoia V. Mesenchymal stem cells in health and disease. *Nat Rev Immunol.* 2008;8(9):726–736.

120. Jones S, Horwood N, Cope A, et al. The antiproliferative effect of mesenchymal stem cells is a fundamental property shared by all stromal cells. *J Immunol.* 2007;179(5):2824–2831.

121. Cho DI, Kim MR, Jeong HY, et al. Mesenchymal stem cells reciprocally regulate the M1/M2 balance in mouse bone marrow-derived macrophages. *Exp Mol Med.* 2014;46:e70. doi:10.1038/emm.2013.135

122. Spaggiari GM, Moretta L. Cellular and molecular interactions of mesenchymal stem cells in innate immunity. *Immunol Cell Biol.* 2013;91(1):27–31.

123. Maggini J, Mirkin G, Bognanni I, et al. Mouse bone marrow-derived mesenchymal stromal cells turn activated macrophages into a regulatory-like profile. *PLOS ONE.* 2010;5(2):e9252. doi:10.1371/journal.pone.0009252

124. Raffaghello L, Bianchi G, Bertolotto M, et al. Human mesenchymal stem cells inhibit neutrophil apoptosis: a model for neutrophil preservation in the bone marrow niche. *Stem Cells.* 2008;26(1):151–162.

125. Maqbool M, Vidyadaran S, George E, et al. Human mesenchymal stem cells protect neutrophils from serum-deprived cell death. *Cell Biol Int.* 2011;35(12):1247–1251.

126. Brown JM, Nemeth K, Kushnir-Sukhov NM, et al. Bone marrow stromal cells inhibit mast cell function via a COX2-dependent mechanism. *Clin Exp Allergy.* 2011;41(4):526–534.

127. Sotiropoulou PA, Perez SA, Gritzapis AD, et al. Interactions between human mesenchymal stem cells and natural killer cells. *Stem Cells.* 2006;24(1):74–85.

128. Zhang W, Ge W, Li C, et al. Effects of mesenchymal stem cells on differentiation, maturation, and function of human monocyte-derived dendritic cells. *Stem Cells Dev.* 2004;13(3):263–271.

129. Nauta AJ, Kruisselbrink AB, Lurvink E, et al. Mesenchymal stem cells inhibit generation and function of both CD34+-derived and monocyte-derived dendritic cells. *J Immunol.* 2006;177(4):2080–2087.

130. Franquesa M, Hoogduijn MJ, Bestard O, et al. Immunomodulatory effect of mesenchymal stem cells on B cells. *Front Immunol.* 2012;3:212. doi:10.3389/fimmu.2012.00212

131. Di Nicola M, Carlo-Stella C, Magni M, et al. Human bone marrow stromal cells suppress T-lymphocyte proliferation induced by cellular or nonspecific mitogenic stimuli. *Blood.* 2002;99(10):3838–3843.

132. Waterman RS, Tomchuck SL, Henkle SL, et al. A new mesenchymal stem cell (MSC) paradigm: polarization into a pro-inflammatory MSC1 or an immunosuppressive MSC2 phenotype. *PLOS ONE.* 2010;5(4):e10088. doi:10.1371/journal.pone.0010088

133. Marigo I, Dazzi F. The immunomodulatory properties of mesenchymal stem cells. *Semin Immunopathol.* 2011;33(6):593–602.

134. Lozito TP, Tuan RS. Mesenchymal stem cells inhibit both endogenous and exogenous MMPs via secreted timps. *J Cell Physiol.* 2011;226(2):385–396.

135. Uccelli A, Moretta L, Pistoia V. Immunoregulatory function of mesenchymal stem cells. *Eur J Immunol.* 2006;36(10):2566–2573.

136. Djouad F, Bouffi C, Ghannam S, et al. Mesenchymal stem cells: innovative therapeutic tools for rheumatic diseases. *Nat Rev Rheumatol.* 2009;5(7):392–399.

137. Giordano A, Galderisi U, Marino IR. From the laboratory bench to the patient's bedside: an update on clinical trials with mesenchymal stem cells. *J Cell Physiol*. 2007;211(1):27–35.

138. Centeno CJ. Clinical challenges and opportunities of mesenchymal stem cells in musculoskeletal medicine. *PM R*. 2014;6(1):70–77.

139. Banfi A, Muraglia A, Dozin B, et al. Proliferation kinetics and differentiation potential of ex vivo expanded human bone marrow stromal cells: implications for their use in cell therapy. *Exp Hematol*. 2000;28(6):707–715.

140. Izadpanah R, Kaushal D, Kriedt C, et al. Long-term in vitro expansion alters the biology of adult mesenchymal stem cells. *Cancer Res*. 2008;68(11):4229–4238.

141. Halleux C, Sottile V, Gasser JA, et al. Multi-lineage potential of human mesenchymal stem cells following clonal expansion. *J Musculoskelet Neuronal Interact*. 2001;2(1):71–76.

142. Ankrum J, Karp JM. Mesenchymal stem cell therapy: two steps forward, one step back. *Trends Mol Med*. 2010;16(5):203–209.

143. Kishk NA, Abokrysha NT, Gabr H. Possible induction of acute disseminated encephalomyelitis (ADEM)-like demyelinating illness by intrathecal mesenchymal stem cell injection. *J Clin Neurosci*. 2013;20(2):310–312.

144. Hatzistergos KE, Blum A, Ince T, et al. What is the oncologic risk of stem cell treatment for heart disease? *Circ Res*. 2011;108(11):1300–1303.

145. Heldman AW, DiFede DL, Fishman JE, et al. Transendocardial mesenchymal stem cells and mononuclear bone marrow cells for ischemic cardiomyopathy: the TAC-HFT randomized trial. *JAMA*. 2014;311(1):62–73.

146. Tarte K, Gaillard J, Lataillade JJ, et al.; Société Française de Greffe de Moelle et Thérapie Cellulaire. Clinical-grade production of human mesenchymal stromal cells: occurrence of aneuploidy without transformation. *Blood*. 2010;115(8):1549–1553.

147. Bernardo ME, Zaffaroni N, Novara F, et al. Human bone marrow derived mesenchymal stem cells do not undergo transformation after long-term in vitro culture and do not exhibit telomere maintenance mechanisms. *Cancer Res*. 2007;67(19):9142–9149.

148. Rubio D, Garcia-Castro J, Martin M, et al. Retraction: spontaneous human adult stem cell transformation [published erratum in: Cancer Res. 2005 Jun 1;65(11):4969. doi:10.1158/0008-5472. CAN-10-1305 PMCID: PMC5363595]. *Cancer Res*. 2010;70:6682.   doi:10.18632/oncotarget.12678. PMID: 20631079.

149. Lalu MM, McIntyre L, Pugliese C, et al.; Canadian Critical Care Trials Group. Safety of cell therapy with mesenchymal stromal cells (safecell): a systematic review and meta-analysis of clinical trials. *PLOS ONE*. 2012;7(10):e47559.

150. Klopp AH, Gupta A, Spaeth E, et al. Concise review: dissecting a discrepancy in the literature: do mesenchymal stem cells support or suppress tumor growth? *Stem Cells*. 2011; 29(1):11–19.

151. Gad SC. *Pharmaceutical manufacturing handbook: regulations and quality*. Hoboken: John Wiley and Sons; 2008.

152. Capelli C, Domenghini M, Borleri G, et al. Human platelet lysate allows expansion and clinical grade production of mesenchymal stromal cells from small samples of bone marrow aspirates or marrow filter washouts. *Bone Marrow Transplant*. 2007;40(8):785–791.

153. Centeno CJ, Schultz JR, Cheever M, et al. Safety and complications reporting update on the re-implantation of culture-expanded mesenchymal stem cells using autologous platelet lysate technique. *Curr Stem Cell Res Ther*. 2011;6(4):368–378.

154. Schallmoser K, Bartmann C, Rohde E, et al. Human platelet lysate can replace fetal bovine serum for clinical-scale expansion of functional mesenchymal stromal cells. *Transfusion*. 2007;47(8):1436–1446.

155. Walenda G, Hemeda H, Schneider RK, et al. Human platelet lysate gel provides a novel three dimensional-matrix for enhanced culture expansion of mesenchymal stromal cells. *Tissue Eng Part c Methods*. 2012;18(12):924–934.

156. Nagata MJ, Messora MR, Furlaneto FA, et al. Effectiveness of two methods for preparation of autologous platelet-rich plasma: an experimental study in rabbits. *Eur J Dent*. 2010;4(4):395–402.

157. Molloy T, Wang Y, Murrell G. The roles of growth factors in tendon and ligament healing. *Sports Med*. 2003;33(5):381–394.

158. Nguyen RT, Borg-Stein J, McInnis K. Applications of platelet-rich plasma in musculoskeletal and sports medicine: an evidence-based approach. *PM R*. 2011;3(3):226–250.

159. Kajikawa Y, Morihara T, Sakamoto H, et al. Platelet-rich plasma enhances the initial

mobilization of circulation-derived cells for tendon healing. *J Cell Physiol*. 2008;215(3):837–845.

160. Freitag J, Bates D, Boyd R, et al. Mesenchymal stem cell therapy in the treatment of osteoarthritis: reparative pathways, safety and efficacy—a review. *BMC Musculoskelet Disord*. 2016;17:230. doi:10.1186/s12891-016-1085-9

161. Saw KY, Anz A, Siew-Yoke Jee C, et al. Articular cartilage regeneration with autologous peripheral blood stem cells versus hyaluronic acid: a randomized controlled trial. *Arthroscopy*. 2013;29(4):684–694.

162. Maniwa S, Ochi M, Motomura T, et al. Effects of hyaluronic acid and basic fibroblast growth factor on motility of chondrocytes and synovial cells in culture. *Acta Orthop Scand*. 2001;72(3):299–303.

163. Matsiko A, Levingstone TJ, O'Brien FJ, et al. Addition of hyaluronic acid improves cellular infiltration and promotes early-stage chondrogenesis in a collagen-based scaffold for cartilage tissue engineering. *J Mech Behav Biomed Mater*. 2012;11:41–52.

164. Zhu H, Mitsuhashi N, Klein A, et al. The role of the hyaluronan receptor CD44 in mesenchymal stem cell migration in the extracellular matrix. *Stem Cells*. 2006;24(4):928–935.

165. Succar P, Medynskyj M, Breen EJ, et al. Priming adipose-derived mesenchymal stem cells with hyaluronan alters growth kinetics and increases attachment to articular cartilage. *Stem Cells Int*. 2016;2016:9364213.

166. Roseti L, Serra M, Tigani D, et al. Cell manipulation in autologous chondrocyte implantation: from research to cleanroom. *Chir Organi Mov*. 2008;91(3):147–151.

167. Halme DG, Kessler DA. FDA regulation of stem-cell-based therapies. *N Engl J Med*. 2006;355(16):1730–1735.

168. Cyranoski D. FDA's claims over stem cells upheld. *Nature*. 2012;488(7409):14.

169. Zarembinski TI, Tew WP, Atzet SK. The use of a hydrogel matrix as a cellular delivery vehicle in future cell-based therapies: biological and nonbiological considerations. In: Eberli D, ed. *Regenerative medicine and tissue engineering—cells and biomaterials*. InTech; 2011.

170. Kim N, Cho SG. Clinical applications of mesenchymal stem cells. *Korean J Intern Med*. 2013;28(4):387–402.

171. Crisan M, Yap S, Casteilla L, et al. A perivascular origin for mesenchymal stem cells in multiple human organs. *Cell Stem Cell*. 2008;3(3):301–313.

172. Oberbauer E, Steffenhagen C, Wurzer C, et al. Enzymatic and non-enzymatic isolation systems for adipose tissue-derived cells: current state of the art. *Cell Regen (Lond)*. 2015;4:7. doi:10.1186/s13619-015-0020-0

173. Wyles CC, Houdek MT, Crespo-Diaz RJ, et al. Adipose-derived mesenchymal stem cells are phenotypically superior for regeneration in the setting of osteonecrosis of the femoral head. *Clin Orthop Relat Res*. 2015;473(10):3080–3090.

174. Schmitt A, van Griensven M, Imhoff AB, et al. Application of stem cells in orthopedics. *Stem Cells Int*. 2012;2012:394962.

175. van der Valk J, Brunner D, De Smet K, et al. Optimization of chemically defined cell culture media–replacing fetal bovine serum in mammalian in vitro methods. *Toxicol in Vitro*. 2010;24(4):1053–1063.

176. Lange C, Cakiroglu F, Spiess AN, et al. Accelerated and safe expansion of human mesenchymal stromal cells in animal serum-free medium for transplantation and regenerative medicine. *J Cell Physiol*. 2007;213(1):18–26.

177. Müller I, Kordowich S, Holzwarth C, et al. Animal serum-free culture conditions for isolation and expansion of multipotent mesenchymal stromal cells from human BM. *Cytotherapy*. 2006;8(5):437–444.

178. Ng F, Boucher S, Koh S, et al. PDGF, TGF-beta, and FGF signaling is important for differentiation and growth of mesenchymal stem cells (MSCs): transcriptional profiling can identify markers and signaling pathways important in differentiation of MSCs into adipogenic, chondrogenic, and osteogenic lineages. *Blood*. 2008;112(2):295–307.

179. Xie X, Wang Y, Zhao C, et al. Comparative evaluation of MSCs from bone marrow and adipose tissue seeded in PRP-derived scaffold for cartilage regeneration. *Biomaterials*. 2012;33(29):7008–7018.

180. Rose RA, Jiang H, Wang X, et al. Bone marrow-derived mesenchymal stromal cells express cardiac-specific markers, retain the stromal phenotype, and do not become functional cardiomyocytes in vitro. *Stem Cells*. 2008;26(11):2884–2892.

CHAPTER 12

HARVESTING TECHNIQUES OF BONE MARROW AND ADIPOSE FOR STEM CELL PROCEDURES

Jay E. Bowen, Raisa Bakshiyev, and Sony M. Issac

A detailed medical evaluation including history of the present condition, medications/supplements, medical/surgical problems, social history, functional status/limitations, physical examination, and diagnostic testing is first necessary to determine an appropriate treatment plan, which may include regenerative treatment options. Considerations need to be made regarding optimizing the health and function of the patient and site for treatment (pre-habilitation), the treatment tissue to be used, best donor site(s), technical aspects of acquisition and deployment of the cells, and posttreatment rehabilitation. Cell therapies for musculoskeletal conditions encompass many issues including ethical and regulatory, which cannot be overlooked.

Mesenchymal stem cells (MSCs) isolated from adipose tissue (AT) or bone marrow (BM) have the potential for multipotency and have been shown to be readily expandable in vitro. AT and BM can be obtained through minimally invasive techniques and can differentiate toward osteogenic, adipogenic, myogenic, chondrogenic, and neurogenic lineages. In order to expand BM, one does not need enzymes or washing. Expansion takes time and is considered more than minimal manipulation, and thus is not approved by the U.S. Food and Drug Administration (FDA) (1).

Autologous cells are derived from the host themselves, whereas allogenic are derived from a related or unrelated matched donor (2). Use of autologous cells enables the avoidance of ethical concerns and graft versus host reactions. The FDA does not allow for more than minimal manipulation of cells or cell expansion as the practice of medicine. BM is a cellular product that can be separated, whereas the separation of adipose, which is a structured tissue, would be considered more than minimal manipulation. Products that are considered to be the results of a process requiring more than minimal manipulation would be required to go through the official FDA process, and thus in lipoaspirate, the stromal vascular fraction (SVF), which is composed of adipose stromal cells, hematopoietic stem cells, and progenitor cells, if manipulated, is considered a drug by the FDA (2). Debate exists regarding whether the method by which cells are obtained, processed, and implanted can stress the cell and ultimately the viability impacting therapeutic outcome.

When deciding on the method by which to obtain the cells, the use of local anesthetic agents can affect cell viability (3–5). Cell properties are also believed to be an important characteristic. In addition to being progenitor cells, additional effects such as paracrine, angiogenesis potential, proliferation ability, resistance to apoptosis, and potential to enhance repair have been described (6).

The stem cell source to use for treatment has also been debated. It has been stated that BM contains a fewer number of cells than AT. The magnitude of difference depends on comparisons such as bone aspirate versus concentration with lipoaspiration versus SVF and many studies expanded cells. MSCs are 0.01% to 0.001% of all nucleated cells (NC) in bone marrow aspirate (BMA), that is, 1/10,000 or 1/100,000. After centrifugation, the NC fraction concentrates by about 20 times, resulting in 1/500 to 1/5,000 MSCs in the sample, but the volume has been reduced from 100 mL. This would be about 0.2% to 0.02% bone marrow (BM)-MSCs. Adipose derived (AD)-MSCs are about 1% to 4% of all the NCs in SVF. Therefore, there is a 20 to 50 times difference. Strem noted ADSC yield was approximately 5,000 CFU-F/g of AT compared to about 100 to 1,000 CFU-F/mL of BM, which is a 5 to 50 times difference (7). These are in contrast to some noting a 1,000-fold difference (8–11). However, BM is usually limited by available volume, whereas adipose stores are larger and have less limitation. Additionally, it is unlikely that the sole benefit is from the MSC, but the potpourri of cells in the injectate. The optimal cell or cells and ratios have yet to be determined.

HISTORY OF BM

Trepanning is one of the oldest known medical procedures, dating back 8,000 to 10,000 years. It was originally performed in the skull to relieve headaches, mental illness, and intracranial pressure (12). Pianese in Italy first harvested BM in 1903 for diagnostic reasons by puncturing the epiphysis of a femur, describing a case of anemia. In 1922, Morris and Falconer introduced BM tibial biopsy using a drill-like instrument. A Russian physician, Anirkin, then published his results of 103 BM biopsies, citing that it stimulated BM activity. In 1950, Rubenstein and Bierman suggested the iliac crest as a BM source, as the sternum was used most often prior to this. Multiple needle advancements were made to aid in the ease of obtaining aspirate and Wakitani et al. expanded MSCs from BM to treat knee osteoarthrosis (OA) in 2002 (13).

Indications for BM Evaluation

Reasons for obtaining BM aspirate may include unexplained anemia, evaluation of iron stores and metabolism, evaluation of leukopenia, thrombocytopenia, or pancytopenia. Additionally, BM biopsies are used to diagnose or stage lymphoma or leukemia, or for confirmation of matched BM in potential allogenic hematopoietic cell donor. Furthermore, BM-derived MSCs have multipotent potential in regenerative medicine with the ability to differentiate into various cell types such as hepatocytes, pancreatocytes, vascular endothelial cells, adipocytes, and osteocytes, among others (14).

Risks of Procurement of BM Aspirate and Treatment

Fortunately, a graft versus host reaction does not exist in an autologous sample and the issue is raised only if there is an allogenic donor. Other potential complications from obtaining a BM aspirate are developing anemia, causing a hematoma, infection, or fracture. The most common complaint related to BM aspiration is pain at the extraction site, which may last up to several days.

Pain may occur from the procedure either from inadequate local anesthesia or negative pressure within the cavity on aspiration. Additional factors include patient's anticipatory anxiety, long procedure duration, procedure difficulty, and the technician's previous BM aspiration experience (15). Education of the patient can minimize anxiety. Grønkjaer et al. reported that

BM specimen quality was better with the "R-technique," a quick pull of the syringe, causing high differential pressure for the duration of the aspiration lasting about 1 second, but was less painful with the "S-technique" which is a slow, low differential pressure technique, and uniform pull of the 10 mL syringe, aspirating for 5 to 15 seconds (16). There is debate on whether one should be gentle to minimize bleeding or pain versus causing microinjury to mobilize more cells potentially causing trauma and more bleeding.

Considering a posterior iliac approach to the pelvis, anatomical structures such as the sciatic nerve, cluneal nerve, lumbar nerve roots, superior gluteal vessels, or the sacroiliac joint can be compromised so one should be familiar with the relevant anatomy (17) (Figure 12.1 A–E). Hernigou et al. noted only eight marrow aspiration (18) complications in 1,800 patient procedures via a parallel approach to the iliac tables, which is reassuring (Figure 12.2). However, an additional study by Hernigou noted 410 cadaveric trocar entries (parallel in various sectors) with 114 medial or lateral table breaches (28%) which are concerning (20). There is a greater risk of complications from this approach if the

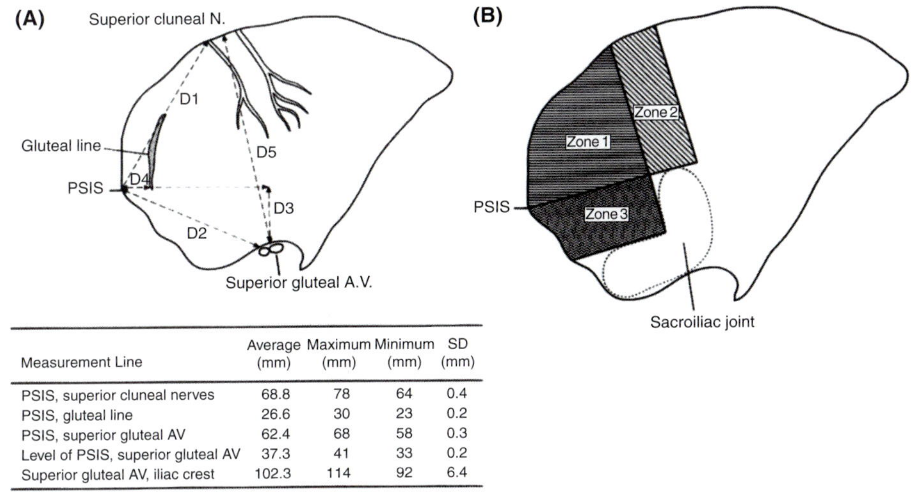

Measurement Line	Average (mm)	Maximum (mm)	Minimum (mm)	SD (mm)
PSIS, superior cluneal nerves	68.8	78	64	0.4
PSIS, gluteal line	26.6	30	23	0.2
PSIS, superior gluteal AV	62.4	68	58	0.3
Level of PSIS, superior gluteal AV	37.3	41	33	0.2
Superior gluteal AV, iliac crest	102.3	114	92	6.4

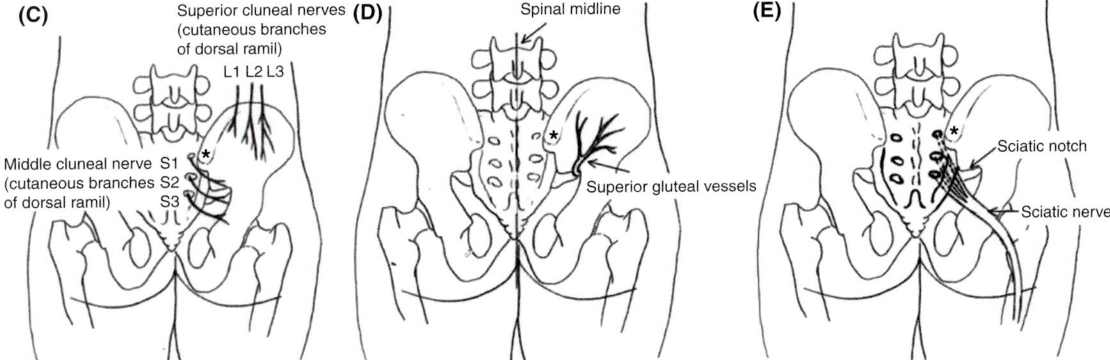

FIGURE 12.1: Measurements from landmarks to vital structures in the posterior pelvis. (A) Anatomic considerations for posterior iliac bone harvesting (19); (B) Schematic representation of the zone dividing the posterior iliac region. Anatomic considerations for posterior iliac bone harvesting (19). (C) The superficial sensory branches represented (17). (D) The path of the vessels is represented (17). (E) The sciatic nerve path is represented (17).

AV, artery and vein; PSIS, posterior superior iliac spine; SD, standard deviation.

Source: Parts A and B from Ref. (19); Parts C–E from Ref. (17).

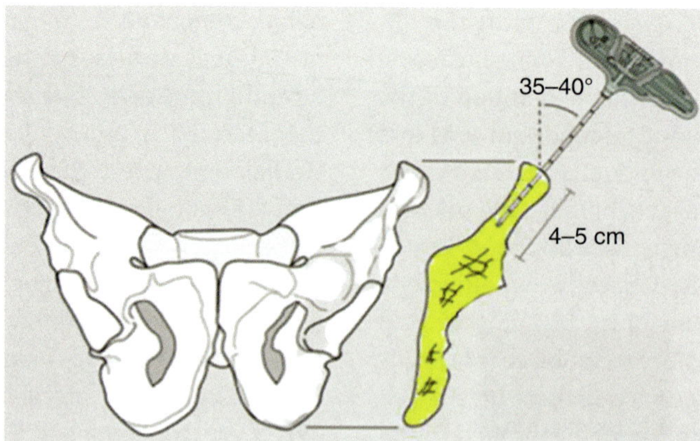

FIGURE 12.2: Trocar introduced between the two tables of the illium. The yellow is a cross section of the pelvis demonstrating the angle needed for a trocar to enter the bone marrow cavity via a parallel approach between the iliac tables.

Source: From Ref. (20). Hernigou J, Alves A, Homma Y, et al. Anatomy of the ilium for bone marrow aspiration: map of sectors and implication for safe trocar placement. *Int Orthop*. 2014;38(12):2585–2590. doi:10.1007/s00264-014-2353-7, with permission of Springer.

practitioner is inexperienced or the patient is obese (body mass index >30). Bain et al. carried out a survey of BM biopsies done by hematologists. Adverse events associated with perpendicular BM biopsy totaled 26 out of 54,890 biopsies (Figure 12.3). The most serious and frequent event was hemorrhage in 14 patients. The risk factor associated with hemorrhage was most often associated with aspirin use, or an underlying myeloproliferative disorder, or both. There was one death from hemorrhage, felt to be attributable to the procedure (21). An additional risk is potential allergy to medications. And the final, and potentially most important point to make, is the risk of obtaining dead cells, because the therapy will not be effective no matter how careful and meticulous the treatment deployment is.

When considering use of anesthesia, it should be noted that although most procedures would be performed with the use of local anesthetic, there are levels of toxicity. For example, a maximum dose of lidocaine is 4.5 mg/kg, up to 300 mg lidocaine without epinephrine, or 7 mg/kg or 500 mg lidocaine with epinephrine. (Depending on the reference chosen, the maximum recommended volume would be between 32 mL and 45 mL of 1% lidocaine without

epinephrine in a 70 kg male (22,23) (Tables 12.1 and 12.2).

There is no concern with cell toxicity and death when obtaining BM, because the anesthetic is outside of the BM cavity. However, with lipoaspirate, anesthetic is infiltrated into the AT; thus it can have negative effects if residual anesthetic is left when the treatment is deployed. As little as 0.03% lidocaine can have a negative effect on adipose-derived stem cells (ASC). Toxicity has been demonstrated in tenofibroblasts, chondrocytes, and human MSCs (24–29). When preparing tumescent (typically 500 mL of injectable saline, 25 mL of 2% lidocaine, 2 ampules of epinephrine 1:1,000, and 10 mL of 8.4% sodium bicarbonate), it is recommended to use 35 mg/kg of lidocaine with lidocaine concentration of 0.8 mg/mL or less to avoid cytotoxicity of the adipose graft. Breu et al. studied local anesthetic cytotoxic effects on MSCs and found that exposure to higher concentrations of bupivacaine, ropivacaine, and mepivacaine caused a decline in viable cells. Additionally, the number of apoptotic cells increased 96 hours after treatment with all the three groups of anesthetics; however, there was no difference after exposure to saline through 1 week after treatment. One can consider a regional nerve block to make the

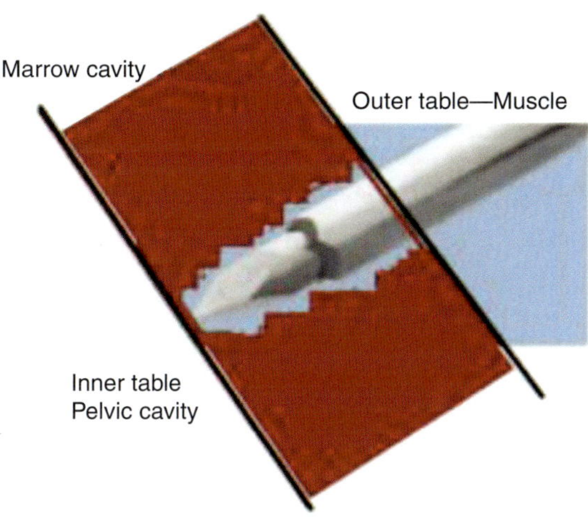

FIGURE 12.3: The trocar is entering the marrow cavity via a perpendicular approach through the outer table and stopped at the inner table.

Source: Reprinted from Ref. (11). Bowen JE. Technical issues in harvesting and concentrating stem cells (bone marrow and adipose). *PMR*. 2015;7(4 Suppl):S8–S18, with permission from Elsevier.

TABLE 12.1 **Toxic Dosages of Various Local Anesthetics**

Agent	Minimum Toxic Dose (mg/kg)
Procaine	19.2
Tetracaine	2.5
Chloroprocaine	22.8
Lidocaine	6.4
Mepivacaine	9.8
Bupivacaine	1.6
Etidocaine	3.4

Source: Reprinted with permission from Ref. (22). Goldfrank LR, Flomenbaum NE, Lewin NA, Weisman RS, eds. Goldfrank's Toxicologic Emergencies. 6th ed. New York, NY: McGraw-Hill; 1998:897–903. https://www.mhprofessional.com/catalogsearch/result/?q=goldfrank%27s McGraw-Hill Education.

procedure be as comfortable as possible. Overall, ropivacaine appears to the least toxic anesthetic (30). One can also consider nitrous oxide analgesic, but the effects on cells or on healing are unknown.

Consent, Preparation, and Testing

As with any procedure, informed consent is mandatory. Patients occasionally are anxious about a BM biopsy, more so than lipoaspiration. The written consent should include the patient's name, date, time, institution, name of procedure, name of practioner(s) involved, risks, benefits, alternative procedures and treatment, statement stating the procedure was explained and that the patient had opportunity to ask questions, signatures of the patient or guardian, witness, and name of person explaining the procedure (11). One should consider an additional statement stating that this is not the standard of care and is experimental, if applicable. Risks including hematoma, infection, or fracture (higher risk in patients with osteoporosis) should be discussed. With regard to lipoaspiration, the occurrence of soft tissue deformities is an additional potential risk.

Once it is determined that the procedure should be performed, the patient should be counseled that use of nonsteroidal anti-inflammatory medications should be stopped at least 5 days prior to the procedure (31). Additionally, corticosteroids have been found to have a

TABLE 12.2 Officially Recommended Highest Doses of Local Anesthetics in Various Countries

	Finland	Germany	Japan	Sweden	United States (mg)
2-Chloroprocaine	–	–	–	–	800
With epinephrine	–	–	1,000 mg	–	1,000
Procaine	–	500 mg	600 mg (epidural)	–	500
With epinephrine	–	600 mg	–	–	–
Articaine	7 mg/kg	4 mg/kg	–	–	–
With epinephrine	7 mg/kg	4 mg/kg	–	–	–
Bupivacaine	175 mg (200 mg![a]) (400 mg/24 h)	150 mg	100 mg (epidural)	150 mg	175
With epinephrine	175 mg	150 mg	–	150 mg	225
Levobupivacaine	150 mg (400 mg/24 h)	150 mg	–	150 mg	150
With epinephrine	–	–	–	–	–
Lidocaine	200 mg	200 mg	200 mg	200 mg	300
With epinephrine	500 mg	500 mg	–	500 mg	500
Mepivacaine	–	300 mg	400 mg (epidural)	350 mg	400
With epinephrine	–	500 mg	–	350 mg	550
Prilocaine	400 mg	–	–	400 mg	–
With epinephrine	600 mg	–	–	600 mg	–
Ropivacaine	225 mg (300 mg![a]) (800 mg/24 h)	No mention	200 mg (epidural) 300 mg (infiltr)	225 mg	225 (300 mg![a])
With epinephrine	225 mg	No mention	–	225 mg	225 (300 mg![a])

[a]For brachial plexus block in adults.

Source: Reprinted with permission from Ref. (23). Rosenberg PH, Veering BT, Urmey WF. Maximum recommended doses of local anesthetics: a multifactorial concept. *Reg Anesth Pain Med.* 2004;29(6):564–575; discussion 524. http://journals.lww.com/rapm/Abstract/2004/11000/Maximum_Recommended_Doses_of_Local_Anesthetics__A.10.aspx.

negative impact on tissues, even with one-time injection or with the use of inhaled steroids for asthma, even though it was once thought they were not systemic (32,33). The procedure should be delayed for at least 8 weeks after a steroid injection and use of inhaled steroids should be discontinued, if possible, prior to the procedure. Furthermore, the U.S. FDA published a labeling alert in July 2016 regarding the black box warning of increased risk of tendinitis and tendon rupture associated with fluroquinolones (34). Concerns have also been raised regarding the effect of proton pump inhibitors and hydroxymethylglutaryl (HMG)-CoA reductase inhibitors on in vitro stem cell growth. HMG-CoA reductase inhibitors do inhibit angiogenesis (35), thus supplementation with coenzyme Q-10 should be considered (36).

The need for baseline laboratory testing has not been determined. A baseline hemoglobin and hematocrit should be considered if harvest of a high volume of aspirate is planned. One may also consider obtaining prothrombin time/partial thromboplastin time (PT/PTT) and hemoglobin A1C. Diabetes may attenuate the aspiration of cells (37,38). There is evidence that abnormal hemoglobin A1C levels will lead to poorer outcomes. Despite some recommendations for infectious disease testing (hepatitis panel and HIV), this is not necessary for an autologous treatment. Pharmaceuticals, especially multiple medications, or poor diet can cause various nutritional deficiencies. Deficiencies can adversely affect tissue healing, which is the goal of regenerative medicine. Thus, screening should include 25-hydroxy vitamin D, albumin, zinc, and free T3, free testosterone, and estradiol (E2) and progesterone in postmenopausal women (39,40). CoQ-10, selenium, RBC-magnesium, and omega fatty acids levels can also be considered.

Contraindications to BM

When considering BM aspiration, one should be aware of the contraindications to the procedure, which include infection at the graft site, hemophilia or decimated intravascular coagulopathy, and related bleeding disorders. If someone is on anticoagulants, the risk of thrombosis by stopping these medications outweighs the risk of bleeding (41). This should be discussed between the patient and the treating physician who prescribed the medication.

BONE MARROW ASPIRATE PROCEDURE

Anatomy

Understanding anatomy is critical for risk minimization, comfort, efficiency, quality of aspirate, and efficacy of treatment. The anatomy of the ilium is well described in anatomical and surgical textbooks. The BM is located between sinusoids of spongy bone, and the porous bone organized into honeycomb trabecular bone (Figure 12.4). At birth, all of the BM is red and as one ages, the red marrow converts to yellow, eventually all converting to fat. BM contains mature NCs, erythrocytes, serum from peripheral blood, hematopoietic marrow, adipocytes from fatty marrow, endothelial cells, and osteogenic progenitor cells. BM aspirate has higher cell concentration closer to the torso of the body, and MSC concentration diminishes quickly toward the extremities. The quantity and concentration of MSCs in BM diminishes from proximal to distal within each structure. The iliac crest has the highest yield of osteogenic progenitor cells compared to the distal tibia or calcaneus, with no significant difference between the tibia

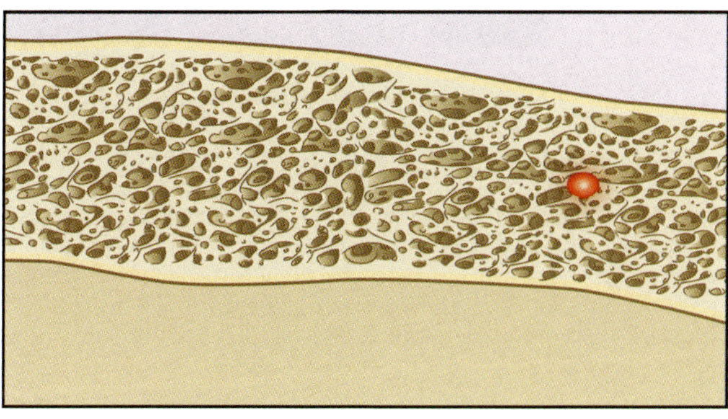

FIGURE 12.4: Honeycomb of trabecular bone.

and the calcaneus (42). Marx et al. reported the yield of total NCs was equal between the posterior and anterior ilium, and more than twice than from the tibial plateau (43).

In regard to BM aspiration, the iliac crest has been divided into six different zones known as "sectors" as described by Hernigou et al. in order to help avoid neurovascular structures (18) (Figure 12.5 A,B). These sectors can be easily drawn between the anterior and posterior superior iliac spines, dividing the iliac crest into six equal sectors. Ninety-four breaches were observed in 480 parallel entry points, and higher risks were identified in thinner sectors of bone, in obese patients, and with less experienced surgeons. The thickest portions of the iliac crest were more posterior, especially in sectors 5 and 6. In sector 1 entries, there was one patient out of 40 who had a lateral femoral cutaneous nerve injury and secondary numbness, and two patients had a hematoma. The risk of a 10 cm trocar reaching the external iliac artery was found to occur when the trocar deviated more than 20° on average; however, this value was different according to sector used and gender (Figure 12.5C). The average distance between the sciatic notch and the iliac crest is 56.6 mm minimally and averages at 70 mm, according to Hernigou's research. This distance varies based on gender and the size of the patient. Thus, if using a parallel approach from the posterior ilium, one may reach the sciatic nerve and the superior gluteal artery (Figure 12.1A,B).

The risk of adverse events, such as bleeding or perforation through the tables of the ilium, appears to be directly related to the anatomy of the ilium. For example, if using an 8-gauge trocar, one cannot safely insert the trocar in the iliac wing where the minimum thickness can be less than 3 mm (Figure 12.6).

Knowledge of the anatomy is crucial in avoiding potential complications such as neural injury (i.e., sciatic nerve injury via posterior approach or lateral femoral cutaneous nerve via anterior approach) and hematoma (resulting from puncture of the external iliac or superior gluteal arteries), as described previously (18).

Equipment and Procedure

Standard procedure supplies for an aseptic technique are obtained. Aseptic technique typically

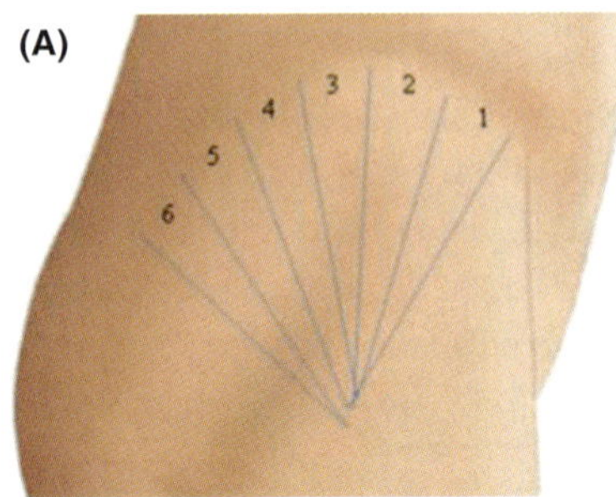

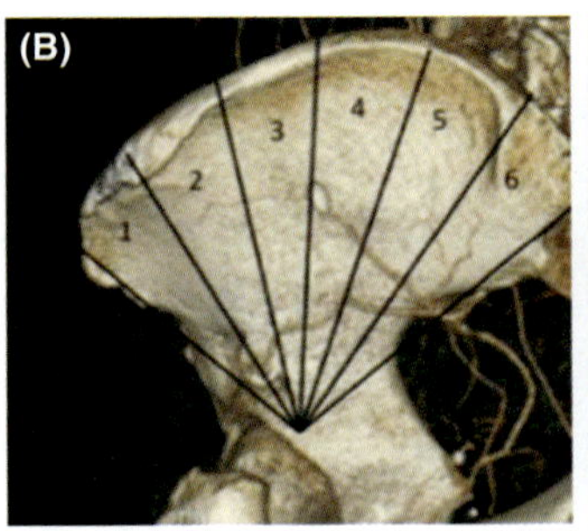

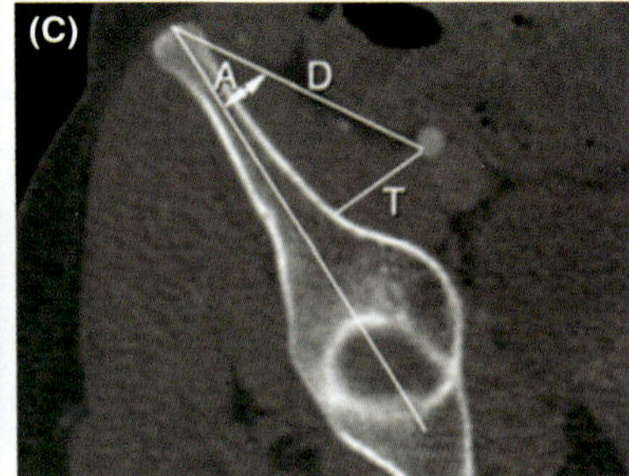

FIGURE 12.5: (A) The corresponding sectors can be found and marked on the patient by using the same technique and correspond in clinical practice to different zones of bone marrow aspiration according to the position of the patient. Three different approaches can be used to harvest bone marrow from the iliac crest: patient supine and anterior crest approach (sectors 1, 2, and 3), patient prone and posterior iliac crest approach (sectors 4, 5, and 6), and patient in the left or right lateral position allowing easier middle iliac crest approach (sectors 3 and 4). (B) The iliac wing (three-dimensional reconstruction) was divided by drawing lines from equidistant points spaced along the rim of the iliac crest to the center of the hip. These lines were approximately perpendicular to the curve of the iliac crest. Six sectors were defined by these lines. Sectors 1 and 2 anterior part of the iliac bone, sectors 3 and 4 center part of the iliac bone, sectors 5 and 6 posterior part of the iliac bone. (C) Radial CT cut of the ilium, showing (A) angle from Iliac bone to external iliac vessel.

Source: Part (B) from Ref. (18). Hernigou J, Picard L, Alves A, et al. Understanding bone safety zones during bone marrow aspiration from the iliac crest: the sector rule. *Int Orthop.* 2014;38(11):2377–2384, with permission of Springer.

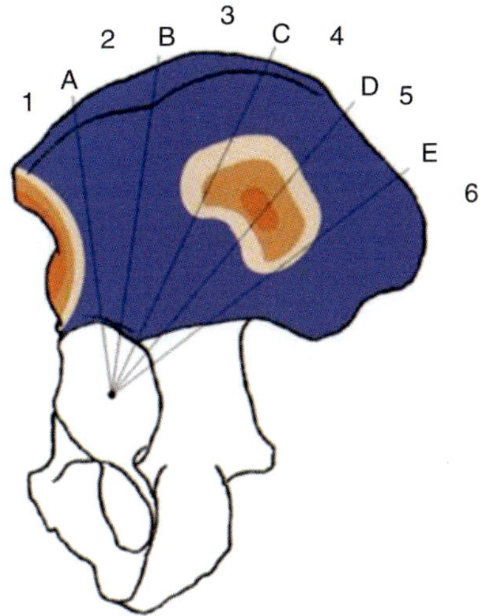

FIGURE 12.6: Map of the ilium. The blue zone is the part of the ilium where the thickness of the spongiousus bone is always >3 mm. The yellow area corresponds to the zone wherein 50% cases of the thickness is <3 mm but >2 mm. The orange area corresponds to the zone wherein 25% cases of the thickness is <2 mm but >1 mm. The red area corresponds to the zone wherein 20% cases of the thickness is <1 mm. The yellow, orange, and red zones are in sectors 1, 4, and 5. Line A is the border between sectors 1 and 2 and line B the border between sectors 2 and 3, and so forth.

Source: From Ref. (20). Hernigou J, Alves A, Homma Y, et al. Anatomy of the ilium for bone marrow aspiration: map of sectors and implication for safe trocar placement. *Int Orthop*. 2014;38(12):2585–2590. doi:10.1007/s00264-014-2353-7, with permission of Springer.

involves the use of sterile gloves and equipment to prevent the spread of pathogens during a procedure. Clean technique uses hand hygiene and non-sterile clean gloves to minimize exposure (44). Additionally, oxygen, a pulse-oximeter monitor, a crash cart, and defibrillator need to be accessible to manage a complication if it occurs. Chlorhexidine–alcohol solution is better than povidone–iodine (Betadine) (45) for superficial incisional and deep incisional infections. After the agent has dried, there are continued antibacterial effects. Standard procedure should also include a face mask, hair cap, sterile gloves, and drapes or towels. If ultrasound is being used, a sterile transducer condom can be applied.

A procedure tray should include an 18-gauge needle to draw up the medication, a 27-gauge ×

1.25 inch needle for a skin wheal, a 22-gauge × 2.75 inch needle for anesthetizing the deeper tissues and periosteum, a 10 mL syringe, syringes for the BM (10 or 30 mL), Luer-lock syringe caps, gauze, a needle stick pad, and a bag(s) to transport the BM sample if needed. Additional supplies include ice packs, sterile 2 × 2 gauze squares and a transparent occlusive dressing cover.

Medications include 1% lidocaine without epinephrine, 50% dextrose, sodium bicarbonate, normal saline solution, and heparin (20,000 units/mL × 2 and 10,000 IU/mL × 1). Additionally, a 1,000 IU/mL solution of heparin should be made to rinse the aspirating trocar and syringes prior to initiating the procedure. Tumescent anesthetic (i.e., 250 mL of injectable saline, 10 mL of 2% lidocaine, 1 ampule of epinephrine 1:1,000, and 5 mL of 8.4% sodium bicarbonate) can be considered as it is better tolerated, faster onset of action, and reduces bleeding.

The patient should be positioned prone on firm surface, the table should have a head cutout, and a pulse-oximeter should be worn (Figure 12.7). A firm surface is especially necessary if using axial force with a manual trocar. The needle placement for optimal harvest site is confirmed with imaging to assist in anesthetizing the skin and periosteum of the desired entry sites (Figure 12.8). When deciding on imaging choice, fluoroscopy or ultrasound can be used.

A fluoroscopic image can be used for initial scout view, followed by 20° to 30° of ipsilateral oblique and caudal tilt to visualize the ilium, iliac crest, and posterior superior iliac spine (PSIS). A radiopaque marker identifies the area 1 cm lateral to the PSIS, and a hub view is obtained once the needle is inserted (Figure 12.9A) for perpendicular approach. A skin wheal of local anesthetic is placed over the harvest site. Only one skin entry site should be necessary. The addition of sodium bicarbonate will normalize the pH to reduce the burning sensation (46). One potential safety feature of a perpendicular approach is, on entering the marrow cavity from the outer table, the inner table can temporarily stop the needle from entering the pelvic cavity. In the parallel method, bone contact can more readily be lost.

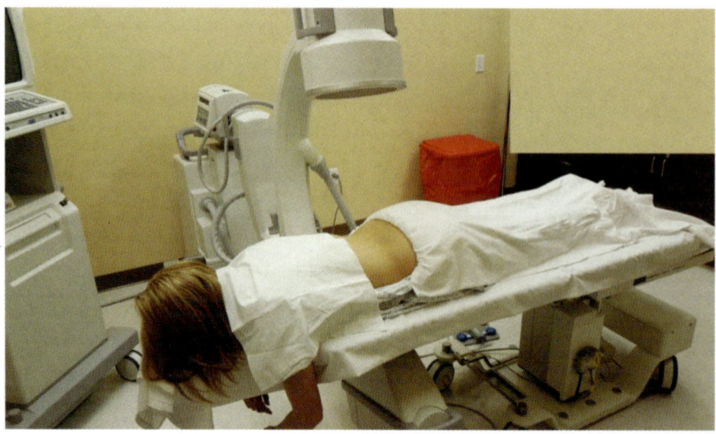

FIGURE 12.7: General prone positioning of patient on fluoroscopic table with face in a table cut out. The patient may have nasal cannula with oxygen in place, blood pressure cuff on the arm, and pulse oximeter on the finger.

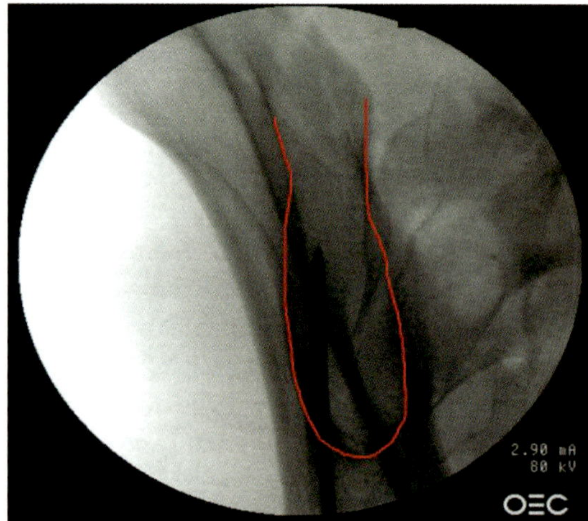

FIGURE 12.8: Fluoroscopic image of the left posterior ilium with outline of the medial and lateral borders in red and the inferior portion being the PSIS. The needle is lying on the skin with the tip marking the entry site. Positioning for imaging and access to the left iliac crest cephalad to the PSIS. The physician is on the ipsilateral side with fluoroscope providing a contralateral oblique at about 20° to 30°.

PSIS, posterior superior iliac spine.

One should not start superolateral to the PSIS to avoid cluneal nerve injury or too inferior to the PSIS to avoid injury to the superior gluteal vessels. To guide the parallel approach, the fluoroscope is moved 20° contralateral (Figure 12.9B). A hub view of the needle will be used to anesthetize and aspirate.

If using ultrasound, the transducer depends on body habitus. Namely, a linear probe can be used for thinner individuals, whereas a curvilinear probe may be necessary if greater depth is needed for osseous imaging. The procedure may be ultrasound guided for a perpendicular or parallel approach to the PSIS, or ultrasound assisted for a parallel approach. In a parallel approach (Figure 12.10A), the PSIS is marked, the width of iliac crest should be taken into account, and about 4 cm anterolateral from the PSIS entering though the skin markings. For an ultrasound-assisted parallel approach, the PSIS, medial and lateral iliac wing are marked on the skin, but there is no direct visualization of the trocar from skin to bone (Figure 12.10B). For a perpendicular approach with ultrasound (Figure 12.10C), the medial part of the probe is placed on the PSIS and the lateral portion points toward the greater trochanter (Figure 12.11A,B). The needle is then inserted from lateral to medial about 1 cm to 2 cm from the iliac crest for marrow entry and can be adjusted to obtain cells from additional sites. Similar to when using fluoroscopy, one potential safety feature of a perpendicular approach is the ability to use the inner table to prevent entry into the pelvic cavity.

When deciding on the aspiration tool, a manual or a mechanical device can be used. If using a powered rotatory device, a specialized needle fits into the battery-powered handle. The

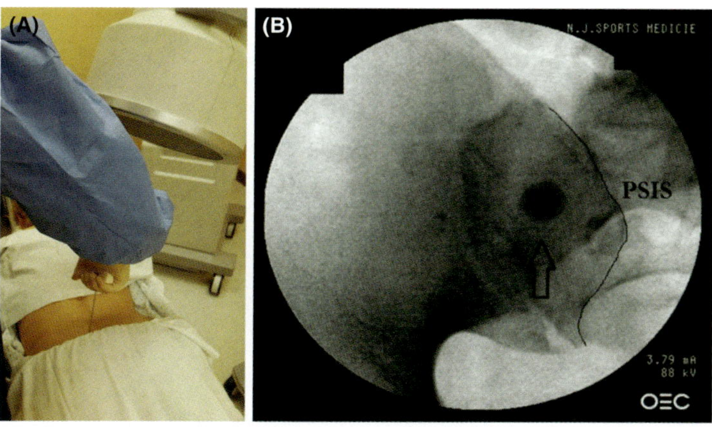

FIGURE 12.9: (A and B) Left pelvis with outline of the medial aspect of the ilium/PSIS (posterior superior iliac spine) and arrow identifying the bone marrow aspirating needle "hub view" for a perpendicular approach. The "hub view" is when the needle and fluoroscopic x-rays are parallel so only the end of the needle can be identified.

PSIS, posterior superior iliac spine.

Source: Reprinted from Ref. (11). Bowen JE. Technical issues in harvesting and concentrating stem cells (bone marrow and adipose). *PMR*. 2015;7(4 Suppl): S8–18, with permission from Elsevier.

rotatory device needle will typically not lose contact as readily as a manual trephine needle (i.e., Jamshidi, a T-handle BMA needle) because limited axial focus is required affording better control. If decided to use a manual trephine needle, the diamond tip is better for preventing loss of bone contact (Figure 12.12). When entering the bone, firm pressure must be applied and 180° of rotation should be used, alternating 90° clockwise and counterclockwise. An option to aid in manual marrow cavity entrance is use of a mallet, which can afford better control. This can be performed by one individual or one can hold the needle, while another person taps the aspirating needle with the mallet. As rotatory devices require less axial force a smaller, 15-gauge needle can be used. This reduces procedure time and the chance of sliding on the iliac crest (47). There is less morbidity with an 11-gauge rotatory needle versus an 11-gauge manual needle, so a 15-gauge needle with rotatory device should afford even less issues. Berenson et al. studied 102 patients who underwent either a powered BM biopsy versus a manual method and found that while pain was not different between the groups, the powered group experienced a shorter procedural time and the aspirate volume was greater. One must be careful to take care not to wrap one's glove

or the patient's skin around the rotating biopsy needle, as these were the only two complications in the drill-powered bone biopsy group (47). Additionally, there appears to be less bone fractures with a rotatory device and there is the additional convenience of having depth markings on the drill needle. A rotatory device can also reduce wrist stress on the physician especially in an individual with dense bone where multiple sites are to be aspirated. Rotatory devices are more costly than simple manual needles, their sound can be undesirable for the patient, and one can run into technical issues such as a dead battery, so having a manual needle available should be considered.

When harvesting the aspirate, the perpendicular approach is generally better tolerated than the parallel approach; however, patient tolerance varies between these two approaches, but a parallel approach generally yields a greater cell volume. Additionally, fractures are less likely to occur posteriorly via the PSIS than with an anterior entry (48). If choosing to do the anterior approach, keep in mind that you will be visible and "on stage" for the patient.

The goal of BMA for regenerative treatments is to obtain the greatest number of NCs. In the marrow cavity, the cells are adherent to the trabeculae. The aspiration technique is important to

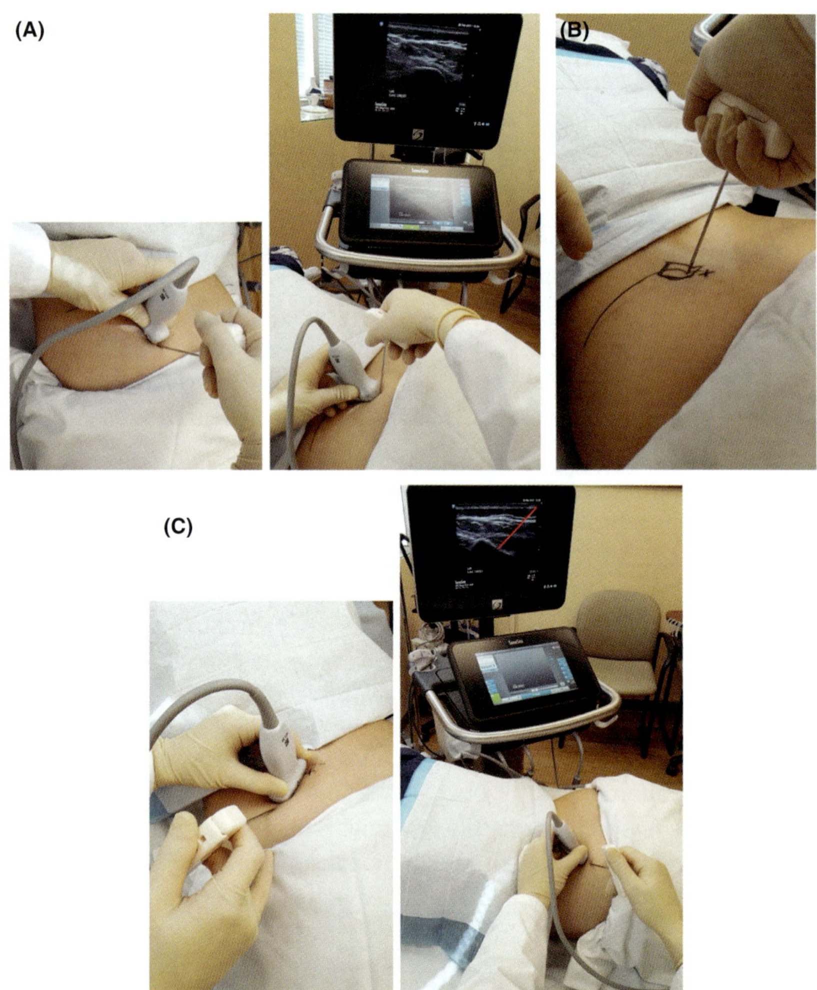

FIGURE 12.10: (A) US-guided entry—parallel. Left image: needle entry and the X mark overlies the PSIS. Right image: needle entry with corresponding US image. (B) Ultrasound assisted—parallel approach. The left iliac crest is outlined. The X overlies the PSIS. The rectangle outlines the medial and lateral portions of the iliac crest. The needle is angled about 30° lateral and 10° to 20° cephalad. (C) Ultrasound-guided entry—perpendicular. Left image: needle entry and the X mark overlies the PSIS. Right image: the red line on the US image denotes the trajectory of the needle.

PSIS, posterior superior iliac spine; US, ultrasound.

maximize the cell yield and minimize the peripheral blood content. Cells need to be harvested from multiple sites to maximize return. Muschler et al. noted 2 mL aspiration from each site was sufficient noting that more than this amount caused peripheral blood dilution (49), although others have aspirated 4 mL (50). However, practically, 5 mL to 10 mL per site is acceptable. Hernigou et al. found that 10 mL syringes provided 300% higher MSC concentration than

50 mL syringes (51). Additionally, the aspiration resulted in higher MSC concentration when the syringe was filled to 10% to 20% of its full volume, suggesting that strong negative pressure provides higher-quality harvesting of MSCs, confirming prior studies. Additionally, a smaller syringe can ease with faster aspiration, whereas a larger syringe can result in a slow pull (52). Slow aspiration may ease discomfort, but may limit cell acquisition. Rapid, short duration aspiration

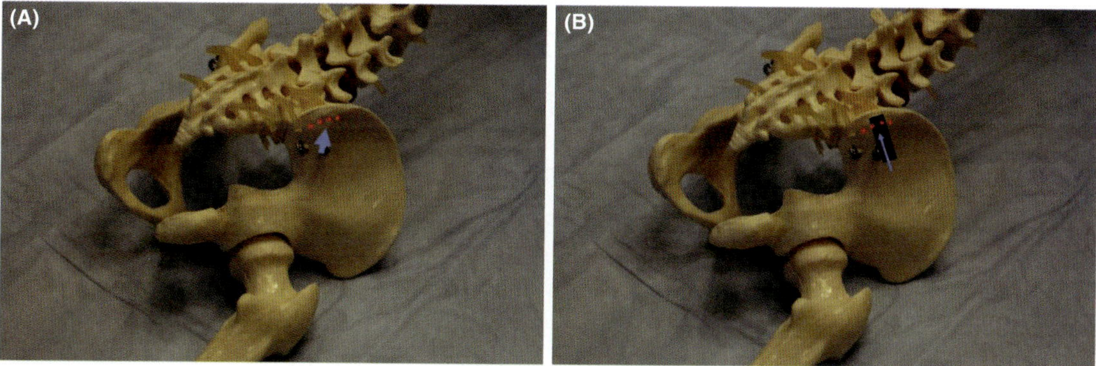

FIGURE 12.11: (A) The osseous entry site in the pelvis for bone marrow aspiration needle via a "perpendicular" approach. The blue arrow represents the needle for aspiration. (B) The black box represents the footprint of the ultrasound probe. The blue arrow represents the needle for aspiration.
Source: Reprinted from Ref. (11). Bowen JE. Technical issues in harvesting and concentrating stem cells (bone marrow and adipose). *PMR.* 2015;7(4 Suppl): S8–18, with permission from Elsevier.

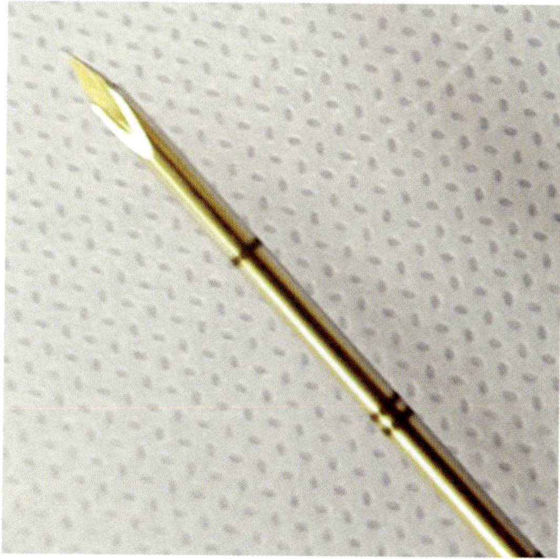

FIGURE 12.12: Diamond needle tip of a bone marrow aspiration trocar.

without sufficient force to cause bubbles is likely optimal to pull cells and minimize peripheral blood while minimizing potential lysis, but this requires additional research.

Postprocedure Care

When the cannula is removed, pressure is applied to the insertion site and a 2 × 2 gauze with or without antibiotic gel with clear occlusive bandage is applied. Ice is applied to the donor site to minimize bleeding and pain and speed recovery; however, ice should not be applied beyond 20 minutes to minimize the risk of thermal injury as local anesthesia was administered. The area should be kept clean and dry for 24 hours with no soaking in a hot tub, pool, or bath for 3 days. Written instructions can be provided to assist in achieving compliance. If there is donor site pain, discharge, erythema, chills, sweating, or fever, this should prompt the patient to return so the area can be inspected for infection. Rehydration should be encouraged and strenuous activity or heavy lifting should be avoided for 5 to 6 hours.

Factors Affecting BM Stem Cell Yield From Harvesting Standpoint

Unfortunately, there is little research available regarding what factors improve cell acquisition or are detrimental to viability. It is a common belief that the quantity and concentration of MSCs in BM diminish from proximal to distal within each structure. The iliac crest has the highest yield of osteogenic progenitor cells compared to the distal tibia or calcaneus, with no significant difference between the tibia and the calcaneus (30). Marx et al. reported the yield of total NCs was equal between the posterior and anterior ilium, and more than twice than from the tibial plateau.

In terms of positioning, a lateral decubitus can be more convenient as it aids in ultrasound guidance as well as ease of aspiration due to the effect of gravity. One can consider a prone position for an obese patient. Large volume aspirations can cause blood dilution, which increases the number of mononucleated cells but does not increase the number of MSCs (53) and multiple aspirations from the same site are associated with reduced concentration of NCs and MSCs (54).

Needle size may also have an effect on yield of BM-MSCs. Li et al. found that an end-holed needle had a mean of 11.35 MSC colonies/mL versus side-holed needle with a closed end, which returned a mean of 17.76 MSC colonies/mL (54). Larger core diameter needles were found to be associated with increased cell density of bone aspiration product (55) and generally people use an 11-gauge needle for manual drawing or an 11-gauge or a 15-gauge if using a rotatory device.

Liposuction

Adipose-derived cells have potentially wide-ranging applications to a variety of clinical disorders. There is a growing body of research regarding treatment of degenerative OA. AT and cells have demonstrated safety and clinical efficacy in most patients treated (56).

History of Liposuction

Liposuction was described by Dr. Fournier (the first physician to complete a syringe liposuction) as "a modeling of the contours, a real artistic job of architecture bound to restore the juvenile and harmonic forms of the body by working with the hypodermic fatty tissues." Dr. Martin was the first physician in the United States to complete liposuction in 1982 and in 1984 Drs. Chrisman and Field published the first report. In 1987, Dr. Klein from the United States was the first to use tumescent anesthesia. In 2001, Zuk et al. published on human adipose as stem cells (57).

Contraindications Particular to Lipoaspiration

The majority of data for lipoaspiration is from cosmetic research with the procedure reserved mainly for healthy individuals. Anticoagulants should be discontinued 2 weeks prior to the procedure, so a discussion with the patient's primary care physician and/or cardiologist may be required to determine if this is possible. History should be elicited for herbs and supplements that may affect bleeding. Allergies to any of the medications would necessitate a substitution. Morbid obesity is a relative contraindication, as it has been used in assistance for weight loss management, and can be treated by suction lipoplasty when combined with other procedures (58).

Equipment

Similar to the BMA procedure, oxygen, a pulse-oximeter, crash cart, defibrillator, chlorhexidine alcohol solution, sterile drapes, optional ultrasound transducer, ice packs, gauze, a #11 blade, Luer-Lok caps, 18-gauge needles, 22-gauge × 4 inch and 27-gauge by 1.25 inch needles, a needle stick pad, ice packs, and a transparent occlusive dressing cover are needed. The medications include 1% lidocaine with epinephrine (1:100,000) or tumescent anesthesia mixture, sodium bicarbonate, normal saline, and anticoagulant citrate dextrose solution (ACD-A) (59).

Low Pressure Lipoaspirate Technique

Depending on the location of the adipose harvest donor site, the patient can be prone, supine, or in the lateral decubitus position. Usually fat is obtained from the lower abdomen, lateral gluteal region, medial/lateral thigh, or flank. Padoin et al. found that the greatest number of viable cells are harvested from the lower abdomen followed by the thigh (60). However, Li et al. did not find a statistically significant difference between different donor sites with respect to graft weight and volume after 12 weeks (61). A study by Lim et al. in 2012 failed to find any significant difference in abdominal versus other fat donor sites (62). A study by Small et al. in 2014 found that volume retention in fat grafting for breast reconstruction was not significantly affected by the donor site (63). A study by Choudhery et al. in 2015 noted that there was similar MSC yield, viability, and growth characteristics of samples taken from various sites in a single donor. Additionally, the differentiation capacity was also unaffected when compared to various sites (64). As should be expected, depending on the gender of the patient, adipose will be best harvested in different areas of the body. Using ultrasound imaging can be considered when first learning or in very thin patients to identify the optimal donor site.

The patient is cleansed and draped in the usual aseptic manner. A 27 g needle can be used to provide a superficial skin wheal of tumescent anesthesia at the entry site. A small skin nick is made with an 18-guage needle or scalpel at the anesthetic injection site to provide access through the skin for a blunt tip cannula which delivers the tumescent solution. Usually 180 to 300 mL of tumescent is delivered but generally speaking, the area has to become tense, so a large area will require additional volume. After this is achieved, 15 to 20 minutes are allowed for diffusion and epinephrine to take effect and minimize bleeding.

The pressure of the fluid and epinephrine in the tumescent solution can limit bleeding. Once the time elapses, insert the cannula and make a few passes to distribute the anesthetic and break down the AT, and aspirate into a 20 mL or 60 mL syringe with locking device to maintain the vacuum (Figure 12.13A,B). Repeat the process until 12 to 20 mL of adipose is obtained. Caution should be taken to obtain a moderate volume as dictated by the aspirating cannula's hole size. A sample that is too large may result in non-viability as a result of central necrosis. With a sample that is too small, there is potential for non-viability as a result of oil release, which is toxic to the cell yield. Then the aspirate is transferred from aspiration syringe to an additional syringe(s) via Luer-lok connector for processing.

Doi noted similar cell acquisition from a manual versus automated technique ($7.01 \pm 2.43 \times 10^5$ and $7.02 \pm 1.89 \times 10^5$ cells/mL aspirated AT by the manual and automated method, respectively, from 50 mL aspirate) (65).

There are multiple devices on the market for obtaining an adipose harvest; however, we recommend against their use for a simple low volume (60–100 mL) aspirate, because they could damage the cells and each would require validation.

Processing the Adipose Aspirate

In the United States, the FDA has determined that more than minimal manipulation of a graft or cells is considered a new drug under their purview. Less than minimal manipulation would be under the jurisdiction of each state's Board of Medical Examiners. Some treatments are rendered under a research protocol with institutional review board monitoring. Do not rely on a commercial company or representative's advice without verification. Processing of the initial aspirate is necessary to remove red blood cells and oil that can interfere with healing and can cause procedural pain, reduce total volume, and concentrate the rare occurring cells that will produce the desired healing effect. The final product should be of a volume sufficient to address the targeted disease

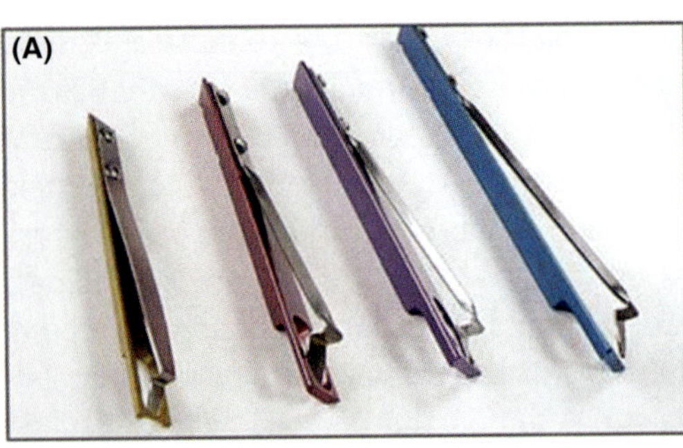
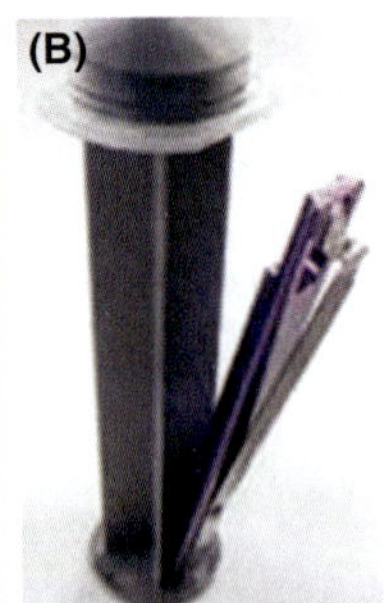
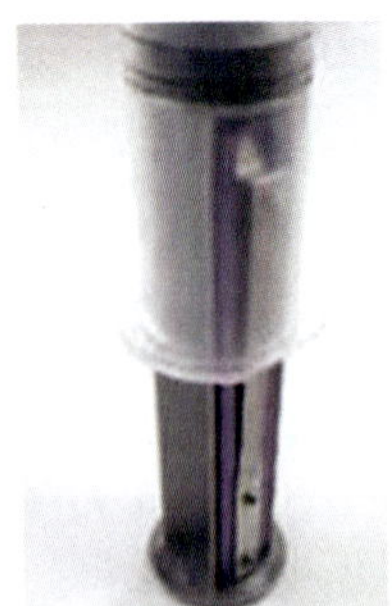
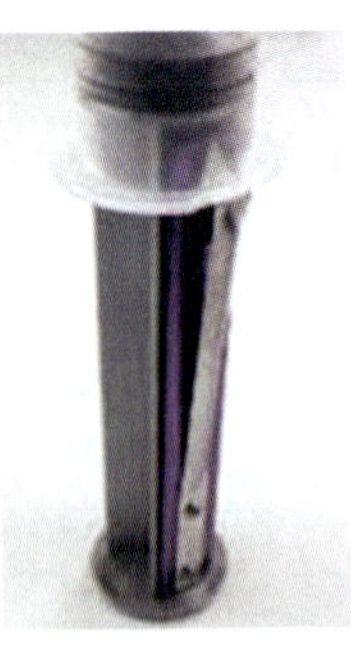

FIGURE 12.13: Snap lok device (Tulip®). (A) Snap lok device in four different sizes to accommodate various syringe sizes. (B) Snap lok device being placed into the plugger with silver spring depressed to return the plunger to an empty syringe position followed by plunger being withdrawn until it snaps/locks into place.

Source: http://www.tulipmedical.com/index.html

and with the maximum amount of multipotent cells and growth factors.

There are a variety of commercial kits and supplies available. Some kits include only aspiration and others both aspiration and processing. The companies that produce kits include, but are not limited to, Alliance Spine Cyclone®, Arthrex Angel System™, Celling® Biosciences ART BMC, DePuy Synthes PROCURE®, EmCyte GenesisCS PureBMC®, Globus Medical RETRIEVE®, Harvest® TerumoBCT BMAC® System, Magellan® MAROMax™, Ranfac Marrow Cellution™, and Zimmer Biomet BioCUE® (Table 12.3). The centrifugation systems generally provide a graft in about 15 to 20 minutes with some companies having different size kits to accommodate larger initial volume to render larger final product volumes.

Companies that produce products to harvest and/or process AT include AdiPrep® from Harvest®, AdiStem™, Lipogems®, Puregraft®, and Tulip®. The AdiPrep® system uses centrifugation to separate the lipids/oil, AT, and blood cells/fluid to isolate concentrated AT for treatment use. AdiStem™ recommends use of their medium, which extracts stromal cells by dissolving lipids and connective tissue from a lipoaspirate. Clinical use of the final product may not be compliant with the U.S. FDA. The final product is then treated with light to signal release of chemicals in the graft. The Lipogems® and Puregraft®

are closed systems and provide autologous fat for lipofilling that can be delivered percutaneously. They do not extract cells from the adipose structure (i.e., SVF) and therefore maintain compliance with the U.S. FDA's minimal manipulation position. Lipogems® provides for manual adipose harvest to process the aspirate in their closed-loop, mechanical device that gently washes, rinses, and resizes the autologous AT, while maintaining the vascular stromal niche. It provides a consistent, uniform final graft size. The Puregraft® product is indicated for transfer of autologous fat tissue for reinjection for aesthetic body contouring. It is designed to filter and wash lipoaspirate of blood cells, free lipids, and contaminants. The system provides for adjustable graft hydration. The Lipogems® and Puregraft® systems have different available sizes, are sterile for use in a surgical suite or an office, and are disposable single use. Lipogems® provides a specific lipoaspiration cannula and supplies for harvest. Tulip® provides various lipoaspiration cannulas and equipment (i.e., syringe locks, syringe connectors, etc.) as well as NanoTransfer™ devices to reduce the size of the graft.

With either the BM or adipose systems, there are few to no human studies published to demonstrate the effectiveness of one of these systems over another. Some of the companies have ongoing research, while others are trying to bring devices to market usually with little clinical

TABLE 12.3 BMA Company Chart

Column 1	Column 2	Column 3	Column 4	Column 5[a]	Column 6	Column 7	Column 8	Column 9	Column 10
					Process		Adjustable		
Company/ System	BMA Approved	Point of Care	Closed	Aspiration Supplies	Centrifuge	Manual Transfer	WBC	RBC	Max. Volume (mL)
Alliance Spine Cyclone®	A	Yes	Yes	A	Yes	Minimal	No	No	240
Arthrex Angel System™	No!b	Yes	Yes	No	Yes	Minimal	Yes	Yes	180
Celling® Biosciences ARTBMC	No!b	Yes	Yes	No	Yes	Minimal	Yes	Yes	60
DePuy Synthes PROCURE®	Yes, only for aspiration	Yes	NA	Yes	NA	NA	NA	NA	NA
EmCyte GenesisCS PureBMC®	Yes	Yes	Yes	Yes	Yes	Yes	Yes	Yes	120
Globus Medical RETRIEVE®	Yes, only for aspiration	Yes	NA	Yes	NA	NA	NA	NA	NA
Harvest® BMAC® System	Yes	Yes	No	Yes	Yes	Yes	No	No	120
Magellan® MAROMax™	No!b	Yes	Yes	Yes	Yes	Minimal	No	No	60

(continued)

TABLE 12.3 BMA Company Chart (*continued*)

Column 1	Column 2	Column 3	Column 4	Column 5[a]	Column 6	Column 7	Column 8	Column 9	Column 10
Ranfac Marrow Cellution™	Yes, only for aspiration	Yes	NA	Yes	No	Minimal	No	No	NA
Zimmer Biomet BioCUE®	No!b	Yes	Yes	Yes	Yes	Yes	Limited		30 BMA (and 60 peripheral blood)
						Minimal means only into a device and removal of final product			

[a]Unclear; !bApproval for PRP from BMA.

BMA, bone marrow aspirate; NA, not applicable; RBC, red blood cell; WBC, white blood cell.

outcomes data available especially for musculoskeletal issues.

ASCs can be divided into several different types. SVF was looked at by Michalek et al., in mainly hip and knee osteoarthritis. A total of 1,856 joints were injected in 1,128 patients and followed for an average of 17 months. Main assessments were Knee injury and Osteoarthritis Outcome Score (KOOS) at 3, 6, and 12 months after treatment. Seventy-five percent improvement was achieved in 63% of the patients and 50% improved in 91% of the patients at 12 months after SVF therapy. Obesity and higher grade OA were associated with slower healing, and no serious side effects, systemic infection, or cancer were associated with SVF therapy (66). Other ASCs can be found in the form of a fat graft transfer, or microfractured raw fat graft. This contains everything that is in an SVF sample, with the addition of pericytes attached to microvasculature, exosomes, collagen from stroma, and intact adipocyte clusters.

Postprocedure Care

After withdrawal of the cannula, apply pressure, and a 2 × 2 gauze with clear Tegaderm. Ice can also be applied to the donor site(s), but less than 20 minutes to avoid thermal injury as the area was anesthetized. Patients should be instructed to keep the area dry and to avoid soaking in a hot tub until the wound has closed, which is about 7 days. Additionally, they should be reassured that the sites may drain for 1 to 2 days if tumescent was used and should be instructed to report any change or worsening condition.

Complication in Liposuction Cases

Complication risks are low in liposuction. Maione et al. studied 1,000 patients in whom there were 2 donor-site hematomas and 83 local deformities (56). In a 2002 survey of 66,000 tumescent liposuction cases, no deaths were reported, and the complication rate was 0.068 per 1,000 cases (67). A 1988 survey of 55 dermatologists and 9,478 liposuction cases, the complication

rate was 0.07% (68). A 1995 survey by Hanke et al. of 66 dermatologists and 15,336 liposuction cases demonstrated no serious complications of death, embolism, hypovolemic shock, or necessity for transfusions with the procedure. The top five complications were scrotal or labial edema or ecchymosis (0.38%), infection (0.34%), permanent skin irregularity such as dimpling or retraction (0.26%), postoperative focal subcutaneous panniculitis-like reaction (0.20%), and hematoma/seroma (0.17%) (69). Prior to the advent of tumescent anesthesia, general anesthesia was used, which did not provide hemostasis, causing severe complications such as hemorrhage, hematoma, skin irregularities, and volume instability. Tumescent, being a diluted solution of lidocaine and epinephrine, allows for hemostasis and anesthesia, improving safety, precision, and less recovery time. It also allows for more uniform adipose removal, making it a safe and effective procedure. Lidocaine, as previously stated, is toxic in high dosages, but lipid-soluble lidocaine is removed with aspirated fat, and vasoconstriction minimizes absorption. Additionally, lidocaine may have antibacterial properties that may also minimize the risk of infection. Epinephrine also may increase cardiac output, which may quicken hepatic metabolism of lidocaine. Globally, the risks of the procedure are infection, anemia, or pulmonary embolism, whereas locally there may be skin irregularity, asymmetry, pain, fibrosis, seroma, skin necrosis, infection, or abdominal perforation. To reduce seroma or hematoma risk, it is recommended to use ice after the procedure (12 hours) and compressive garments for 7 days. There is a risk of obtaining dead cells despite careful and meticulous acquisition and treatment deployment. In regenerative medicine, using dead cells may yield less than optimal results.

Factors Affecting Cell Harvesting: Lipoaspiration

Local anesthetics are known to affect ASC survival. Wang studied tumescent versus local anesthesia and both groups had lower ASC survival than saline (70); however, Shoshani et al. found that tumescent consisting of lidocaine and epinephrine did not alter the take of fat grafts and furthermore did not influence the viability of adipocytes (71).

Moore et al. studied the difference between fat obtained by blunt syringe suction lipectomy versus AT from elective surgery. The cells did not differ functionally, responded similarly to insulin stimulation, and preserved the same growth pattern in culture. Lidocaine inhibited adipocyte growth, but this effect was resolved with cell washing (72). Moore et al. hypothesized that lidocaine inhibits the growth of adipocytes in culture by slowing glucose transport and lipolysis and that the use of epinephrine in the anesthetic solution inhibits the lidocaine from diffusing and therefore exacerbates the local effects of lidocaine-induced impairment on adipocyte function. However, clinical practice does not incubate local anesthetics in culture for treatment.

Agostini et al. compared viability of adipocytes harvested through the dry technique versus with tumescent in 65 healthy women. Fat was collected through a two-hole Coleman blunt cannula attached to a Luer-Lock 10 mL syringe. Their study found that fat collected through the wet technique is more preserved than through the dry technique, but the results were not significant, indicating no histomorphometric or cell viability variations between either lipoaspirate harvesting techniques (73). Keck et al. studied SVF isolation in vitro and exposed it to different anesthetic agents. It was found that different anesthetics and pH can affect quantity and quality of viable adipocytes and the highest cell viability was reported with use of bupivacaine (74).

A 2012 study by Livaoglu et al. compared angiogenesis and volumetric measurements by performing adipose harvests in rats using either lidocaine with epinephrine, prilocaine, or a saline control. This study noted no significant difference between these three groups (75). Weichman et al. reviewed Livaoglu's article and noted limitations of using a new grafting model, the variation of harvest and processing from common clinical practice, and the amount of time of anesthetic to tissue exposure. Despite these findings, they concluded continued support for use of tumescent solution (76).

In conclusion, there is limited data on the effect of local anesthetics on autologous fat grafts or local anesthetics with epinephrine and less regarding isolated epinephrine. The few studies are limited including in vitro technique and prolonged anesthetic contact time, which is not representative of clinical practice. There is no standard process as of yet in obtaining and processing cells; however, at this time, using tumescent anesthesia at the time of adipose harvest does not appear to have a detrimental effect on adipocyte viability.

Pressure effects and cannula type and size can also alter cell viability; however, no clear consensus has yet been reached. Nguyen et al. noted 90% adipocyte injury at −760 mmHg (77). Cheriyan et al. looked at abdominal lipoaspiration at high and low pressures (−760 mmHg and −250 mmHg, respectively), and its effect on viability of the surviving cells in three patients (78). Tumescent solution was used with both systems. Adipocyte count was immediately higher with low pressure when compared to high pressure. Furthermore, the fat was more homogeneous without an oil layer, indicating less fat cell lysis during aspiration. Although cell viability decreased in both groups at day 7, the low pressure group was higher at day 7 with the low-pressure group having a better concentration nevertheless. A 2012 study by Herold et al. demonstrated significant pressure changes inside a 10 mL syringe from −42 mmHg at the 1 mL plunger position to −392 mmHg at the 10 mL position. Therefore, negative pressure at 10 mL was nearly nine times greater than the pressure measured at 1 mL (79). A 2008 study by Ferguson et al. compared a commercial system with standard syringe adipose harvest and noted greater viability from the commercial device that was set at a negative pressure no greater than 762 mmHg (80). The premise was that at higher pressures (more negative), the cells undergo a mechanical insult leading to damage in membrane integrity and thus cell death (81).

As with negative pressure lysing cells, smaller cannula size may disrupt cell membranes leading to reduced viability and greater oil contamination. But, this may not be the case. Alharbi et al. noted that a 2 mm blunt tip cannula with multiple perforations increased cell yield by 22.4% compared to the standard 3 mm blunt tip Coleman cannula. Additionally, the 3 mm cannula aspirate included higher levels of vascular endothelial growth factor (VEGF) and insulin-like growth factor (IGF)-1, which would likely be washed away in the cleaning process and could have a negative impact on outcomes. There was also a loss of aspirate vitality from the 3 mm cannula 48 hours after harvest compared to the 2 mm cannula (80). However, in 2012, Nguyen et al. demonstrated good viability with a 3 mm Coleman cannula when compared to a multi-perforated cannula (82). In 2009, Erdim et al. performed a study of liposuctions on adult females under general anesthesia without the use of a tumescent solution using pyramid tipped 2, 3, and 6 mm cannulas and a 50 mL syringe. Results demonstrated that there was a significantly higher viability of adipocytes from use of the 6 mm cannula compared to the 2 mm and 4 mm cannulas (83). Charles-de-Sá et al. studied the effect on viable adipocyte mesenchymal stem cells (AMSCs) and found neither type of device, nozzle, diameter tip, nor pressure regimen produced a significant effect in the number of viable AMSCs extracted during harvesting (84). Despite clear consensus, it is recommended that a low-pressure system be used with a blunt-tipped multi-perforated 3 to 4 mm cannula to yield viable aspirate.

Osinga et al. looked at whether mechanical processing the lipoaspirate between two inter-connected 10 mL syringes would affect the viability, structure, or differentiation of the isolated SVF. They shuffled the fat 0, 5, or 30 times in six healthy donors, and when examining under immunofluorescent staining, the microscopic structure of the lipoaspirate did not change, nor did the viability, cell number, adipogenic differentiation, or ratio of cell composition (85).

McCurdy's commentary of Berdegeuer's leg fat contouring results (86) noted that the donor site should be of low vascularity, recipient of high vascularity, adipocyte aspiration should be performed at low pressure, harvested adipocytes should be properly handled, injection into recipient should be performed with cannula of sufficient size to minimize adipocyte injury, implantation technique should be multilayered for a large volume-to-surface rather than large volume in the same region, and the site should be overcorrected and that a subsequent transplantation will be required to achieve the desired cosmetic result.

Onishi et al. looked at AMSCs and their viability under different needle conditions. The control group did not use a needle, and the other two used an 18-gauge needle, and a 30-gauge needle. All three groups demonstrated similar growth in culture up to day 4 with a similar metabolic profile. Interestingly, their results also showed that AMSCs mount a cytoprotective response, which is a genetic upregulation to counteract stresses emerged during handling of the cells (87). Erdim's study also used aspirate from a 6 mm cannula to inject through 14, 16, and 20-gauge needles noting no difference in viability of adipocytes from any needle (83).

Peripheral Circulation Mobilization of Cells

Mobilization can be defined as the release of hematopoietic stem and progenitor cells to the peripheral blood following treatment with cytokines and/or chemotherapy. Proteases like elastase and catephsin play a role in mobilization from BM into the blood, as they downregulate adhesion molecules and chemokine receptors to drive these cells into the blood. These anchorage proteins are absent in the peripheral blood, suggesting their role in mobilization. Plerixafor is an inhibitor of some of these anchorage proteins and their receptors, and has been shown to have significant stem cell mobilizing activity. Research has shown that the cells mobilized with Plerixafor are more primitive than those mobilized with granulocyte-colony stimulating factor (G-CSF), and additionally there is an absolute increase in overall CD34$^+$ cells. When sampling peripheral blood, the concentration of CD34$^+$ cells correlates with a better stem cell count. Peripheral blood stem cells (PBSCs) offer advantages such has decreased pain during harvesting, and it is associated with more rapid engraftment. PBSCs have replaced BM in autologous stem cell transplants (autoSCT). AutoSCT has become the standard of care for patients with multiple myeloma, and has been used successfully in long-term cure in those with recurrent or refractory non-Hodgkin's lymphoma (88). Additional agents can mobilize stem cells including SCF, growth hormone, possibly parathormone, stromal cell-derived factor 1 (SDF-1) analogs especially with G-CSF, and 4F-benzoyl-TN14003 (T-140) and T134 in mouse models (89).

Although used in cancer, peripheral mobilization is not approved by the FDA to be used in regenerative therapies. Currently, there have been studies of autologous/allogenic cell vascular infusions for chronic obstructive pulmonary disease (COPD) (90,91), acute respiratory distress syndrome (ARDS) (92,93), diabetes (94), multiple sclerosis (95), and inflammatory bowel disease (96), but no infusion therapy research for musculoskeletal pathology. However, the aforementioned studies demonstrate systemic effect including immunomodulatory effects that may be of benefit in rheumatologic diseases, and so on, that involve joints or other systems (97).

Whether to assist in peripheral blood cell number or enhance BM yield, endurance exercise and caloric restriction have demonstrated the ability to increase the number of hematopoietic stem/progenitor cells in both regions (98,99). Additional research will be required to determine how best to harness the effect for clinical benefit such as before and/or after a treatment.

REFERENCES

1. Minimal manipulation of human cells, tissues, and cellular and tissue-based products—draft guidance for industry and Food and Drug Administration staff. December 2014.

2. Types of stem cell transplants for cancer treatment. American Cancer Society. http://www.cancer.org/treatment/treatmentsandsideeffects/treatmenttypes/bonemarrowandperipheralbloodstemcelltransplant/stem-cell-transplant-types-of-transplants

3. Peng L, Jia Z, Yin X, et al. Comparative analysis of mesenchymal stem cells from bone marrow, cartilage, and adipose tissue. *Stem Cells Dev.* 2008;17(4):761–773.

4. Cox B, Durieux ME, Marcus MA. Toxicity of local anaesthetics. *Best Pract Res Clin Anaesthesiol.* 2003;17(1):111–136.

5. Zink W, Graf BM. The toxicity of local anesthetics: the place of ropivacaine and levobupivacaine. *Curr Opin Anaesthesiol.* 2008;21(5):645–650.

6. Breu A, Scheidhammer I, Kujat R, et al. Local anesthetic cytotoxicity on human mesenchymal stem cells during chondrogenic differentiation. *Knee Surg Sports Traumatol Arthrosc.* 2015;23(4):937–945.

7. Strem BM, Hicok KC, Zhu M, et al. Multipotential differentiation of adipose tissue-derived stem cells: review. *Keio J Med.* 2005;54(3):132–141.

8. Mizuno H, Tobita M, Uysal AC. Concise review: adipose-derived stem cells as a novel tool for future regenerative medicine. *Stem Cells.* 2012;30(5):804–810.

9. Strioga M, Viswanathan S, Darinskas A, et al. Same or not the same? Comparison of adipose tissue-derived versus bone marrow-derived mesenchymal stem and stromal cells. *Stem Cells Dev.* 2012;21(14):2724–2752.

10. Yoshimura K, Suga H, Eto H. Adipose-derived stem/progenitor cells: roles in adipose tissue remodeling and potential use for soft tissue augmentation. *Regen Med.* 2009;4(2):265–273.

11. Bowen JE. Technical issues in harvesting and concentrating stem cells (bone marrow and adipose). *PM R.* 2015;7(4 Suppl):S8–S18.

12. Parapia LA. Trepanning or trephines: a history of bone marrow biopsy. *Br J Haematol.* 2007;139(1):14–19.

13. Wakitani S, Imoto K, Yamamoto T, et al. Human autologous culture expanded bone marrow-mesenchymal cell transplantation for repair of cartilage defects in osteoarthritic knees. *Osteoarthr Cartil.* 2002;10:199–206. doi:10.1053/joca.2001.0504

14. Konno M, Hamabe A, Hasegawa S, et al. Adipose-derived mesenchymal stem cells and regenerative medicine. *Dev Growth Differ.* 2013;55(3):309–318.

15. Degen C, Christen S, Rovo A, et al. Bone marrow examination: a prospective survey on factors associated with pain. *Ann Hematol.* 2010;89(6):619–624.

16. Grønkjær M, Hasselgren CF, Østergaard AS, et al. Bone marrow aspiration: a randomized controlled trial assessing the quality of bone marrow specimens using slow and rapid aspiration techniques and evaluating pain intensity. *Acta Haematol.* 2016;135(2):81–87.

17. Sittitavornwong S, Falconer DS, Shah R, et al. Anatomic considerations for posterior iliac crest bone procurement. *J Oral Maxillofac Surg.* 2013;71: 1777–1788.

18. Hernigou J, Picard L, Alves A, et al. Understanding bone safety zones during bone marrow aspiration from the iliac crest: the sector rule. *Int Orthop.* 2014;38(11):2377–2384.

19. Xu R, Ebraheim NA, Yeasting RA, et al. Anatomic considerations for posterior iliac bone harvesting. *Spine.* 1996;21(9):1017–1020.

20. Hernigou J, Alves A, Homma Y, et al. Anatomy of the ilium for bone marrow aspiration: map of sectors and implication for safe trocar placement. *Int Orthop.* 2014;38(12):2585–2590. doi:10.1007/ s00264-014-2353-7

21. Bain BJ. Bone marrow biopsy morbidity: review of 2003. *Br J Haematol.* 2003;58(4):406–408. doi:10.1136/jcp.2004.022178

22. Goldfrank LR, Flomenbaum NE, Lewin NA, et al. (eds) *Goldfrank's toxicologic emergencies*, 6th ed. New York, NY: McGraw-Hill; 1998:897–903.

23. Rosenberg PH, Veering BT, Urmey WF. Maximum recommended doses of local anesthetics: a multifactorial concept. *Reg Anesth Pain Med.* 2004;29(6):564–575; discussion 524.

24. Carragee EJ, Lincoln T, Parmar VS, et al. A gold standard evaluation of the "discogenic pain" diagnosis as determined by provocative discography. *Spine.* 2006;31(18):2115–2123.

25. Ohmura S, Kawada M, Ohta T, et al. Systemic toxicity and resuscitation in bupivacaine-, levobupivacaine-, or ropivacaine-infused rats. *Anesth Analg.* 2001;93 (3):743–748.

26. Scott DB, Lee A, Fagan D, et al. Acute toxicity of ropivacaine compared with that of bupivacaine. *Anesth Analg.* 1989;69(5):563–569. doi:10.1213/ 00000539-198911000-00003

27. Baeszwkra P. Cytotoxicity of local anesthetics on human mesenchymal stem cells in vitro. *Arthroscopy.* 2013;29(10):1676–1684.

28. Jacobs TF, Vansintjan PS, Roels N, et al. The effect of lidocaine on the viability of cultivated mature human cartilage cells: an *in vitro* study. *Knee Surg Sports Traumatol Arthrosc.* 2011;19(7):1206–1213.

29. Dragoo JL, Braun HJ, Kim HJ, et al. The in vitro chondrotoxicity of single-dose local anesthetics. *Am J Sports Med.* 2012;40(4):794–799. doi:10.1177/ 0363546511434571

30. Dony P, Dewinde V, Vanderick B, et al. The comparative toxicity of ropivacaine and bupivacaine at equipotent doses in rats. *Anesth Analg.* 2000;91(6):1489–1492.

31. van Esch RW, Kool MM, van As S. NSAIDs can have adverse effects on bone healing. *Med Hypotheses.* 2013;81(2):343–346. doi:10.1016/ j.mehy.2013.03.042

32. Gogia PP, Brown M, al-Obaidi S. Hydrocortisone and exercise effects on articular cartilage in rats. *Arch Phys Med Rehabil.* 1993;74(5):463–467.

33. Lipworth BJ. Systemic adverse effects of inhaled corticosteroid therapy: a systematic review and meta-analysis. *Arch Intern Med.* 1999;159(9):941–955.

34. FDA updates warnings for fluoroquinolone antibiotics. U.S. Food and Drug Administration. http://www.fda.gov/NewsEvents/Newsroom/ PressAnnouncements/ucm513183.htm

35. Vincent L, Chen W, Hong L, et al. Inhibition of endothelial cell migration by cerivastatin, an HMG-CoA reductase inhibitor: contribution to its anti-angiogenic effect. *FEBS Lett.* 2001;495(3):159–166.

36. Kalén A, Appelkvist EL, Dallner G. Age-related changes in the lipid compositions of rat and human tissues. *Lipids.* 1989;24(7):579–584.

37. Westerweel PE, Teraa M, Rafii S, et al. Impaired endothelial progenitor cell mobilization and dysfunctional bone marrow stroma in diabetes mellitus. *PLOS ONE.* 2013;8(3):e60357.

38. Albiero M, Poncina N, Tjwa M, et al. Diabetes causes bone marrow autonomic neuropathy and impairs stem cell mobilization via dysregulated p66Shc and Sirt1. *Diabetes.* 2014;63(4): 1353–1365.

39. Singh G, Bonham AJ. A predictive equation to guide vitamin D replacement dose in patients. *J Am Board Fam Med.* 2014;27(4):495–509.

40. Lindenfeld T, Wojtys E, Husain A. Instructional course lectures, The American Academy of Orthopaedic Surgeons. *J Bone Jt Surg.* 1999;63(March 2014):

2152–2157. http://www.ejbjs.org/cgi/content/extract/81/12/1772

41. Yoon SH, Lee HY, Lee HJ, et al. Optimal dose of intra-articular corticosteroids for adhesive capsulitis: a randomized, triple-blind, placebo-controlled trial. *Am J Sports Med.* 2013;41(5):1133–1139.

42. Hyer CF, Berlet GC, Bussewitz BW, et al. Quantitative assessment of the yield of osteoblastic. *J Bone Jt Surg.* 2013;95:1312–1316. doi:10.2106/JBJS.L.01529

43. Marx RE, Tursun R. A qualitative and quantitative analysis of autologous human multipotent adult stem cells derived from three anatomic areas by marrow aspiration: tibia, anterior ilium, and posterior ilium. *Int J Oral Maxillofac Implants.* 2013;28(5):e290–e294.

44. Preventing central line–associated bloodstream infections: useful tools, an international perspective. The Joint Commission. https://www.jointcommission.org/assets/1/6/CLABSI_Toolkit_Tool_3-8_Aseptic_versus_Clean_Technique.pdf

45. Miller HJ, Awad SS, Crosby CT, et al. Chlorhexidine–alcohol versus povidone–iodine for surgical-site antisepsis. *N Engl J Med.* 2010;362:18–26.

46. Auletta MJ. Local anesthesia for dermatologic surgery. *Semin Dermatol.* 1994;13(1):35–42.

47. Berenson JR, Yellin O, Blumenstein B, et al. Using a powered bone marrow biopsy system results in shorter procedures, causes less residual pain to adult patients, and yields larger specimens. *Diagn Pathol.* 2011;6:23. doi:10.1186/1746-1596-6-23

48. Bischoff-Ferrari HA, Willett WC, Orav EJ, et al. A pooled analysis of vitamin D dose requirements for fracture prevention. *N Engl J Med.* 2012;367(1):40–49.

49. Muschler GF, Boehm C, Easley K. Aspiration to obtain osteoblast progenitor cells from human bone marrow: the influence of aspiration volume. *J Bone Joint Surg Am.* 1997;79(11):1699–1709. doi:10.1002/jcp.1041530205

50. Hernigou P, Mathieu G, Poignard A, et al. Percutaneous autologous bone-marrow grafting for nonunions: surgical technique. *J Bone Joint Surg Am.* 2006;88(Suppl 1):322–327. doi:10.2106/JBJS.F.00203

51. Hernigou P, Homma Y, Flouzat Lachaniette CH, et al. Benefits of small volume and small syringe for bone marrow aspirations of mesenchymal stem cells. *Int Orthop.* 2013;37(11):2279–2287.

52. Kuznetsov SA, Mankani MH, Leet AI, et al. Circulating connective tissue precursors: extreme rarity in humans and chondrogenic potential in guinea pigs. *Stem Cells.* 2007;25(7):1830–1839.

53. Fennema EM, Renard AJ, Leusink A, et al. The effect of bone marrow aspiration strategy on the yield and quality of human mesenchymal stem cells. *Acta Orthop.* 2009;80(5):618–621.

54. Li J, Wong WHS, Chan S, et al. Factors affecting mesenchymal stromal cells yield from bone marrow aspiration. *Chinese J Cancer Res.* 2011;23(1):43–48. doi:10.1007/s11670-011-0043-1

55. Teraa M, Schutgens RE, Sprengers RW, et al.; Juventas Study Group. Core diameter of bone marrow aspiration devices influences cell density of bone marrow aspirate in patients with severe peripheral artery disease. *Cytotherapy.* 2015;17(12):1807–1812.

56. Maione L, Vinci V, Klinger M, et al. Autologous fat graft by needle: analysis of complications after 1,000 patients. *Ann Plast Surg.* 2015;74(3):277–280. doi:10.1097/SAP.0000000000000050

57. Zuk PA, Zhu M, Mizuno H, et al. Multilineage cells from human adipose tissue: implications for cell-based therapies. *Tissue Eng.* 2001;7(2):211–228.

58. Perez RA. Liposuction and diabetes type 2 development risk reduction in the obese patient. *Med Hypotheses.* 2007;68(2):393–396.

59. Ostad A, Kageyama N, Moy RL. Tumescent anesthesia with a lidocaine dose of 55 mg/kg is safe for liposuction. *Dermatol Surg.* 1996;22(11):921–927.

60. Padoin AV, Braga-Silva J, Martins P, et al. Sources of processed lipoaspirate cells: influence of donor site on cell concentration. *Plast Reconstr Surg.* 2008;122(2):614–618.

61. Li K, Gao J, Zhang Z, et al. Selection of donor site for fat grafting and cell isolation. *Aesthetic Plast Surg.* 2013;37(1):153–158.

62. Lim AA, Fan K, Allam KA, et al. Autologous fat transplantation in the craniofacial patient: the UCLA experience. *J Craniofac Surg.* 2012;23(4):1061–1066.

63. Small K, Choi M, Petruolo O, et al. Is there an ideal donor site of fat for secondary breast reconstruction? *Aesthet Surg J.* 2014;34(4):545–550.

64. Choudhery MS, Badowski M, Muise A, et al. Subcutaneous adipose tissue-derived stem cell utility is independent of anatomical harvest site. *Biores Open Access.* 2015;4(1):131–145.

65. Doi K, Tanaka S, Iida H, et al. Stromal vascular fraction isolated from lipo-aspirates using an automated processing system: bench and bed analysis. *J Tissue Eng Regen Med.* 2012;7(11):864–870.

66. Michalek AJ, Moster R, Lukac L, et al. Autologous adipose tissue-derived stromal vascular fraction

cells application in patients with osteoarthritis. *Cell Transplant.* 2015;20:1–36. doi:10.3727/096368915X686760

67. Housman TS, Lawrence N, Mellen BG, et al. The safety of liposuction: results of a national survey. *Dermatol Surg.* 2002;28(11):971–978.

68. Zens M, Niemeyer P, Ruhhammer J, et al. Length changes of the anterolateral ligament during passive knee motion: a human cadaveric study. *Am J Sports Med.* 2015;43(10):2545–2552.

69. Hanke CW, Bernstein G, Bullock S. Safety of tumescent liposuction in 15,336 patients. National survey results. *Dermatol Surg.* 1995;21(5):459–462.

70. Wang WZ, Fang XH, Williams SJ, et al. Lidocaine-induced ASC apoptosis (tumescent vs. local anesthesia). *Aesthetic Plast Surg.* 2014;38(5):1017–1023.

71. Shoshani O, Berger J, Fodor L, et al. The effect of lidocaine and adrenaline on the viability of injected adipose tissue: an experimental study in nude mice. *J Drugs Dermatol.* 2005;4(3):311–316.

72. Moore JH Jr, Kolaczynski JW, Morales LM, et al. Viability of fat obtained by syringe suction lipectomy: effects of local anesthesia with lidocaine. *Aesthetic Plast Surg.* 1995;19(4):335–339.

73. Agostini T, Davide L, Alessandro P, et al. Wet and dry techniques for structural fat graft harvesting. *Plast Reconstr Surg.* 2012;130(2):331e–339e. doi:10.1097/PRS.0b013e3182589f76

74. Keck M, Zeyda M, Gollinger K, et al. Local anesthetics have a major impact on viability of preadipocytes and their differentiation into adipocytes. *Plast Reconstr Surg.* 2010;126(5):1500–1505.

75. Livaoğlu M, Buruk CK, Uraloğlu M. Effects of lidocaine plus epinephrine and prilocaine on autologous fat graft survival. *J Craniofac Surg.* 2012;23(4):1015–1018.

76. Weichman KE, Warren SM. Effects of lidocaine plus epinephrine and prilocaine on autologous fat graft survival. *J Craniofac Surg.* 2012;23:1019.

77. Nguyen A, Pasyk KA, Bouvier TN, et al. Comparative study of survival of autologous adipose tissue taken and transplanted by different techniques. *Plast Reconstr Surg.* 1990;85(3):378–386; discussion 387.

78. Cheriyan T, Kao HK, Qiao X, et al. Low harvest pressure enhances autologous fat graft viability. *Plast Reconstr Surg.* 2014;133(6):1365–1368.

79. Herold CP, Utz M, Pflaum M, et al. Negative pressure of manual liposuction with Coleman technique is highly dependent on the position of plunger of the syringe. *J Plast Reconstr Aesthet Surg.* 2012;65(7):983–984.

80. Alharbi Z, Opländer C, Almakadi S, et al. Conventional vs. micro-fat harvesting: how fat harvesting technique affects tissue-engineering approaches using adipose tissue-derived stem/stromal cells. *J Plast Reconstr Aesthet Surg.* 2013;66(9):1271–1278.

81. Ferguson RE, Cui X, Fink BF, et al. The viability of autologous fat grafts harvested with the LipiVage system: a comparative study. *Ann Plast Surg.* 2008;60(5):594–597.

82. Nguyen PS, Desouches C, Gay AM, et al. Development of micro-injection as an innovative autologous fat graft technique: the use of adipose tissue as dermal filler. *J Plast Reconstr Aesthet Surg.* 2012;65(12):1692–1699.

83. Erdim M, Tezel E, Numanoglu A, et al. The effects of the size of liposuction cannula on adipocyte survival and the optimum temperature for fat graft storage: an experimental study. *J Plast Reconstr Aesthet Surg.* 2009;62(9):1210–1214.

84. Charles-de-Sá L, Gontijode Amorim NF, Dantas D, et al. Influence of negative pressure on the viability of adipocytes and mesenchymal stem cell, considering the device method used to harvest fat tissue. *Aesthet Surg J.* 2015;35(3):334–344. doi:10.1093/asj/sju047

85. Osinga R, Menzi NR, Tchang LA, et al. Effects of inter-syringe processing on adipose tissue and its cellular components: implications in autologous fat grafting. *Plast Reconstr Surg.* 2015;135(6):1618–1628.

86. McCurdy JA Jr. Five years of experience using fat for leg contouring (commentary). *Am J Cosmet Surg.* 1995;12:228–233.

87. Onishi K, Jones DL, Riester SM, et al. Human adipose-derived mesenchymal stromal/stem cells remain viable and metabolically active following needle passage. *PM R.* 2015;8(9):844–854. doi:10.1016/j.pmrj.2016.01.010

88. Mohty M, Ho AD. In and out of the niche: perspectives in mobilization of hematopoietic stem cells. *Exp Hematol.* 2011;39(7):723–729.

89. Civriz Bozdag S, Tekgunduz E, Altuntas F. The current status in hematopoietic stem cell mobilization. *J Clin Apher.* 2015;30(5):273–280.

90. Ribeiro-Paes JT, Bilaqui A, Greco OT, et al. Unicentric study of cell therapy in chronic obstructive pulmonary disease/pulmonary emphysema. *Int J Chron Obstruct Pulmon Dis.* 2011;6:63–71.

91. Weiss DJ, Casaburi R, Flannery R, et al. A placebo-controlled, randomized trial of mesenchymal stem cells in COPD. *Chest.* 2013;143(6):1590–1598.

92. Zheng G, Huang L, Tong H, et al. Treatment of acute respiratory distress syndrome with allogeneic adipose-derived mesenchymal stem cells: a randomized, placebo-controlled pilot study. *Respir Res.* 2014;15:39. doi:10.1186/1465-9921-15-39

93. Simonson OE, Mougiakakos D, Heldring N, et al. *In vivo* effects of mesenchymal stromal cells in two patients with severe acute respiratory distress syndrome. *Stem Cells Transl Med.* 2015;4(10):1199–1213.

94. Thakkar UG, Trivedi HL, Vanikar AV, et al. Insulin-secreting adipose-derived mesenchymal stromal cells with bone marrow–derived hematopoietic stem cells from autologous and allogenic sources for type 1 diabetes mellitus. *Cytotherapy.* 2015;17(7):940–947.

95. Connick P, Kolappan M, Patani R, et al. The mesenchymal stem cells in multiple sclerosis (MSCIMS) trial protocol and baseline cohort characteristics: an open-label pre-test: post-test study with blinded outcome assessments. *Trials.* 2011;12:62. doi:10.1186/1745-6215-12-62

96. Garcia-Olmo D, Schwartz DA. Cumulative evidence that mesenchymal stem cells promote healing of perianal fistulas of patients with Crohn's disease: going from bench to bedside. *Gastroenterology.* 2015;149(4):853–857.

97. Wang LT, Ting CH, Yen ML, et al. Human mesenchymal stem cells (MSCs) for treatment towards immune- and inflammation-mediated diseases: review of current clinical trials. *J Biomed Sci.* 2016;23(1):76. doi:10.1186/s12929-016-0289-5

98. Marycz K, Mierzejewska K, Smieszek A, et al. Endurance exercise mobilizes developmentally early stem cells into peripheral blood and increases their number in bone marrow: implications for tissue regeneration. *Stem Cells Int.* 2016;2016:5756901.

99. Mazzoccoli G, Tevy MF, Borghesan M, et al. Caloric restriction and aging stem cells: the stick and the carrot? *Exp Gerontol.* 2014;50: 137–148.

CHAPTER 13

TECHNIQUES FOR PERFORMING REGENERATIVE PROCEDURES FOR ORTHOPEDIC CONDITIONS

Imran James Siddiqui, Timothy J. Mazzola, and Brian J. Shiple

In this chapter, we present a manual to teach our readers how to perform the most common musculoskeletal regenerative injections such as plate-rich plasma (PRP), bone marrow concentrate (BMC), and lipoaspirate (LA). Although there are unique aspects to most injections, there are general guidelines one should always apply based on the characteristics of both the tissue and pathology being treated. Later in the chapter, we present specific injection techniques for those most commonly performed; however, these general guidelines outlined in the introduction can be applied to any tissue structure and pathology relating to tendon, muscle, ligament, joint, and bone pathology. For a greater breadth of specific ultrasound (US)-guided injection set up and approaches, we recommend an injection atlas, such as the "Atlas of Ultrasound Guided Injections" (1). However, it is important to note that such atlases describe US-guided techniques for corticosteroid injection. There are important technical distinctions when one is performing a regenerative injection, which this chapter describes.

GENERAL JOINT INJECTION GUIDELINES

Pertinent Anatomy and Pathology

Joints consist of two or more articulating bones with hyaline cartilage at each interface. In addition to hyaline cartilage, some joints have a fibrocartilage component such as the meniscus in the knee or the labrum in the shoulder. Joints have a surrounding synovial membrane and a capsule that isolates the joint from the rest of the body. They also have supporting ligaments to provide stability. Common pathologic findings include hyaline cartridge loss, osteophytes, joint effusion, fibrocartilage tear, capsular tears/instability, and synovial hypertrophy or inflammation.

Indications for Regenerative Treatments

Common joint pathology where regenerative therapies are beneficial include: mild-moderate-joint effusion/synovitis, hyaline cartilage degeneration, and fibrocartilage tears/degeneration. A relative contraindication to regenerative treatments is severe osteoarthritis (OA) with osteophytes causing bony impingement and osteocartilagenous loose bodies resulting in the loss of range of motion (ROM), as outcomes are poor. A period of physical therapy to regain ROM should be attempted before proceeding with regenerative procedures. If ROM limitation is secondary to capsular adhesions, consider joint lavage with capsular hydroexpansion and manual therapy or manipulation under anesthesia using nerve blocks before regenerative therapy. If ROM is restricted secondary to small bony osteophyte(s), consider percutaneous debridement and lavage or surgical resection for larger lesions and loose bodies resulting in mechanical block.

A red blood cell-free, leukocyte-poor PRP (LP-PRP) product is preferred over leukocyte-rich PRP (LR-PRP) for intra-articular use as it induces greater chondrocyte proliferation and has lower counts of inflammatory cytokines (2). In general, BMC is preferred over other stem cell-rich tissues such as adipose for hyaline cartilage regeneration, as it is most homologous. However, there is increasing literature to support the effectiveness of adipose-derived stem cells (ADSC) for cartilage pathology including OA. In addition, whole LA may be beneficial as a structural scaffold for larger fibrocartilage tears or hyaline defects. There is building evidence that stem cell-rich tissues, such as BMC and minimally processed LA can heal cartilage defects and reverse OA (3–5).

Technical Considerations

Hydroexpansion may be beneficial if there is a component of capsular adhesions contributing to ROM deficits, but take care as to not overextend the joint with too much volume as it can cause increased pain, capsular laxity, or even capsular rupture. This can be done with normal saline and perhaps a very dilute anesthetic agent such as 0.5% lidocaine. It should be noted that anesthetic agents are toxic to tenocytes and chondrocytes. Retesting of the joint ROM should be performed with the goal of trying to achieve 50% to 75% of the motion of the opposite unaffected joint. If there is significant fibrocartilage degeneration, or tearing, fenestrate the fibrocartilage, depositing microdoses of the biologic, then deposit the remaining injectate into the joint. If there is joint laxity, consider treating the associated ligaments in conjunction with or in isolation of treating intra-articularly. This may require a prolotherapy/dextrose injection of these tissues before injection of the orthobiologic agent sometime later. When treating ligaments, one should deposit a portion of the injectate into the ligament before injecting the rest into the joint space. If there is a tear or stretch injury of the ligament, consider injecting microdoses into the ligament with fenestration.

GENERAL TENDON INJECTION GUIDELINES

Pertinent Anatomy and Pathology

Tendons provide the connection between muscles and bones. Each muscle has a tendon origin and a tendon insertion. Many tendons have a tendon sheath, but some do not, such as the Achilles tendon. Specific tendons may also overlay a fat pad that provides nutrients to the tendon, such as the patella and Achilles. Common pathologic findings include tendinosis, tenosynovitis, partial, and full thickness tears. Some tendons are supported by an overlying retinaculum, which if damaged can result in tendon subluxation, which may be associated with tendinopathy.

Indications for Regenerative Therapy

Common tendon pathology where regenerative treatments are indicated include: tendinosis and partial thickness tears. There is some debate about whether orthobiologic procedures are effective for many larger thickness tears in the absence of some type of surgical repair. In these cases, some type of scaffold to "fill in the gap" is generally felt necessary. The treatment of chronic, refractory tendinosis has been one of the most widely studied and proven uses of PRP (6,7). Clinical studies have found no significant difference in LR-PRP versus LP-PRP for tendinopathy (8). However, LP-PRP has been shown to create a stronger fibrin matrix, while LR-PRP stimulates greater inflammation and vascular proliferation (9,10). There has been some evidence in animal models for using PRP with a fibrin or LA graft for large partial thickness tears or even larger thickness tears without significant retraction (11). In general LA is preferred more than BMC for larger tears as it is a more homologous tissue source and provides a structural tissue graft to support the healing defect.

Technical Considerations

When treating tendons, one should fenestrate the tendinosis or partial thickness tear as one deposits microdoses into the tendon. There is no consensus on the number of fenestrations that are necessary. In cases of partial thickness tears, the main target is the granulation tissue around the tear rather than the tear itself. Although one should also deposit some of the biologic into the tear, great care should be taken not to overdistend the tear. While injecting, look for extension of the tear being treated, as well as other tears that were not previously seen and have been uncovered by the injection. Ensure that these areas are treated as well. The remaining injectate should be deposited into the adjacent tendon sheath, peritenon, or bursa. Consider immobilization if extensive needling with a larger gauge needle (ie, 18 G) is performed, especially in active individuals.

GENERAL MUSCLE INJECTION GUIDELINES

Pertinent Anatomy and Pathology

Muscles provide locomotion and are attached to bones via tendons. They are composed of fascicles of myofibers that are prone to rupture if overloaded. The other common pathologies seen in muscles include fibrosis, atrophy, and heterotopic ossification, as well as central tendon defects and partial or full thickness tears.

Indications for Use

Muscle rupture is the most commonly seen pathology where regenerative treatments are indicated. While the evidence is mixed, PRP has been shown to improve muscle regeneration, reduce scar formation, and accelerate healing in acute muscle tears (12–14). Thus, treating with PRP may accelerate return to sport and theoretically improve performance posttear. Additionally, in vitro research conducted by Dr. Dragoo on human skeletal muscle myoblasts demonstrated that platelet-poor plasma (PPP) causes better muscle differentiation than PRP, while PRP showed better muscle proliferation. Thus, the combination of PRP and PPP is likely better than PRP alone in muscle regeneration.

Technical Considerations

One should first aspirate the hematoma associated with the muscle tear. If subacute, the hematoma may be thrombosed and difficult to aspirate. One may attempt lavage with saline to try to increase the aspirate yield. Then inject 6 to 8 mL of the PRP and PPP product into the tear noting filling of the defect. Currently, in vitro results indicate that LP-PRP with a moderate increase in platelet concentration 8 to 10× is most effective for myocyte proliferation (15).

GENERAL BONE INJECTION GUIDELINES

Pertinent Anatomy and Pathology

Bones provide structural support for the body. They are classified according to their shape including: long, short, flat, sesamoid, irregular, and sutured. Common pathologies seen are stress fractures, acute or chronic fractures, occult fractures, bone contusion, periostial inflammation, and tumors.

Indications for Use

Both BMC and PRP have been shown to be effective in the treatment of fractures with delayed healing or nonunion (16–19). Most of the evidence lies within long bone fractures (20,21). However, there is evidence supporting the use in rib fractures (22) and mandibular fractures (23). Fractures with greater than 4 mm of gapping do not show improvement with regenerative treatments (24). These cases would require bone graft.

Technical Considerations

Either US or fluoroscopy can be used to guide the injection. Most studies use a large volume of injectate, 10 to 20 mL for nonunions, but it remains to be seen how much volume is necessary. For stress fractures use smaller volumes, 2 to 5 mL. Needle placement should be directly into the fracture site, with some deposited over it at the periostium as well. There is in vitro evidence to suggest that LP-PRP is most effective for osteoblast proliferation (2).

SHOULDER

Here we present the most commonly treated areas in the shoulder including the glenohumeral (GH) joint, posterior labrum, rotator cuff tendons, and long head biceps tendon (BT). Other areas that can be treated, but are not presented, include the acromioclavicular joint and its ligaments, as well as the anterior labrum, the superior labrum anterior to posterior (SLAP) area, and the rotator interval with the biceps' cables. One can use the general guidelines discussed earlier in the chapter in conjunction with a manual on how to perform US-guided injections to assist in treating these areas.

Glenohumeral Joint and Posterior Labrum

Pertinent Anatomy

The GH joint is a ball and socket joint where the humeral head (ball) meets the glenoid of the scapula (socket). It is stabilized statically by the glenoid labrum, joint capsule, and intrinsic ligaments. It is stabilized dynamically by the rotator cuff muscles and tendons.

US Findings

Imaging of the GH joint is best conducted in long-axis to the joint, posteriorly in long-axis to and over the infraspinatus musculotendinous junction (Figure 13.1). Common findings include hyaline cartridge loss, osteophytes, joint effusion, and labral degeneration/tears. Dynamic testing with external and internal rotations can put stress on the labrum to better visualize small tears and/or subluxation. An effusion around the BT without biceps tendinopathy can be a secondary indicator of GH inflammation as the tendon's sheath communicates with the joint.

Indications for Use

Common GH joint pathology with indication and efficacy for regenerative injections includes mild-to-moderate GH hyaline cartilage degeneration and labrum degeneration or small tears. A relative contraindication to regenerative treatments is severe OA with osteophytes causing bony impingement and loss of ROM, as outcomes are poor. Consider a trial of physical therapy to regain ROM. One can also consider surgical referral for acromioplasty before regenerative treatment. If ROM limitation is because of capsular adhesions, consider GH lavage with capsular hydroexpansion before regenerative therapy. It is important to screen for concomitant rotator cuff tears that are likely to also contribute to dysfunction, and thus need to be treated concomitantly.

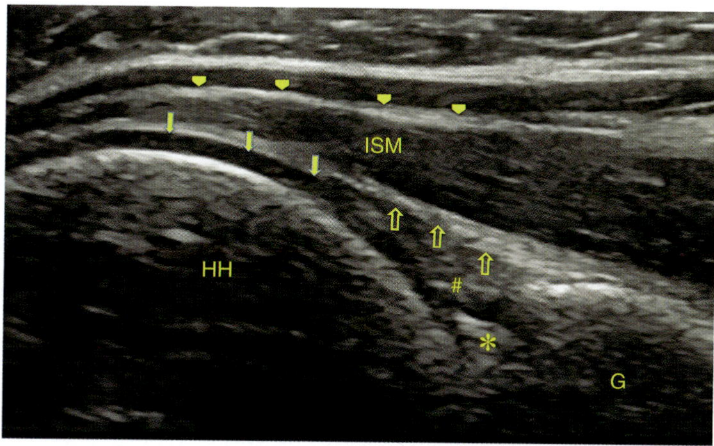

FIGURE 13.1: Posterior shoulder, LAX to glenohumeral joint.

Arrow heads, infraspinatus tendon; arrows, hyaline cartilage of humerus; asterisk, posterior labrum; G, glenoid; HH, humeral head; ISM, infraspinatus muscle; open arrows, posterior joint capsule; pound, glenohumeral joint.

Preferred Technique

1. Equipment
   a. 20 to 25 G 1.5- to 3.5-inch needle
   b. Approximately 5 to 10 mL of injectate
   c. LP-PRP or BMC, for intra-articular injection
2. Patient position
   a. Lateral recumbent position
   b. Target side up
   c. Patient holding side of table (shoulder adducted with internal rotation)
3. Transducer position
   a. Over the posterior GH space in long-axis to the infraspinatus
   b. Identify area of the posterior labrum with greatest degeneration
   c. Use external/internal rotation to identify the joint and to better identify labrum pathology
4. Needle orientation
   a. In-plane
5. Target
   a. Posterior GH space and labrum
   b. Enter lateral to medial
   c. Slip needle tip under the capsule and anterior lip of posterior labrum
   d. Deposit the injectate into the GH joint with bevel down toward joint

6. Special considerations
   a. If treating posterior labrum fenestrate labrum before injection GH joint

Supraspinatus and Infraspinatus Tendons

Pertinent Anatomy

The supraspinatus tendon (SST) travels from the supraspinatus muscle in the supraclavicular fossa under the acromion to insert on the superior and middle facets of the greater tuberosity of the humerus. The subacromial-subdeltoid bursa lies just superficial to the tendon, deep to the deltoid muscle. The infraspinatus tendon (IST) travels from the infraspinatus muscle in the infraclavicular fossa over the posterior GH joint and inserts on the middle facet of the greater tuberosity.

US Findings

Imaging of the supraspinatus is best conducted in both long and short-axis to the tendon, while the patient is in the Crass or modified Crass position with the shoulder in extension and internal rotation (Figure 13.2) (25). This brings the SST out from underneath the acromion. Common findings include tendinosis, bursal side partial tears,

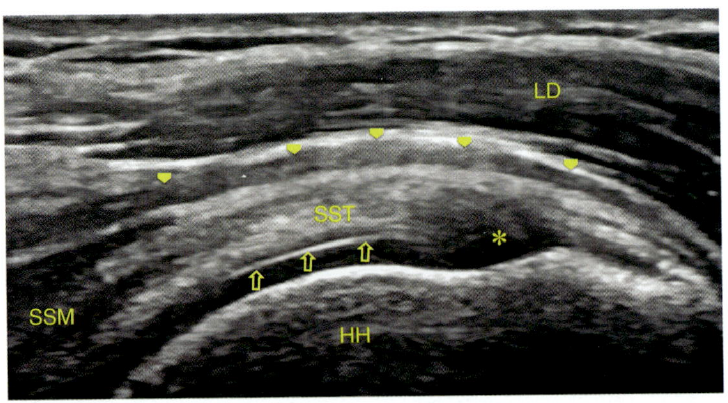

FIGURE 13.2: Lateral shoulder, LAX to supraspinatus tendon (patient in Crass position).

Arrow heads, subacromial-subdeltoid bursa; asterisk, hypoechoic tendon because of anisotropy; HH, humeral head; LD, lateral deltoid; open arrows, hyaline cartilage of humerus (hypoechoic) with cartilage interface sign (hyperechoic); SSM, supraspinatus muscle; SST, supraspinatus tendon.

cortical side partial tears, full thickness tears, calcific tendinosis, and subacromial-subdeltoid bursa abnormalities (calcified or inflamed). Cortical irregularities are secondary indicators of former or active cortical side partial tears. Cartilage interface sign, which is a hyperechoic signal, that appears superficially on the surface of the hyaline cartilage that signifies a through transmission sign of the sound wave going through a partial to full thickness rotator cuff tear. It is important to use dynamic testing for acromial impingement with shoulder abduction in a neutral position. It is important to scan the entire width of the spraspinatus tendon in short-axis from anterior to posterior. This is best assessed with the rotator interval view where you can best visualize the anterior free edge of the tendon, the most common area of tendon tears. The IST should also be examined as a part of a comprehensive US scanning of the shoulder. It is uncommon to find IST tears in isolation without concomitant SST pathology, but IST tears can commonly extend from posterior SST tears. Isolated partial IST tears may also be associated with posterior labrum tears (26).

tendinosis (Figures 13.3A–C) (27). In supraspinatus tears repaired surgically, PRP with or after surgery can decrease re-tear rate (28,29). Currently, full thickness tears should be first treated with primary surgical repair. If surgery is contraindicated, a fibrin or LA graft may be used with PRP or BMC if there is limited retraction. A minimally processed ADSC product can also be used. This is attractive as ADSC contains not only cellular products for tissue healing but can also act to fill in the defect, that is, act as a scaffold. It is important to screen for redundant biceps tendinopathy or other rotator cuff tendinopathy, which should be treated concomitantly. If either calcific tendinopathy or adhesive capsulitis are present, these should be treated before a regenerative treatment.

There is no literature regarding the benefit of using amniotic membrane or umbilical cord blood products for this pathology, although there are tissue collagen, heavy chain hyaluronic acid, various growth factors, and tissue inhibitors of metalloproteases (TIMPs) in amniotic membrane products that could support its potential usefulness for this condition.

Indications for Use

Common pathology seen in the SST that have indications for and efficacy with regenerative injections include partial thickness tears and

Preferred Technique

1. Equipment
   a. 20 to 25 G, 1.5- to 2-inch needle (an 18-G needle may be needed for injecting adipose)

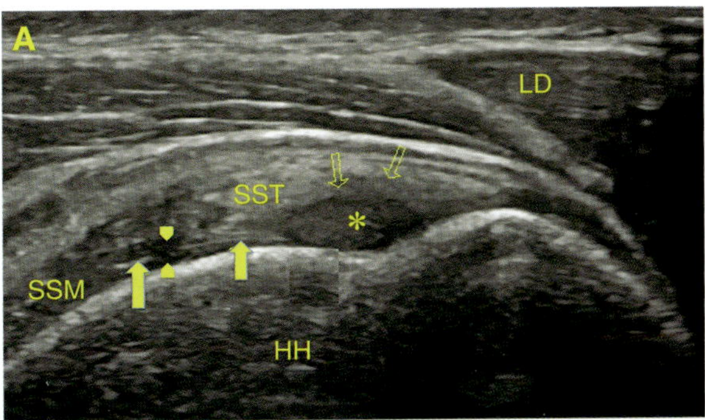

FIGURE 13.3A: Supraspinatus partial tear and tendinosis.

Arrowheads, tendon defect with loss of cartilage interface sign; arrows, hyaline cartilage of humerus (hypoechoic) with cartilage interface sign (hyperechoic); asterisk, Insertional tendinosis; HH, humeral head; LD, lateral deltoid; open arrows, tendon/tendinosis interface; SSM, supraspinatus muscle; SST, supraspinatus tendon.

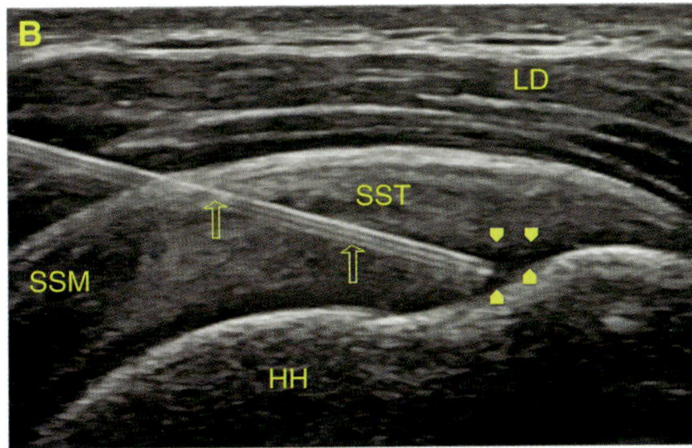

FIGURE 13.3B: Supraspinatus partial tear and tendinosis treatment.

Arrowheads, needle tip inserted into area of tendinosis; HH, humeral head; LD, lateral deltoid; open arrows, needle; SSM, supraspinatus muscle; SST, supraspinatus tendon.

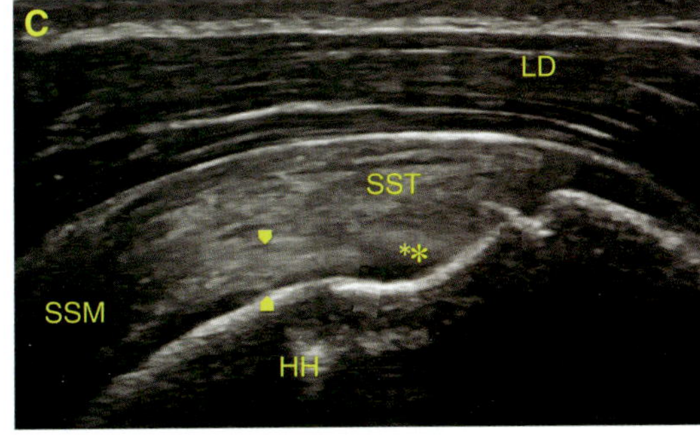

FIGURE 13.3C: Supraspinatus partial tear and tendinosis posttreatment.

Arrowheads, healed tendon defect with retained small area of cartilage loss; asterisk: normal tendon replaced prior tendinosis; HH, humeral head; LD, lateral deltoid; SSM, supraspinatus muscle; SST, supraspinatus tendon.

b. 3 to 5 mL of injectate

c. LR-PRP, LP-PRP, BMC, or ADSC

d. Consider fibrin, amniotic membrane graft (AMG), or fat graft for larger tears

2. Patient position

a. Lateral decubitus position with pathologic side up

b. Modified Crass position with supinated arm in back pocket or over posterior buttock

3. Transducer position

a. Over the supraspinatus in long or short-axis

b. Identify area of pathology (tear or tendinosis)

4. Needle orientation

a. In-plane or out-of-plane

5. Target

a. Fenestrate the tear or tendinosis, depositing microdoses of PRP into the tendon; take care not to overdistend tears with the injectate

b. Deposit the remaining injectate into the subacromial-subdeltoid bursa

6. Special considerations

a. Depending on the location and size of the pathology, an out-of-plane approach

may be more effective in treating the entire length of the tear or tendinosis
    b. Start gentle ROM right away to prevent adhesive capsulitis
    c. Can start gentle resistance strengthening at 2 to 4 weeks depending on tear size
    d. Can apply these principles to both subscapularis and infraspinatus tears

Proximal Biceps and Subscapularis Tendons

Pertinent Anatomy

The proximal long-head BT originates from the supraglenoid tubercle and superior labrum. Its tendon sheath communicates with the GH joint. It then continues distally between the subscapularis and SST through the rotator interval. Here the BT is stabilized by the coracohumeral ligament dorsally, the superior GH ligament laterally, and the medial GH ligament medially. As the BT enters the bicipital groove between the greater and lesser tuberosities, it is secured by the transverse humeral ligament superficially. It then travels under the pectoralis major tendon as it becomes the biceps muscle. The subscapularis tendon (SSCT) arises from the subscapularis muscle on the anterior scapula and travels anteriorly along the anterior scapula to insert on the lesser tuberosity of the humerus. The subcoracoid bursa lies superficial to the SSCT and deep to the anterior deltoid, just lateral to the coracoid process.

US Findings

Imaging of the BT tendon is best conducted in short-axis to the tendon with the patient upright with the elbow flexed to 90° and the palm up (Figure 13.4). The entire portion of the tendon should be evaluated from the pectoralis major tendon inferiorly to the acromion superiorly. Any pathology should be confirmed in long-axis. Common findings include tendinosis and partial split tears. Proximal split tears can extend intra-articularly and indicate a likely SLAP tear. Dynamic testing with internal and external rotation should be performed to look for BT subluxation. Lateral subluxation is common with SSCT tears that include tearing or stretch injury to the transverse humeral ligament. Medial subluxation occurs with injury to the biceps pulley system. The SSCT is best visualized in both long and short-axis with the shoulder in external rotation. It has characteristic fingerlike tendon bundles at the musculotendinous junction, which should not be confused for tendinopathy. Common findings include partial tears, full-thickness tears, calcific tendinosis, and subcoracoid bursal effusion. Isolated subscapularis tears are rare, and are often associated with both supraspinatus and biceps tendinopathy (30).

Indications for Use

Common pathology seen in the BT that have indication for and efficacy with regenerative injections include partial split tears and tendinosis (31). It is important to screen for concomitant SLAP tears if a split tear continues intra-articularly. In addition with biceps split tears, screen for SST and SSCT tendinopathy. Fluid around the biceps without BT pathology indicates a concomitant supraspinatus tear or a GH source. Biceps subluxation is a relative contraindication to regenerative treatments, as stabilizing ligaments need to be repaired to prevent re-tear form recurrent subluxation.

Preferred Technique

1. Equipment
    a. 20 to 25 G, 1.5- to 2-inch needle
    b. 3 to 5 mL of injectate
    c. LP-PRP (as tendon communicates intra-articularly), BMC, or ADSC
2. Patient position
    a. Supine position
    b. Palm up
    c. For SSCT have the patient externally rotate

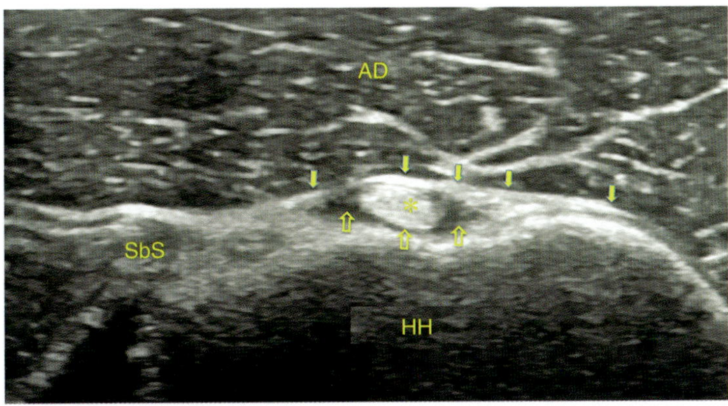

FIGURE 13.4: Anterior shoulder, SAX to biceps tendon.

AD, anterior deltoid; arrows, transverse humeral ligament; asterisk, biceps tendon; HH, humeral head; open arrows, physiologic intrasheath fluid; SbS, subscapularis tendon.

3. Transducer position
   a. Over BT in short axis
   b. Over the SSCT in long-axis and/or short-axis
   c. Identify area of pathology (tear or tendinosis)

4. Needle orientation
   a. Out-of-plane for BT lateral to medial approach to avoid the anterior humeral circumflex artery found in the lateral aspect of the biceps groove
   b. In-plane and/ or out-of-plane for SSCT

5. Target
   a. Fenestrate the tear or tendinosis, depositing microdoses of PRP into the tendon
   b. Take care not to overdistend tears with the injectate
   c. Deposit the remaining injectate into the BT sheath for BT injections or subcoracoid bursa for SSCT injections

6. Special considerations
   a. If a small SLAP tear is suspected, perform the BT injection in long-axis with an in-plane needle orientation to ensure flow of the injectate intra-articularly
   b. Start gentle ROM within 2 to 3 days
   c. Can start gentle resistance strengthening at 2 weeks
   d. If BT subluxation, medial or lateral, consider surgical referral

ELBOW

Here, we present the most commonly treated areas in the elbow including the common flexor and extensor tendons, and the ulnar and radial collateral ligaments. The other areas that can be treated, but are not presented, include the elbow joint, triceps tendon, and distal BT. One can use the general guidelines earlier in the chapter in conjunction with a manual on how to perform US-guided injections to assist in treating these areas.

Common Extensor Tendon and Radial Collateral Ligament Complex

Pertinent Anatomy

The common extensor tendon (CET) originates at the lateral epicondyle and runs distally along the posterior radius and ulna forming the extensor carpi radialis brevis (ECRB), extensor carpi ulnaris (ECU), extensor digitiorum communis and extensor digiti minimi. The radial collateral ligament complex (RCLC) provides stability between the radius and both the humerus and ulna. It is composed of the radial collateral ligament proper (RCL), annular ligament (AL), and the lateral ulnar collateral ligament (LUCL). The RCL lies just deep to the CET and runs from the lateral epicondyle to the AL. The AL encircles the head of the radius at the radio-humeral articulation. The LUCL runs from the posterior lateral epicondyle to the supinator crest on the ulna. It is relatively indistinguishable from the RCL and is often referred to as the posterior band of the RCL.

US Findings

Imaging of the CET is best conducted in long-axis to the tendon to visualize the entire footprint of the origin (Figure 13.5). The patient's elbow flexed to 90° and the forearm pronated. Common pathologic findings include tendinosis, partial thickness tears, and calcific enthesophytes. One should always interrogate the RCL to look for partial tears especially in the posterior aspect of the lateral epicondyle. One should perform dynamic testing during supination and pronation to look for radial head subluxation as a secondary indicator to LUCL and RCL tears (22). This is also an important dynamic test to find AL tears, which can mimic lateral epicondylosis. One should also examine the radial nerve at the level of the arcade of Frohse as a mild compression can mimic lateral epicondylosis, which is hallmarked by a deep branch of the radial nerve of greater than 1 mm area squared in circumference.

Indications for Use

Common pathology seen in the CET that have indication for and efficacy with regenerative injections include partial thickness tears and tendinosis. Lateral epicondylosis is the most widely studied condition for use of PRP and there is level 1 evidence that supports its efficacy (3,4). Consider debriding enthesophytes before regenerative treatments if one feels they are symptomatic, which is uncommon. It is important to screen for concomitant RCL and/or LUCL tears and stretch injuries, which should be treated concomitantly.

There is no literature regarding the benefit of using amniotic membrane or umbilical cord blood products for this pathology, although there are numerous growth factors in these products that could support its potential usefulness for this condition.

Preferred Technique

1. Equipment
   a. 27 to 20 G (generally 22 G), 1.25- to 1.5-inch needle
   b. 3 to 4 mL of injectate
   c. LR-PRP or LP-PRP, BMC, LA, AMG
2. Patient position
   a. Supine position
   b. Elbow flexed and neutral pronation/supination with internal shoulder rotation to rest the arm and elbow on the patient's abdomen
3. Transducer position
   a. Over the CET in long-axis and short axis
   b. Identify area of pathology (tear or tendinosis)
4. Needle orientation
   a. In-plane and check out-of-plane to make sure the A/P diameter of the pathologic area has been fully treated with the needling and injection technique
5. Target
   a. Fenestrate the tear or tendinosis, depositing microdoses of PRP into the tendon
   b. Take care not to overdistend tears with the injectate
6. Special considerations
   a. If there are multiple sites of pathology (e.g., CET, RCL, LUCL, AL), an out-of-plane approach may be more effective in treating all areas thoroughly with one entry point
   b. Start gentle ROM in 48 hours
   c. Start or restart pain-free physical therapy exercises (especially eccentrics) at 2 weeks

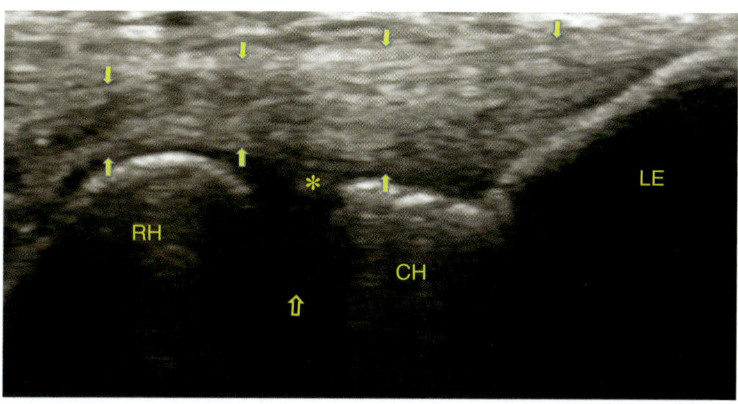

FIGURE 13.5: Lateral elbow, LAX to common extensor tendon.

Arrows, common extensor tendon; asterisk, annular ligament of the radius; CH, capitulum of the humerus; LE, lateral epicondyle; open arrow, humeroradial joint space; RH, radial head.

Common Flexor Tendon, Ulnar Collateral ligament

Pertinent Anatomy

The common flexor tendon (CFT) originates at the medial epicondyle and runs distally along the ulna forming the flexor carpi radialis, palmaris longus, flexor digitorum superficialis, and flexor carpi ulnaris. The pronator teres (PT) muscle has two heads: the humeral head and the ulnar head. The two heads of the PT connect the ends of the humerus and the ulna to the radius. The humeral head is larger than the ulnar portion. The humeral head begins above the medial epicondyle, on the medial supracondylar ridge and proximal to the CFT. The ulnar head originates below the elbow joint on the inside of the coronoid process of the ulna. The two heads approximate, cross the forearm diagonally, and insert halfway down the lateral surface of the radius via a common tendon.

The ulnar collateral ligament (UCL) provides stability between the ulna and the humerus. It is composed of an anterior band from the medial epicondyle to the coronoid process and the posterior band from the medial epicondyle to the olecranon. At this level, the ulnar nerve is just posterior to the CFT lying between the medial epicondyle and the olecranon in the cubital tunnel.

US Findings

Imaging of the CFT is best conducted in long-axis to the tendon to visualize the entire footprint of the origin (Figure 13.6). The patient's elbow flexed to 90° with the shoulder abducted and externally rotated. Common pathologic findings include tendinosis, partial thickness tears, and calcific enthesophytes. One should always interrogate the UCL to look for partial tears. Dynamic imaging with a valgus force can help establish UCL incompetency, which is greater than 0.5 mm of gapping in normal patients and greater than 2 mm in overhead throwing athletes (32). One should also examine the ulnar nerve along common entrapment points, as a mild compression (nerve cross sectional area of greater than 8 mm²) can mimic medial epicondylosis.

Indications for Use

Common pathology seen in the CFT that have indication for and efficacy with regenerative injections include partial thickness tears and tendinosis. Consider debriding enthesophytes before regenerative treatments if one feels they are symptomatic. It is important to screen for concomitant UCL tears and chronic stretch injuries, which should be treated concomitantly.

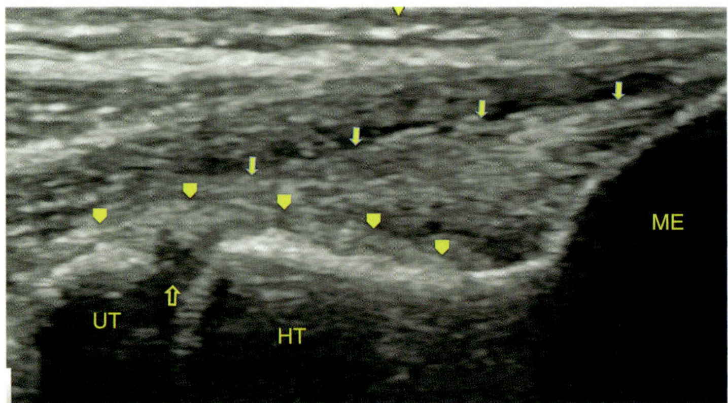

FIGURE 13.6: Medial elbow, LAX to common flexor tendon.

Arrowheads, ulnar collateral ligament; arrows, common flexor tendon; HT, humeral trochlea; ME, medial epicondyle; open arrow, humeroradial joint space; UT, ulnar trochlea.

Preferred Technique

1. Equipment
   a. 27 to 20 G (generally 22 G), 1.25- to 1.5-inch needle
   b. 2 to 4 mL of injectate
   c. LR-PRP or LP-PRP, BMC, LA, AMG

2. Patient position
   a. Supine position
   b. Elbow flexed to 90° with the shoulder abducted and externally rotated

3. Transducer position
   a. Over the CFT in long-axis and/or short-axis
   b. Identify area of pathology (tears or tendinosis)

4. Needle orientation
   a. In-plane or out-of-plane

5. Target
   a. Fenestrate the tear or tendinosis, depositing microdoses of PRP into the tendon
   b. Take care not to overdistend tears with the injectate

6. Special considerations
   a. If there are multiple sites of pathology (e.g., CFT, PT, UCL), an out-of-plane approach may be more effective in treating all areas thoroughly with one entry point
   b. Start gentle ROM in 48 hours

   c. Start or restart pain-free physical therapy exercises (especially eccentrics) at 2 weeks

WRIST AND HAND

Here, we present the most commonly treated areas in the wrist and hand including the first carpometacarpal (CMC) joint, carpal joint and ligaments, wrist extensor tendons, and the triangular fibrocartilage complex (TFCC). Other areas that can be treated, but are not presented, include the interphalangeal (IP) joints, other (2 to 5) CMC joints, and flexor tendons. One can use the general guidelines earlier in conjunction with an atlas of US-guided injections to assist in treating these areas.

First CMC Joint

Pertinent Anatomy
The first CMC joint is the articulation between the first metacarpal and the trapezium. The dorsal joint lies at the distal aspect of the anatomic snuffbox. The volar joint is at the base of thenar eminence. It is a saddle joint that allows for abduction, adduction, flexion, extension, circumduction, and opposition. Thus, the joint is prone to OA.

US Findings

Imaging of the CMC joint is best interrogated on the palmar surface in long-axis to the metacarpal, but the entire joint should be scanned palmar to dorsal (Figure 13.7). Common findings include cortical irregularities, osteophytes, effusion, and joint space narrowing and dorsal subluxation of the trapezium.

Indications for Use

Regenerative therapy for CMC arthritis is indicated for mild to moderate degenerative joint disease with at least moderate preservation of ROM. Consider debridement of mild to moderately sized osteophytes before regenerative treatments if there is restriction in ROM or symptomatic. It is important to screen for median neuropathy at the wrist (carpal tunnel syndrome) as it can mimic first CMC joint pain or coexist with it.

Preferred Technique

1. Equipment
   a. 25 to 27 G, 0.5- to 1.5-inch needle
   b. 0.5 to 2 mL of injectate
   c. LP-PRP or BMC
2. Patient position
   a. Supine or seated position
   b. Hand in neutral position with ulnar side down, resting on the table (radial up)

3. Transducer position
   a. Over CMC in long-axis to the 1st metacarpal on the dorsal side of the hand/wrist
4. Needle orientation
   a. Out-of-plane
5. Target
   a. CMC joint space
6. Special considerations
   a. Overdistention of the joint capsule causes increased postprocedure pain and can cause rupture of the capsule
   b. If the CMC joint is subluxed more than 25% dorsally, this may be a common reason for regenerative injection treatment failure and surgical reconstruction may be indicated

Carpal Bones and Articulation

Pertinent Anatomy

There are 15 bones and 20 articulations that make up the carpal joints. The bones include the distal radius and ulna, the eight carpal bones, and the five metacarpals. The radius and ulna articulate with the first row of metacarpals from radial to ulnar: scaphoid, lunate, triquetrium, and pisiform. These proximal carpal bones articulate

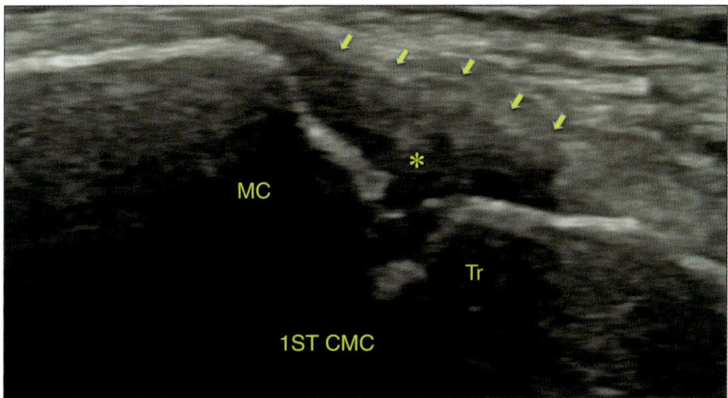

FIGURE 13.7: First carpometacarpal joint.

Arrows, joint capsule; asterisk, joint space; MC, first metacarpal; Tr, trapezium.

with the distal row from radial to ulnar: trapezium, trapezoid, capitate, and hamate, which articulate with the five metacarpals. Important articulations for treatment purposes include the distal radioulnar, scapholunate, scaphotrapeziotrapezoidal, lunocapitate, and carpometacapal joints.

US Findings

Imaging of the carpal joint(s) is best performed in long-axis to the joint being interrogated. One should palpate these joints for instability and/or pain to focus one's exam. The joints should be examined on both the dorsal and volar aspect. Common findings include cortical irregularities, fractures, osteophytes, effusion, ligament injury, and joint space narrowing. Common areas to find an effusion are the radioulnar, radiotriquetral (radiocarpal joint recess), and lunocapitate joints (midcarpal recess). Common areas of instability from ligament injury are the scapholunate (Figure 13.8) and scaphotrapeziotrapezoidal. One may also find osteonecrosis of the lunate.

Indications for Use

Regenerative therapy in the carpal region is indicated for mild to moderate degenerative joint disease with at least moderate preservation of ROM, as well as ligamentous injury. Consider debridement of small osteophytes that may be limiting ROM before regenerative therapy. Delayed or nonunion fractures also respond well to both PRP and BMC (16,17). (See general bone guidelines in the beginning of chapter.)

Preferred Technique

1. Equipment
   a. 25 to 30 G, 0.5- to 1.5-inch needle
   b. 1 to 3 mL of injectate
   c. LP-PRP or BMC
2. Patient position
   a. Supine
   b. Hand pronated with palmar side resting on a bolster on the table

3. Transducer position
   a. Long-axis over the carpal joint that is being treated
4. Needle orientation
   a. Out-of-plane
5. Target
   a. Carpal joint space
   b. Carpal ligaments (if necessary)
6. Special considerations
   a. If there is a suspicion for concomitant joint and ligament pathology, inject the joint first leaving some injectate left in the syringe. Layer the remaining injectate on top of the ligaments as one withdraws the needle. If one treats the more superficial ligaments first, there is a risk of injecting air into the tissue, obstructing the view of the joint.

Wrist Extensor Tendons

Pertinent Anatomy

There are nine extensors of the wrist and hand, whose tendons are composed of six separate compartments on the dorsum of the wrist and hand. The six dorsal compartments are as follows from radial to ulnar: (a) abductor pollicis longus (APL) and extensor pollicis brevis (EPB), (b) extensor carpi radialis longus (ECRL) and brevis (ECRB), (c) extensor pollicis longus (EPL), (d) extensor digitorum (ED) and extensor indicis (EI), (e) extensor digiti minimi, and (f) ECU.

US Findings

Imaging of the dorsal compartments of the wrist (DCW) is best conducted in short-axis. Use Lister's tubercle of the radius as a landmark that separates the second and third compartments. Scan radial from Lister's tubercle to identify the second and then the first dorsal compartments. Scan ulnar from Lister's tubercle to identify the third through sixth compartments. Use dynamic movements such as isolated digit extension to aid in proper identification of the compartment.

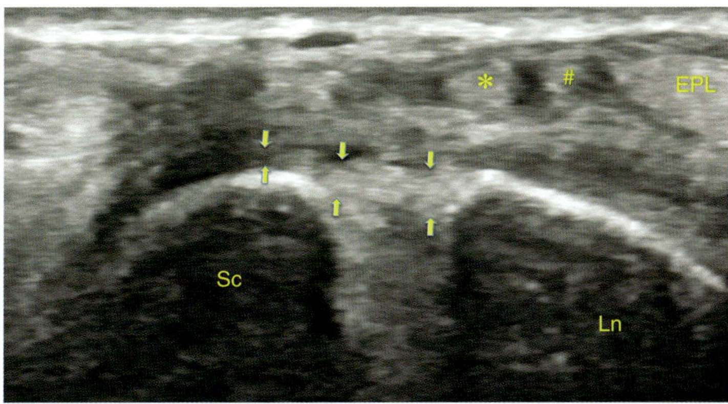

FIGURE 13.8: Dorsal wrist, LAX to scapholunate joint.

Arrows, scapholunate ligament; asterisk, extensor carpi radialis brevis; EPL, extensor pollicis longus; Ln, Lunate; pound, extensor carpi radialis longus; Sc, scaphoid.

Once the compartments are identified, image proximally and distally on the compartments that correlate with the patient's anatomical pain and dysfunction and also image in long-axis. Common findings include partial tears, tendinosis, and tenosynovitis. Dequervian's tenosynovitis involves the first dorsal compartment. Intersection syndrome is a tenosynovitis that occurs 4 to 8 cm proximal to Lister's tubercle where the first and second dorsal compartments intersect. The ECU tendon can also sublux from its groove in the ulna. This is associated with a tear in the tendon sub-sheath and often involves tearing to the tendon itself. It is important to interrogate the triangular fibrocartilage complex (TFCC) (see later) as it can mimic ulnar-sided pain as in ECU tendinopathy. The UCL in the TFCC complex can harbor split tears in gripping sports such as golf and tennis, and can mimic a TFCC or ECU pathology as well.

Indications for Use

Common pathology seen in DCW that has indication and efficacy for regenerative treatments includes partial tears (commonly split tear) and tendinosis. Full thickness tears with retraction are rare, but a relative contraindication to regenerative therapy. If there is solely tenosynovitis without tendinosis or tear consider conservative treatment and corticosteroid injection, and would recommend referral to rheumatology.

Preferred Technique

1. Equipment
   a. 25 to 30 G, 0.5- to 1.5-inch needle
   b. 0.5 to 3 mL of injectate
   c. LP-PRP, LR-PRP or BMC, AMG

2. Patient position
   a. Supine
   c. For compartments 1 to 2, hand in neutral position with ulnar side down, resting on the table (radial up)
   d. For compartments 3 to 6, hand in pronation with palmar side resting on a bolster on the table

3. Transducer position
   a. Over tendon being treated in short axis
   b. Identify area of pathology (tear or tendinosis)

4. Needle orientation
   a. In-plane or out-of-plane

5. Target
   a. Fenestrate the tear or tendinosis, depositing microdoses of injectate only when withdrawing the needle
   b. Do not distend tears with the injectate
   c. Deposit the remaining injectate into the tendon sheath

6.   Special considerations
   a.   Consider starting injection in short-axis then turning in long-axis to ensure all areas of tendinopathy have been treated
   b.   Consider wrist splint for 7 days then transition to only at night and during strenuous activities (e.g., typing)
   c.   Start gentle ROM in 2 to 3 days
   d.   Can start gentle resistance strengthening at 2 weeks
   e.   This technique can also be used for the flexor tendons of the wrist.

Triangular Fibrocartilage Complex

Pertinent Anatomy
The triangular fibrocartilage complex (TFCC) is composed of the articular disc, dorsal and volar radioulnar ligaments, meniscus homolog, ECU tendon sheath, and the ulnocarpal ligaments. The disc lies at the distal end of the ulna and articulates with the ulnar border of the radius. The meniscus homologue originates from the distal ulna and merges with the ECU tendon sheath and ulnocarpal ligaments to attach to the lunate and triquetrium. The TFCC stabilizes the radioulnar and ulnar carpal joints.

US Findings
Imaging of the TFCC is best performed in long-axis over the ulnocarpal joint. One should be able to produce an image with the ulna proximally and triquetrium distally. The TFCC lies between superficial ECU tendon and the lunate deep (Figure 13.9). The disc is distal to the base of the distal ulna while the meniscus and associated ulnocarpal ligaments are more superficial and distal. The most common findings include degenerative tears of the disc, tendinopathy of the ECU, and ligamentous injury to the radioulnar ligaments. However, ligament sprains/tears can be seen in the meniscus homologue and ulnocarpal ligaments.

Indications for Use
Degenerative and partial tears to any portion of the TFCC are indicated for regenerative therapies before surgical treatment. It is important to interrogate all structures that compose the TFCC as more than one area may have pathology.

Preferred Technique
1.   Equipment
   a.   25 to 30 G, 0.5- to 1.5-inch needle
   b.   1 to 2 mL of injectate
   c.   LP-PRP, LR-PRP, BMC, LA or AMG

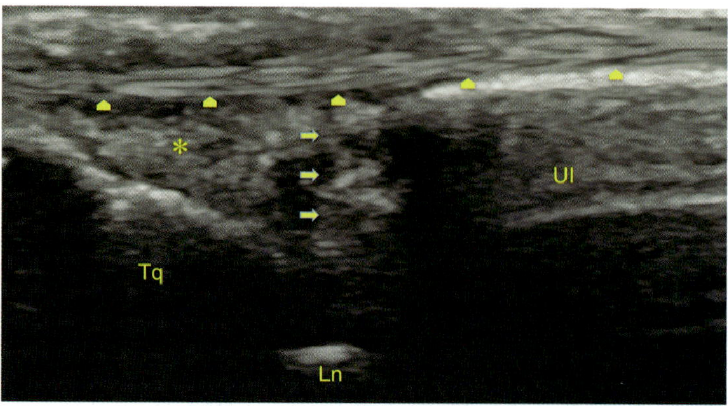

FIGURE 13.9: Ulnar wrist, LAX to ulno-triquetral joint.

Arrowheads, extensor carpi ulnaris; arrows, articular disc; asterisk, meniscus homologue; Ln, l; Tq, triquetrium; Ul, ulna.

2. Patient position
   a. Supine
   b. Palmar side down with forearm pronated and resting on a bolster
3. Transducer position
   a. Dorsally and/or ulnar over TFCC in long-axis to the ECU (as described in US findings)
   b. Identify area of pathology
4. Needle orientation
   a. Out-of-plane
5. Target
   a. Fenestrate the partial and degenerative tears, depositing microdoses of injectate only when withdrawing the needle
   b. Take care as to not extend tears with the injectate
   c. Deposit the remaining injectate between the ECU and TFCC
6. Special considerations
   a. Consider wrist splint for 7 days then transition to only at night and during strenuous activities (e.g., typing)
   b. Start gentle ROM in 2 to 3 days
   c. Can start gentle resistance strengthening at 2 weeks

HIP

Here, we present the most commonly treated areas in the hip including the femoroacetabular joint, acetabular labrum, and gluteus medius and minimus tendons. Other areas that can be treated, but are not presented, include the iliopsoas tendon, hamstring tendons, adductor tendons, pubic symphysis, and external rotator tendons. The hamstring tendons are treated similarly in theory to the gluteal tendons. One can use the general guidelines in this chapter's introduction in conjunction with a manual on how to perform US-guided injections to assist in treating these areas.

Femoroacetabular Joint

Pertinent Anatomy and Indications for Treatment

The femoroacetabular joint is a classic ball and socket joint in which both surfaces are lined with hyaline cartilage and the rim of the acetabulum is lined with a fibrocartilaginous labrum. The femoroacetabular joint is at risk of early chondral degeneration in cases of hip joint deformity. The types of deformity include developmental dysplasia of the hip (DDH) and femoroacetabular bony impingement anatomy (either cam, pincer, or both). Early arthritis can also result from posttraumatic causes, Legg-Calve-Perthes disease, slipped capital femoral epiphysis (SCFE), and avascular necrosis. Although regenerative techniques for hip OA have been shown to help clinically (33–35), in the authors' experience they have been less effective than for other joints. This may be related to the complexity of the hip and lumbopelvic region in general, later presentation, severe loss of ROM at presentation, lack of proximal migration of injectate with classic US or fluoroscopic injection techniques, historical difficulty with offloading the joint, and/or related untreated pathology.

US Findings

The femoroacetabular joint and its labrum are best visualized in a long-axis view over the anterior hip (Figure 13.10). In this view the acetabulum is superior or proximal, the anterior labrum extends distally from the acetabulum over the proximal femoral head. The femoral neck then slopes away from the transducer moving deep as it extends distally. Simple joint injections target the joint at the femoral neck to avoid chondral injury, whereas labral treatment is performed more proximally. The key target of the needle placement for a successful hip joint injection is deep to the overlying joint capsule where the recess of the femoral head neck junction creates a small pouch for the lumen of the needle to penetrate ensuring the injectate is inside the joint cavity. If too proximal, the lumen of the needle may be outside the joint capsule or injure the

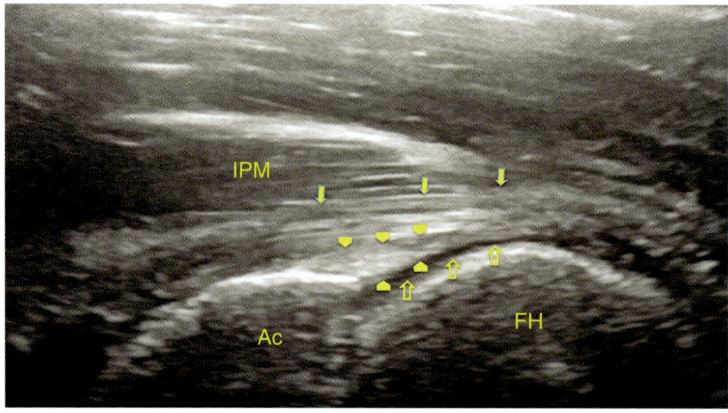

FIGURE 13.10: Anterior hip joint, LAX to femoral–acetabular joint.

Ac, acetabulum; arrowheads, anterior labrum; arrows, Iliopsoas tendon; FH, femoral head; IPM, iliopsoas muscle; open arrows, hyaline cartilage of femoral head.

hyaline cartilage surface. If too distal, the needle tip may rest in the redundant fold of the joint capsule that is not part of the synovial joint cavity.

Preferred Technique

1. Equipment:
   a. 25 G, 2 inch for a thin patient
   b. 22 G, 3.5- to 4-inch needle for a thick patient
   c. For LA use a styleted 20 G, 3.5-inch spinal needle
   d. Injectate: 4 to 8 mL LP-PRP, BMC, AMG for intra-articular injection

2. Patient position
   a. Supine

3. Transducer position
   a. Long-axis over femoroacetabular joint

4. Needle orientation
   a. In-plane from distal to proximal

5. Target
   a. Hip IA injection only: head–neck junction proximal to redundant fold of distal hip capsule
   b. If treating the labrum as well: one can also inject at the femoral acetabular articulation, slipping under the labrum

6. Special considerations
   a. Avoid needling femoral head cartilage. As degenerative labral changes are common in early hip OA, one should consider treating both the labrum, hip capsule, and joint. Off-loading of the joint for 1 to 2 days with nonweight bearing (NWB) and transition to partial weight bearing (PWB) for 2 to 5 days is advisable. Use of a hip unloading brace (such as Ossur unloading hip brace, that can be worn under clothing) can be considered while healing is ongoing, theoretically for 4 to 6 weeks.

Acetabular Labrum

Pertinent Anatomy and Indications

As mentioned earlier, the femoroacetabular joint and labrum are at risk of early chondrolabral degeneration or frank symptomatic tearing in cases of hip joint deformity. The types of deformity include developmental DDH and femoroacetabular bony impingement anatomy (either cam, pincer, or both). In most cases, the labrum is the first structure to degenerate, followed by the hyaline cartilage adjacent to it. US allows good visualization of the labrum and capsule, which consists of the iliofemoral ligaments anteriorly. Regenerative treatments of the labrum would be specific for fibrocartilage and would likely benefit most from LA + PRP or amniotic membrane (36). BMC could be considered, but lacks the extracellular matrix (ECM) needed to best fill defects. Hauser, in 2013, also found positive results with dextrose prolotherapy (37). Choice of treatment would be based on the type of labral pathology (i.e., partial, degenerative, calcific, or detached tear) and large detached labral tears would be the most likely to not respond to nonsurgical regenerative treatments. However, the authors have had small- to medium-sized full thickness tears heal quite effectively in many cases with cellular grafting techniques. Experience and judgment must be used to decide candidacy for regenerative treatment versus surgical excision or repair. There is no literature regarding the potential benefit of using amniotic membrane for this pathology although there are numerous growth factors and collagen scaffolding in this product that could support its usefulness for this condition.

US Findings

Labral degeneration and partial tears typically appear hypoechoic in the anterior femoroacetabular labrum. The tears can be vertically oriented, horizontal, or stellate in appearance. Others include calcifications, impinging exostosis type spurs, thickening and myxoid degeneration of the labrum, as well as paralabral cysts.

Preferred Technique

1. Equipment

a. Styleted 25 G, 2 inch

b. 18 to 21 G, 3.5-inch needle for ADSC

c. Injectate: LP-PRP, LR-PRP (RBC+), ADSC, BMC, AMG or a combination of these products

2. Patient position

   a. Supine

3. Transducer position

   a. Long-axis over the femoroacetabular joint and labrum parallel to the femoral neck

4. Needle orientation

   a. In-plane, with medial–lateral treatment coverage confirmed out-of-plane

   b. Alternatively, if tear involves acetabular origin, can use an out-of-plane approach from lateral to medial. The tear(s) can be interrogated and filled with a cellular graft technique minimizing any intrusion into the hyaline cartilage area of the joint.

5. Target

   a. Acetabular labrum

6. Special considerations

   a. Vascular supply of the labrum arises equally from the bony acetabulum proximally and the anterior capsule overlying the distal labrum. Use a Doppler time out technique to make sure to avoid overlying vessels and femoral head cartilage during injection.

   b. Offloading the hip with crutches, NWB followed by PWB for 2 to 5 days and/or a hip unloading brace such as the Ossur unloading hip brace can be considered for 4 to 6 weeks postinjection, although there is no literature to answer the question if offloading the joint makes a difference in outcomes.

Gluteus Medius, Gluteus Minimus, and Iliotibial Tract

Pertinent Anatomy

Three important tendons are noted about the lateral hip. Most superficial is the tensor fascia lata and its iliotibial (IT) band which extends distally along the lateral thigh to its insertion onto Gerdy's tubercle of the anterolateral tibia. The tendons of the gluteus medius and gluteus minimus lie deep to the IT band in the lateral hip and insert onto the lateral and anterior facets of the greater trochanter, respectively. The gluteus medius insertion is quite large with a footprint on the lateral facet over a 3.5 cm rectangular area that is oriented 37° oblique to the long-axis of the femur (38). The anterior portion of the tendon is thus found more medial and distal, while the superoposterior portion of the glut med insertion is found laterally and proximally, with its distinct thick, stout fibers.

Pathology of all four areas can be identified, and treatment depends on the pathology encountered. PRP of the gluteus tendon insertions has shown promise (39), but needling, prolotherapy, and other treatments are reasonable options (40). Larger tears may require a scaffold or ADSC. There is no literature regarding the potential benefit of using amniotic membrane or umbilical cord products for this pathology, although there are numerous growth factors in these products that could support its potential usefulness for this condition.

US Findings

The gluteus medius and minimus are best found in short-axis where the peak of the greater trochanter separates the anterior from the lateral facet (Figure 13.11). Accurate understanding of the earlier discussed anatomy helps the clinician to better identify treatable tendon pathology, which would include tendinosis, partial tears, calcifications, and enthesopathies. Thickening and/or calcifications of the IT band, full thickness tears, and bursitis can also be seen.

KNEE

Here, we present the most commonly treated areas in the knee including the knee joint, quadriceps and patella tendons, ACL, and medial and lateral meniscus and collateral ligaments. Other areas that can be treated, but are not presented, include distal hamstring tendons, popliteus tendon or muscle, posterior cruciate ligament, and pes anserine tendons. One can use the general guidelines in this chapter's introduction in conjunction with a manual on how to perform US-guided injections to assist in treating these areas.

Suprapatellar Recess of the Knee Joint

Pertinent Anatomy and Indications

The knee joint comprises three compartments, the medial, lateral, and patellofemoral. For intra-articular injections, the lateral suprapatellar pouch of the knee joint is perhaps the most accurate means of successful intra-articular injection (Figure 13.12) (41–43). The suprapatellar recess is

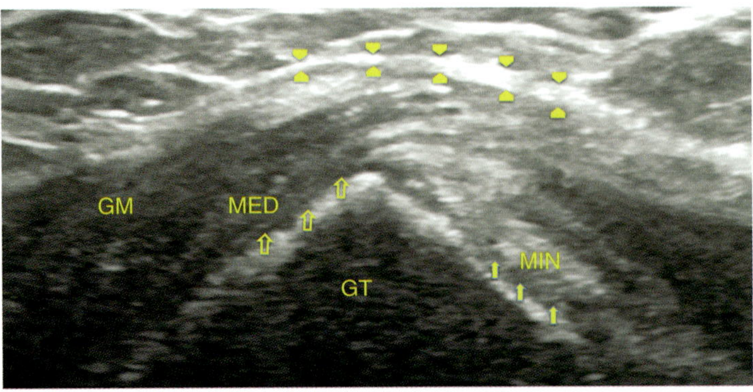

FIGURE 13.11: Lateral hip, SAX over the femur over the greater trochanter.

Arrowheads, iliotibial band; arrows, subgluteus minimus bursa; GM, gluteus maximus muscle; GT, greater trochanter; MED, gluteus medius tendon (hypoechoic form anisotropy); MIN, gluteus minimus tendon; open arrows, subgluteus medius bursa.

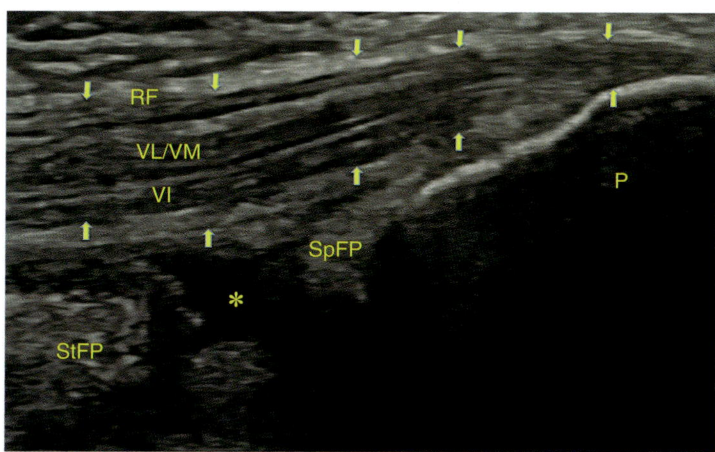

FIGURE 13.12: Anterior knee, LAX to the quadriceps tendon.

Arrows, quadriceps tendon; asterisk, suprapatellar recess; P, patella; RF, rectus femoris portion of quad tendon; SpFP, suprapatellar fat pad; StFP, supratrochlear fat pad; VI, vastus intermedius portion of quad tendon; VL/VM, vastus lateralis and medialis portion of quad tendon.

an extension of the knee joint proximally and lies between the deeper supratrochlear (or prefemoral) fat pad and the more superficial suprapatellar fat pad.

A significant body of literature has emerged worldwide regarding the regenerative treatments for knee OA. There are multiple meta-analyses showing superiority of PRP to traditional treatments such as steroids and viscosupplementation in terms of both pain and function in both short and long term (44–48). Stem cell-rich tissues, including BMC and ADSC, have also been shown to regenerate cartilage defects on both MRI and on second look arthroscopy (3–5). There is no literature regarding the benefit of using amniotic membrane or umbilical cord blood products for this pathology although there are numerous growth factors in these products that could support its potential usefulness for this condition.

US Findings

The knee joint can be difficult to visualize in a dry knee, but is very simple to find when effusion is present. Key landmarks to help ensure intra-articular injection are to distinguish between the fat pads and the suprapatellar recess. With the transducer in long-axis over the distal quadriceps tendon, first look between the suprapatellar and prefemoral fat pads for a hypoechoic line of fluid (Figure 13.12). When found, turn the transducer short-axis and approach that fluid line from lateral to medial with needle in-plane with transducer. In case no fluid exists, one can have the patient perform a quad contraction to visualize this interface. If still unsure, the examiner can push the prefemoral fat pad or lateral patella with a finger from lateral to medial to see the interface between the fat pad and the quadriceps tendon as they slide past one another. An alternative option is to look at the medial and lateral parapatellar recesses where a thin hypoechoic line can often be found that represents an extension of the knee joint. This can be remarkably superficial. This recess can be augmented by pushing the patella laterally, which opens up the parapatellar recess gapping the lateral patellofemoral joint (Figure 13.13). The target is the anechoic joint fluid, taking care to avoid the retropatellar cartilage (49).

Preferred Technique

1. Equipment
    a. 18 (for ADSC injection) to 25 G, 1.5- to 2-inch needle
    b. Injectate: LP-PRP, BMC, ADSC, AMG

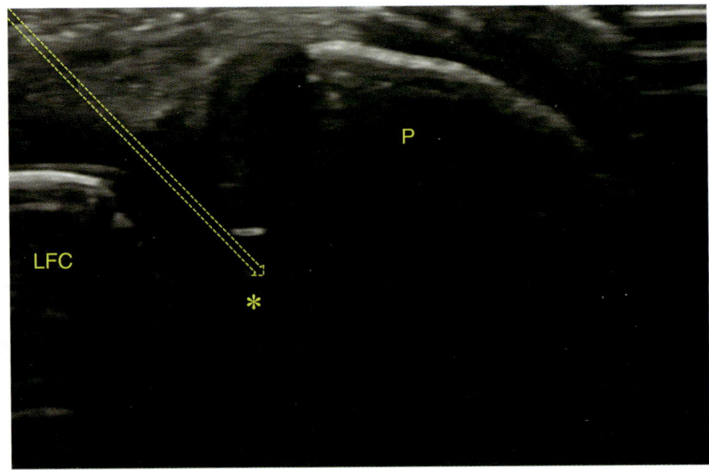

FIGURE 13.13: Lateral approach to intra-articular knee injection (with lateral patella traction).

Asterisk, knee joint; dashed arrows, needle trajectory; LFC, lateral femoral condyle; P, patella.

2. Patient position
    a. Supine with knee on a small bolster or in full relaxed extension

3. Transducer position
    a. Short axis over the distal quadriceps or the parapatellar recess
    b. For patellofemoral approach, the probe is placed short-axis over the lateral patellofemoral joint to view the parapatellar recess (Figure 13.13)

4. Needle orientation
    a. In-plane

5. Target:
    a. Suprapatellar recess of the knee joint
    b. Parapatellar recess of the knee joint

6. Pearls:
    a. A dilute (less than or equal to 0.2% lidocaine) anesthetic injection before helps anesthetize the needle path and localize the true joint space as fluid can be seen shooting across the joint from lateral to medial or disappear into the joint space.
    b. If the injectate expands the fat pad or the quadriceps tendon especially with increased pain, then the needle is not in the joint space and the needle position should be readjusted.

c. If the suprapatellar recess is difficult to visualize, the lateral parapatellar recess can be used or other techniques, such as the medial patellofemoral recess.

Quadriceps and Patellar Tendons

Pertinent Anatomy and Indications

The rectus femoris, vastus lateralis, vastus medialis, and vastus intermedius converge to form the quadriceps tendon. The tendon inserts on the proximal patella, the largest sesamoid bone in the human body. The patellar tendon originates from the distal patella and inserts on the tibial tubercle. The quadriceps and patellar tendons are readily accessible with US guidance and can suffer from partial tears, tendinosis, calcifications, and postoperative scarring. Pathology typically involves deep proximal tendinosis and partial tears, less commonly the distal insertion and more rarely, the entire tendon can be involved. There is evidence to support the use of PRP in these tendons (38,50,51).

US Findings

The quadriceps and patella tendons are best initially visualized in long-axis. The three layers of the quadriceps tendon can be differentiated, with the superficial arising from the rectus femoris, the middle arising from the vastus medialis and lateralis, and the deep layer arising from the vastus intermedius (Figure 13.12). The suprapatellar recess is deep to the quad tendon, while Hoffa's fat pad is deep to the patella tendon (Figure 13.14). The primary diagnosis of quadriceps and patellar tendinosis demonstrate hypertrophic and hypoechoic tendon thickening potentially with calcifications, partial tears, and enthesopathy.

Preferred Technique

1. Equipment
   a. 18 to 25 G, 1.5-inch needle
   b. Injectate: PRP, ADSC, BMC, AMG
2. Patient position
   a. Supine with knee bent 30° flexion supported by a rolled towel or pillow
3. Transducer position
   a. Start in short-axis to the tendon at largest area to the lesion
   b. During treatment switch to long-axis to ensure treatment of the entire three-dimensional pathology
4. Needle orientation
   a. Start in-plane, but ensure three-dimensional treatment medial to lateral including short-axis views

5. Target
   a. Area of tendinopathy
6. Pearls:
   a. After tendon fenestration with injectate, consider hydrodissection of the patella tendon with remaining injectate

Anterior Cruciate Ligament

Pertinent Anatomy and Indications

A partial tear of the ACL can heal, and regenerative techniques may help facilitate that healing. Complete tears of the ACL are an obviously greater challenge, and it is interesting to see if regenerative techniques are able to prove helpful going forward. In the authors' experience, when a patient's exam and MRI are at odds, new in-office mini-arthroscopy has often found partial tears in the ACL, where the MRI suggested a full thickness complete tear. These patients then had the opportunity to be treated with a regenerative medicine injection treatment instead of a surgical reconstruction. This work is in its infancy and currently, full thickness ACL tears should definitely be treated with surgical reconstruction. Animal studies in porcine and canine models have found that a collagen-PRP hydrogel enhanced primary ACL suture repairs as compared to suture repair alone (52,53). Likewise, a human in vitro study of PRP effect on ACL cells

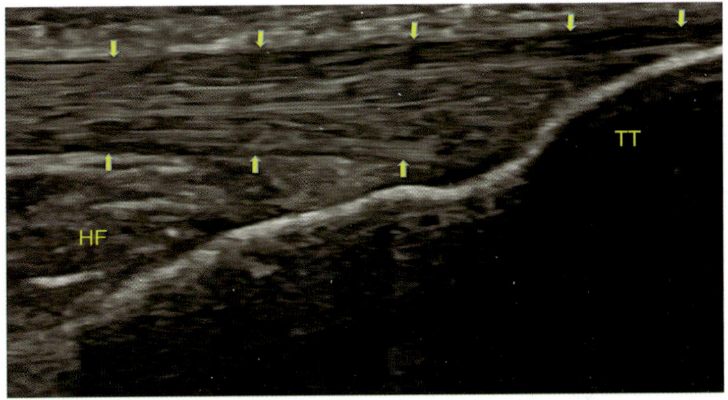

FIGURE 13.14: Anterior knee LAX to the distal patellar tendon.

Arrows, patella tendon; HF, Hoffa's fat pad; TT, tibial tuberosity.

showed significant increases in cell number and collagen production (54).

There is no literature regarding the benefit of using amniotic membrane or umbilical cord blood products for this pathology although there are numerous growth factors in these products that could support its potential usefulness for this condition.

US Findings

ACL tears are much better delineated with MRI than on US. Once the nature and location of the ACL sprain is ascertained from the MRI, it is possible to direct treatment to either the proximal or distal end of the ACL or both ends, as well as a midsubstance targeted treatment. Both fluoroscopic and US-guided procedures have been described (55,56).

Preferred Technique

1. Equipment
   a. 25 G, 2-inch needle
   b. Injectate: PRP, ADSC, or BMC
2. Patient position
   a. Distal ACL: supine with knee bent about 90°
   b. Proximal ACL: prone with knee extended
3. Transducer position
   a. Distal ACL: both long- and short-axis views are helpful. In short-axis, angle the beam posteroinferiorly at about a 45° angle to find the round fibers of the ACL overlying the proximal tibia. This appears as a hyperechoic round ball of ligament fibers when the probe is perpendicular to the ACL fibers and hypoechoic when anisotropic.
   b. Proximal ACL: short-axis view shows the proximal ACL just medial to the LFC along the lateral wall of the intercondylar notch superiorly and directly lateral to the PCL insertion. The PCL has a round ball hyperechoic appearance at its origin and the ACL has a thinner elliptical appearance at its origin. When injured, the ACL origin appears ill-defined, hypoechoic, and swollen compared to its normal compact appearance.

4. Needle orientation
   a. Distal ACL: start with probe in long-axis to the ligament and needle approach out-of-plane to ACL insertion, then switch to out-of-plane with short-axis to ensure needle is within the ACL, treating from medial to lateral
   b. Proximal ACL: short-axis views to the ACL are key to ensure safe passage to the origin of the ACL, while avoiding the neurovascular bundle of the posterior knee. The key safety measure is to visualize the popliteal artery and decide whether its location permits safe passage from a medial to lateral approach or a more vertical short-axis approach if the artery lies more medial.
5. Target:
   a. Distal ACL, target is the distal insertion of the ACL onto the tibia and up proximally as far as one can see.
   b. For proximal ACL, target is the proximal origin of the ACL on the lateral wall of the intercondylar notch and distally as is visible.
6. Pearls:
   a. A partially torn ACL is pressure sensitive. Caution the patient and consider pretreating the ligament injection site with a small amount of anesthesia to facilitate a comfortable injection.
   b. A specific functional rehabilitation program should be reviewed with the patient and treating physical therapist. This would likely include a short period, (1 week) of limited weight-bearing following the procedure. Temporary ACL bracing postprocedure should be considered for 6 weeks postinjection as well.

Medial Meniscus and Medial Collateral Ligament

Pertinent Anatomy and Indications

The fibrocartilaginous medial meniscus lies deep to the medial collateral ligament (MCL). Both should be evaluated when treating medial compartment knee OA as they can contribute to joint line pain. Dynamic US with valgus stress of the extruded medial meniscus is helpful in determining the utility of a medial unloading brace, particularly if it allows the meniscus to reseat into the joint. In such cases, treat the coronary ligament attaching the meniscus to the tibia and the meniscus itself, followed by a short period of NWB and up to 6 weeks of medial unloading bracing. Regarding the MCL, most tears are seen proximally and many are occult, meaning they are only discovered during the hydrostatic injection of treatments or preanesthesia before treatment.

For the meniscus, in vivo and in vitro animal studies show superior histological scores and DNA and ECM synthesis in rabbits that received PRP in a gelatin hydrogel versus platelet-poor plasma (PPP) or the hydrogel alone (57). More recent in vitro and meniscal cell culture study suggests 10% human serum to be superior to 5% PRP or ACP (58), but previous studies have shown optimal meniscal cell culture growth is achieved with 10% to 20% PRP solution (59); therefore, the comparison of human serum to PRP study should be repeated with a higher PRP concentration. Unfortunately, not all in vitro and animal studies have shown beneficial outcomes of PRP in the meniscus (60,61). BMC, however, looks promising in improving healing acute meniscal tears in sheep (62,63). ADSCs have the advantage of providing structural scaffolding, pluripotent cells, and a cellular nest to protect those cells. They have shown excellent promise in rabbit menisci (64) and could help improve survivability of allograft meniscal transplants in surgical patients (65). In horses, both bone marrow and ADSCs implanted on collagen scaffolds led to an improved healing of meniscal tears a year after implantation (66). Clinical data in the MCL are limited to case reports in humans (67), yet there are studies in rabbits suggesting PRP leads to favorable histological and structural properties (68–70).

There is no literature regarding the benefit of using amniotic membrane or umbilical cord blood products for this pathology, although there are numerous growth factors in these products that could support its potential usefulness for this condition.

US Findings

US of the medial meniscus is best performed in long-axis to the MCL (Figure 13.15). The meniscus is deep to the collateral ligament. The MCL has two distinct bands, superficial and deep, with the

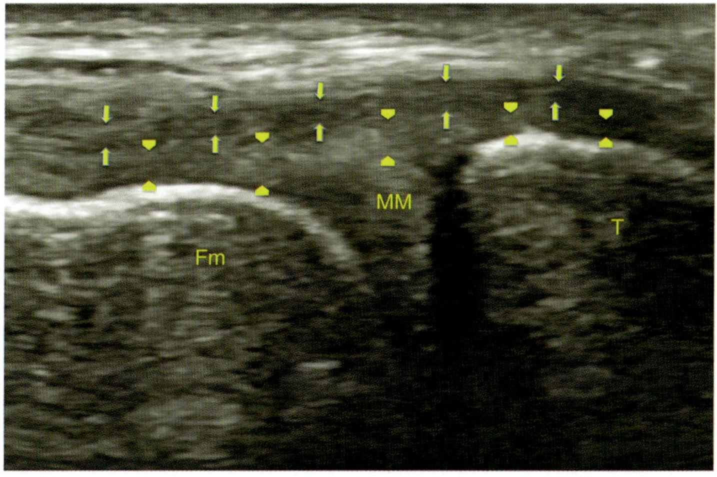

FIGURE 13.15: Medial knee, LAX to the medial collateral ligament.

Arrow heads, deep medial collateral ligament; arrows, superficial medial collateral ligament; Fm, femur; MM, medial meniscus; T, tibia.

deep adhered to the medial meniscus. Meniscus tears will appear anechoic, while myxoid degeneration makes the meniscus generally hypoechoic. It is also important to look for meniscus extrusion with more evidence on knee extension. An MCL partial tear appears anechoic, while a stretch injury has a hypoechoic region of the ligament.

Preferred Technique

1. Equipment:
    a. 18 (for ADSC) to 25 G, 1.5- to 2-inch needle
    b. Injectate: PRP, BMC, ADSC, and amniotic membrane
2. Patient position
    a. Supine with knee slightly bent and leg externally rotated
3. Transducer position
    a. Long-axis over the MCL and confirm anterior to posterior treatment with short axis
4. Needle orientation
    a. Out-of-plane is preferred for meniscus treatment
    b. In-plane or out-of-plane for MCL
5. Target:
    a. For medial meniscus, target plane between MCL and medial meniscus, as well as into the degenerative portions of the meniscus itself.
    b. It is very important to target the coronary ligament defects that accompany many torn and extruded meniscus tears, and then deep into the joint when treating the joint as well.
6. Pearls:
    a. Injecting the MCL and medial meniscus can be very sensitive. Consider a deep obturator nerve block at the distal obturator canal or medial geniculate nerve blocks.
    b. Pulsatility of the medial geniculate artery with Doppler appears to be helpful in predicting the healing potential of the medial meniscus.

Lateral Meniscus and Lateral Collateral Ligament

Pertinent Anatomy and Indications

Lateral compartment arthritis does not respond as well to regenerative treatments of the joint, and especially if the lateral meniscus is involved. This is due to the fact that the lateral meniscus is more fixed to the tibial plateau compared to the medial meniscus. When torn it is more susceptible to shear stress, making it harder to treat and heal with a regenerative treatment. Even when meticulous care of surrounding static and dynamic stabilizers is taken, if the lateral meniscus is discoid, badly torn, unstable, truncated, and significantly extruded, regenerative techniques here are less predictable. As discussed with medial joint and meniscus, lateral unloading bracing following the joint and/or meniscus treatments is wise to avoid excessive shear forces across the joint. As with the medial joint line, evaluation of the lateral geniculate artery for pulsatility before meniscal treatment is advised.

The primary ligament to evaluate in the lateral knee is the fibular collateral ligament (FCL), also known as the "lateral collateral ligament" (LCL) (Figure 13.16). Insertional enthesopathies, calcifications, and partial strains can be identified on US and treated, typically first with prolotherapy or PRP.

See the medial meniscus and medial collateral ligament section for treatment recommendations that can be applied to the lateral joint, meniscus, and collateral ligament.

ANKLE

Here, we present the most commonly treated areas in the ankle including the tibiotalar joint, posterior tibial tendon, subtalar joint, anterior talofibular (ATFL) calcaneofibular and anterior inferior tibiofibular ligaments (AITFL). Other areas that can be treated, but are not presented, include the peroneal, tibialis anterior, flexor digitorum, and flexor hallucis tendons. All of these tendons are treated similarly in theory to the tibialis

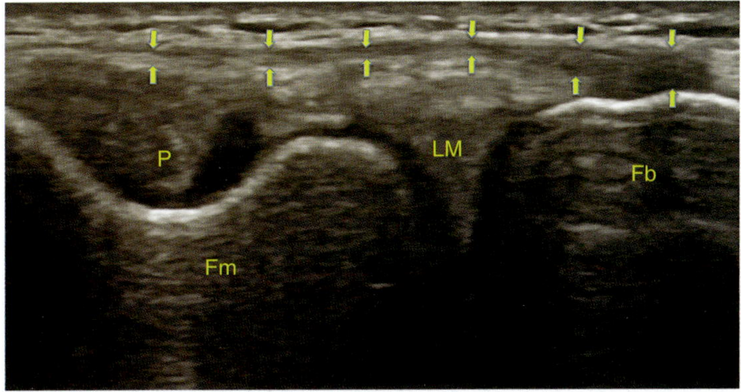

FIGURE 13.16: Lateral knee, LAX to the lateral collateral ligament.

Arrows, lateral collateral ligament; Fb, fibula; Fm, femur; LM, lateral meniscus; P, popliteus.

posterior tendon. One can use the general guidelines at the beginning of the chapter in conjunction with a manual on how to perform US-guided injections to assist in treating these areas.

Tibiotalar Joint

Pertinent Anatomy and Indications

Useful routes for tibiotalar injection are deep to the tibialis anterior tendon and in the anterolateral gutter of the ankle deep to the ATFL (Figure 13.17). Care must be exercised to avoid unintentional intrachondral needling. Offloading via heel wedges, customized shoe modifications or a period of NWB should be considered especially if a significant varus or valgus deformity of the tibiotalar joint is noted on standing x-rays.

Biomechanical realignment and injection of ADSCs have improved outcomes compared to microfracture alone in varus ankle OA (71,72). Bone marrow-derived cells also benefited patients receiving ankle scope debridement for OA with osteochondral lesions of the talus (73). Not surprisingly, in this study, better results were obtained with earlier stages of OA and lower BMI.

Preferred Technique

1. Equipment
   a. 20 to 25 G, 1.5-inch needle
   b. Injectate: LP-PRP, BMC, ADSC, AMG

2. Patient position
   a. Supine for anterior approach
   b. Side lying with lateral ankle up for sub-ATFL technique with pillow or buttress under distal tibia to allow the ankle to invert to help open up the lateral tibiotalar joint space

3. Transducer position
   a. For anterior approach, long-axis over the tibiotalar joint
   b. For lateral recess, transducer should be in long-axis over the ATFL (Figure 13.16)

4. Needle orientation
   a. In-plane or out-of-plane

5. Target
   a. Intra-articular space deep to the anterior fat pad over tibiotalar joint
   b. Deep to the ATFL on ATFL view

6. Pearls:
   a. Use care to avoid needling the talar dome cartilage by using a slight distal to proximal approach, keeping bevel away from the talar dome cartilage.
   b. Because of the risk of injuring talar hyaline cartilage in the anterior approach, the authors' preferred technique is the sub-ATFL technique.
   c. As with other weight-bearing joints, a period of NWB to PWB can be considered.

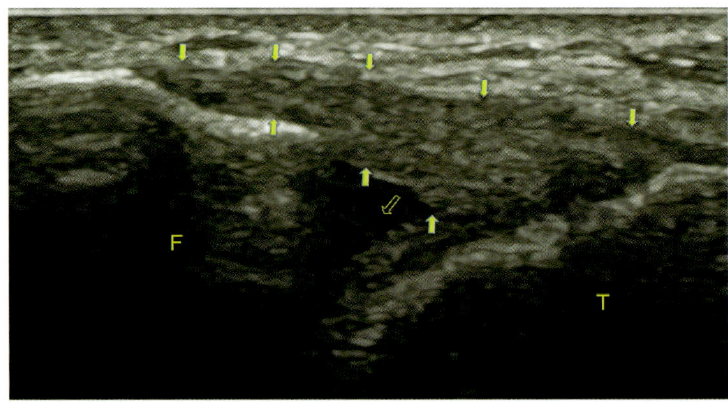

FIGURE 13.17: Lateral ankle joint in LAX.

Arrows, anterior talofibular ligament; F, fibula; open arrow, ankle joint; T, talus.

Posterior Tibial Tendon

Pertinent Anatomy and Indications

Treatment of the posterior tibial tendon (PTT) is typically performed at its insertion onto the navicular bone or more proximally where tendinosis and interstitial partial split tears are found in patients with chronic planovalgus hind foot. When treating partial tears of the PTT, the authors advise a period of NWB for a few days followed by PWB for 7 to 14 days depending on the severity of the injury. In addition, an arch support inside a boot for the first 2 weeks posttreatment is advised, followed by in-shoe consistent arch support or even permanent custom orthotics posttreatment, depending on the severity of the biomechanical misalignment.

Preferred Technique

1. Equipment
   a. 20 to 25 G, 1.5-inch needle
   b. Injectate: PRP, ADSC, amniotic membrane, and BMC

2. Patient position
   a. Supine with knee slightly bent and leg externally rotated

3. Transducer position
   a. Short- and long-axis views over the PTT where greatest area of tendinopathy lies

4. Needle orientation
   a. Out-of-plane to get needle into the tendon then in-plane to treat its length and depth

5. Target:
   a. Pathologic areas of the PTT
   b. Deposit remaining injectate into tendon sheath

6. Pearls:
   a. Postprocedure protocol to offload the chronically overloaded tendon is imperative.
   b. In some cases intrasubstance calcifications can cause pain and can be removed with the Tenex device if the calcification is not too large.

Subtalar Joint

Pertinent Anatomy and Indications

The authors' favored access point for the subtalar joint is through the lateral portal. Just distal to the calcaneofibular ligament (CFL; one probe's width), the peroneal tendons slide inferiorly over the calcaneus, allowing access to the subtalar joint (74). It is best accessed with a distal to proximal, out-of-plane approach with the transducer maintained in the plane of the CFL just one transducer's width distal to it.

Preferred Technique

1. Equipment
   a. 20 to 25 G, 1.5-inch needle
   b. Injectate: LP-PRP, BMC, ADSC
2. Patient position
   a. Side lying with the affected lateral ankle up
3. Transducer position
   a. In-plane of the CFL, one transducer's width distal to the CFL
4. Needle orientation
   a. Out-of-plane coming from distal to proximal
5. Target
   a. Lateral subtalar joint
6. Pearls:
   a. Avoid peroneal tendons and use Doppler to ensure intra-articular flow

ATFL, Calcaneofibular, and AITFL

Pertinent Anatomy and Indications

If any of the previous ligaments are not appropriately healed 6 to 12 weeks after injury, one should consider treatment. In the case of high-level athletes, the timing may be shorter. The ATFL responds well to regenerative treatments and can completely heal (Figures 13.18A,B). The high-ankle sprain, however, deserves special attention in that it typically takes twice as long to heal compared to an ATFL with or without CFL sprain. If the syndesmosis is widened by more than 1 mm on a mortise view of an ankle x-ray or is grossly unstable with AITFL dynamic stress testing on US, a regenerative treatment should be delayed and the patient should be referred to surgery for a syndesmotic screw to stabilize the ankle mortise.

US Findings

Sprains or tears of these ligaments show as hypoechoic, thickened partial, or complete tears with ligamentous laxity on dynamic stress testing (Figure 13.18A). Chronic inadequate healing may show as "ligamentosis," akin to tendinosis, with thickening, hypoechoic changes, and calcific changes.

Preferred Technique

1. Equipment:
   a. 25 G, 1.5-inch needle
   b. Injectate: PRP, BMC, LA, AMG
2. Patient position:
   a. Side lying
   b. Affected lateral ankle up
3. Transducer and needle position:
   a. ATFL
      i) Long-axis over the ATFL with needle coming in-plane from distal to proximal

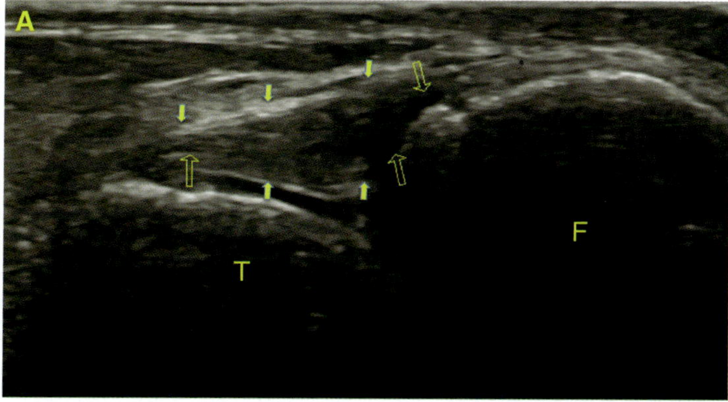

FIGURE 13.18A: Anterior talofibular ligament tear.

Arrows, anterior talofibular ligament; F, fibula; open arrows, partial tearing; T, talus.

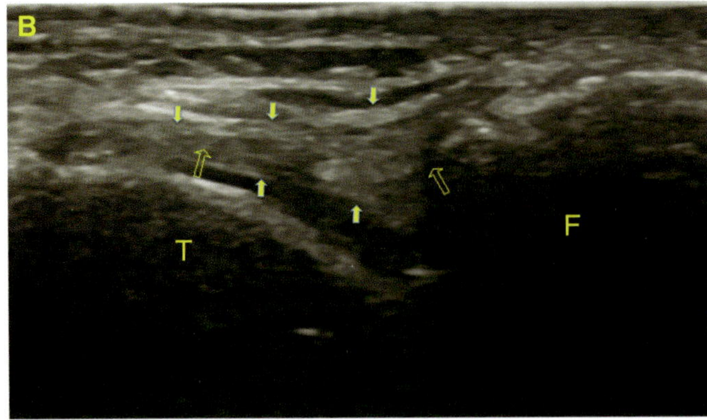

FIGURE 13.18B: Anterior talofibular ligament posttreatment.

Arrows, anterior talofibular ligament; F, fibula; open arrows, resolved partial tears; T, talus.

    b. CFL
       i) Long-axis over the CFL with needle coming in-plane from inferior to superior
    c. AITFL
       i) Long-axis over the AITFL with needle coming in out-of-plane

4. Target
    a. Each of the respective ligamentous tears and/or scar tissue
    b. Consider depositing some injectate into the tibiotalar joint or distal tibiofibular joint for when treating the ATFL and AITFL, respectively

Achilles Tendon

Pertinent Anatomy and Indications

The Achilles tendon is the culmination of the triceps surae and inserts onto the posterior calcaneus with Kager's fat pad deep (Figure 13.19). Treatment of the Achilles tendon is performed differently depending on the location of the tendinopathy: midsubstance or insertional. Treatments for midsubstance Achilles tendon are aimed at healing of the interstitial partial tears, which are readily visualized during the anesthesia portion of the procedure. This helps the physician formulate the treatment plan for which portions of the tendon must be targeted. With regard to insertional calcific tendinosis, regenerative therapies are more likely effective in the absence of a Haglund's deformity. This deformity causes an impingement of the deep fibers of the Achilles at the calcaneus, with resulting retrocalcaneal bursitis.

US Findings

The trademarks of midsubstance Achilles tendinosis are fusiform thickening, interstitial hypoechoic changes, and potentially neovascularization. Diagnostic tenogram during anesthesia is critical in delineating the typically multiple interstitial split tears to target. Insertional hypoechoic thickening is characteristic of tendinosis, and hyperechoic calcifications are common. They can occur together. Sonopalpation is the key in determining which of the areas is most symptomatic. A significant inflammatory retrocalcaneal bursitis and/or pre-Achilles bursitis may lower the effectiveness of regenerative techniques.

Preferred Technique

1. Equipment:
    a. 25 G, 1.5- to 2-inch needle
    b. Injectate
       i) Midsubstance: PRP (75,76), BMC, and amniotic membrane
      ii) Insertional: US-guided needle tenotomy with debridement of calcifications

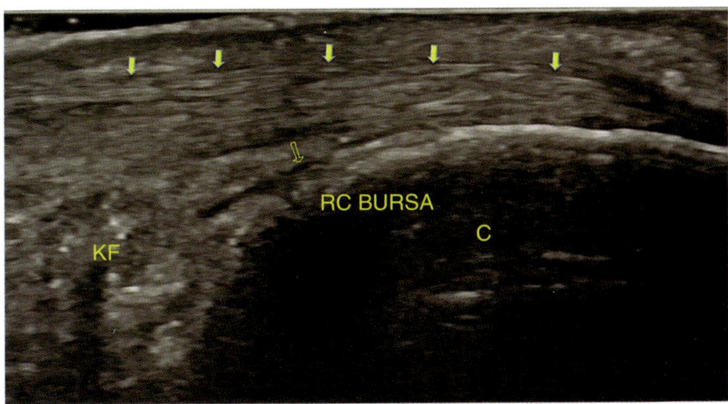

FIGURE 13.19: Achilles tendon in LAX.

Arrows, achilles tendon; C, calcaneus; KF, Kager's fat pad; open arrow, retrocalcaneal bursa.

perhaps with the Tenex tool or larger needle, followed by PRP, LA, amniotic membrane, or BMC

2. Patient position

a. Prone with Achilles up

b. Ankles resting on pillow or bolster

3. Transducer position

a. Start in long-axis to the tendon to identify the areas of tendinopathy

b. Turn to short-axis to the largest area to the lesion and begin the injection at this position

c. During treatment switch back to long-axis to ensure treatment of the entire three-dimensional pathology

4. Needle orientation

a. Start in-plane, in the short-axis view of the tendon, from medial to lateral to avoid the sural nerve. Treat lesions from medial to lateral, and superficial to deep. Re-image in long-axis view of tendon and treat the lesions from proximal to distal, ensuring all lesions are treated in three dimensions.

5. Target

a. Midsubstance: the various interstitial split tears noted at diagnostic tenogram should all be targeted, requiring a fairly large volume of injectate.

b. Insertional: calcifications, interstitial tears, and tendinosis of the distal Achilles; may need to treat the retrocalcaneal bursa in these cases as well. Recommend debridement of calcifications prior to injecting regenerative substance.

6. Pearls:

a. After tendon fenestration with injectate, consider hydrodissection of the Achilles tendon with remaining injectate.

b. Care should be taken to avoid the sural nerve which lies just lateral to the Achilles tendon approximately 4 cm proximal to the lateral malleolus. Recommend debridement of calcifications prior to injecting regenerative substance.

c. Recommend off-loading the tendon with bilateral heel lift, boot, and PWB.

FOOT

Here, we present the most commonly treated areas in the foot including the plantar fascia and metatarsophalangeal (MTP) joints. Other areas that can be treated, but are not presented, include the plantar plate, extensor tendons (i.e., EHL and EDL) of the toes, spring ligament, metatarsal fractures, and all other small joints of the foot. One can use the general guidelines in this chapter's introduction in conjunction with a manual on how to perform US-guided injections to assist in treating these areas.

Plantar Fascia

Pertinent Anatomy and Indications

The plantar fascia is a tendon-like structure that inserts both medially and laterally onto the plantar calcaneus and is prone to fasciosis and tears. If failing 2 to 3 months of appropriate conservative measures including physical therapy with an Alfredson's protocol for gastroc-soleus eccentric and soft tissue mobilization, one can consider regenerative intervention. To date, the most comprehensively studied procedure is the US-guided percutaneous fasciotomy with the Tenex tool. However, there is evidence that dextrose prolotherapy and PRP injections can relieve pain as well (77,78).

There is limited literature regarding the benefit of using amniotic membrane products for this pathology, although there are numerous growth factors in these products that could support its potential usefulness for this condition.

US Findings

Plantar fasciosis consists of thickening (greater than 0.5 cm), hypoechoic changes, and potentially hyperechoic calcifications and scar tissue. Anechoic split tears can be seen and will inflate with fluid during diagnostic tenogram at time of anesthesia.

Preferred Technique

1. Equipment
   a. 20 to 25 G, 1.5- to 2-inch needle
   b. Injectate: PRP, ADSC, BMC, AMG
2. Patient position
   a. Patient supine, leg externally rotated with knee bent and foot on pillow with medial ankle up
   b. Alternate position: patient prone on body pillows and ankle is propped up on pillow to allow a proximal to distal needle injection approach allowing an in-plane approach with a stout needle to approach the diseased tissue
3. Transducer position
   a. Short-axis views over the plantar fascia with needle coming from medial aspect of heel
   b. Alternate plantar approach: long-axis approach from a proximal to distal (or distal to proximal approach)
4. Needle orientation
   a. In-plane to treat plantar fasciopathy
5. Target
   a. All areas of pathology, debriding scar tissue and calcifications, and infiltrating partial tears with regenerative injectate
6. Pearls:
   a. Strongly recommend a tibial nerve block 3 to 4 cm proximal to the medial malleolus (to ensure the medial calcaneal branch of the tibial nerve is anesthetized as well) for patient comfort during this procedure, which can be very painful
   b. Recommend off-loading the fascia with a CAM walker for 1 to 2 weeks

MTP Joints

Pertinent Anatomy and Indications

The MTP joints can be affected with OA, and the first MTP is the most commonly affected, known as "hallux rigidus." The second MTP is the next most common site of MTP OA. IP joints can be affected, but are much less common and most likely posttraumatic when painful.

US Findings

The MTP joint is best viewed in long-axis (Figure 13.20). Common US findings include dorsal osteophytes, joint space narrowing, and effusion. Consider percutaneous debridement of small dorsal osteophytes if clinically symptomatic.

Preferred Technique

1. Equipment
   a. 25 to 30 G, 1- to 1.5-inch needle
   b. Injectate: LP-PRP, BMC. Although all regenerative treatments for hyaline cartilage can help, the authors have found hyaluronic viscosupplementation works well for mild-moderate first MTP OA

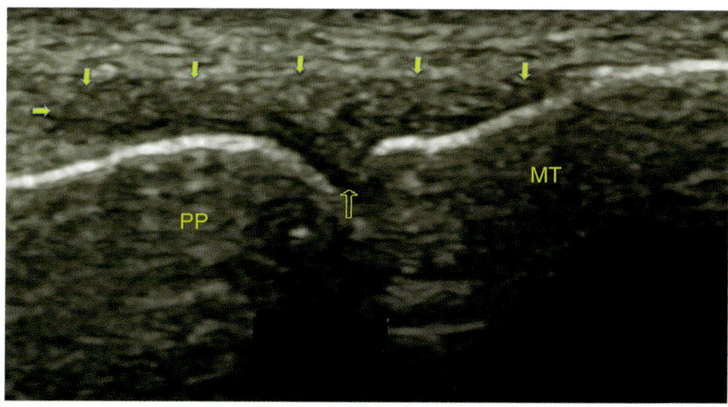

FIGURE 13.20: Dorsal first toe, LAX to metatarsophalangeal joint.

Arrows, MTP joint capsule; MT, metatarsal; open arrow, MTP joint space; PP, proximal phalanx.

2. Patient position
   a. Supine with knee bent and foot flat on table
3. Transducer position
   a. Long-axis over the MTP joint
4. Needle orientation
   a. Out-of-plane
5. Target
   a. Intra-articular joint
6. Pearls:
   a. Avoid the metatarsal head cartilage.
   b. Consider volume distension to break adhesions of the first MTP joint first if adhesive capsulitis is suspected.
   c. Counselling is advised as overdistension of any MTP or IP joint with >0.5–1 mL increases the risk for a postinjection flare that can be quite painful and prolonged.

REFERENCES

1. Malanga G, Mautner K. *Atlas of ultrasound guided injection*. New York: McGraw-Hill Education 2014.
2. Cavallo C, Filardo G, Mariani E, et al. Comparison of platelet-rich plasma formulations for cartilage healing: an *in vitro* study. *J Bone Joint Surg Am*. 2014;96(5):423–429.
3. Bornes TD, Adesida AB, Jomha NM. Mesenchymal stem cells in the treatment of traumatic articular cartilage defects: a comprehensive review. *Arthritis Res Ther*. 2014;16(5):432.
4. Vega A, Martín-Ferrero MA, Del Canto F, et al. Treatment of knee osteoarthritis with allogeneic bone marrow mesenchymal stem cells: arandomized controlled trial. *Transplantation*. 2015;99(8):1681–1690.
5. Michalek J, Moster R, Lukac L, et al. Autologous adipose tissue-derived stromal vascular fraction cells application in patients with osteoarthritis. *Cell Transplant*. 2015. Jan 20. doi: 10.3727/096368915X686760. [Epub ahead of print]
6. Arirachakaran A, Sukthuayat A, Sisayanarane T, et al.. Platelet-rich plasma versus autologous blood versus steroid injection in lateral epicondylitis: systematic review and network meta-analysis. *J Orthop Traumatol*. 2016;17(2):101–112.
7. Murray DJ, Javed S, Jain N, et al. Platelet-rich plasma injections in treating lateral epicondylosis: a review of the recent evidence. *J Hand Microsurg*. 2015;7(2):320–325.
8. Fitzpatrick J, Bulsara M, Zheng MH. Effectiveness of platelet-rich plasma in the treatment of tendinopathy: response. *Am J Sports Med*. 2016;44(10):NP55–NP56. doi:10.1371/journal.pone.0121713.
9. Anitua E, Zalduendo M, Troya M, et al. Leukocyte inclusion within a platelet rich plasma-derived fibrin scaffold stimulates a more pro-inflammatory environment and alters fibrin properties. *PLOS ONE*. 2015;10(3):e0121713.

10. Kobayashi Y, Saita Y, Nishio H, et al. Leukocyte concentration and composition in platelet-rich plasma (PRP) influences the growth factor and protease concentrations. *J Orthop Sci.* 2016;21(5):683–689.

11. Hankemeier S, Hurschler C, Zeichen J, et al. Bone marrow stromal cells in a liquid fibrin matrix improve the healing process of patellar tendon window defects. *Tissue Eng Part A.* 2009;15(5):1019–1030.

12. Zanon G, Combi F, Combi A, et al. Platelet-rich plasma in the treatment of acute hamstring injuries in professional football players. *Joints.* 2016;4(1):17–23.

13. Cianforlini M, Mattioli-Belmonte M, Manzotti S, et al. Effect of platelet rich plasma concentration on skeletal muscle regeneration: an experimental study. *J Biol Regul Homeost Agents.* 2015;29(4 Suppl):47–55.

14. Hamid MS, Mohamed Ali MR, Yusof A, et al. Platelet-rich plasma injections for the treatment of hamstring injuries: a randomized controlled trial. *Am J Sports Med.* 2014;42(10):2410–2418.

15. Mazzocca AD, McCarthy MB, Chowaniec DM, et al. The positive effects of different platelet-rich plasma methods on human muscle, bone, and tendon cells. *Am J Sports Med.* 2012;40(8):1742–1749.

16. Lee DH, Ryu KJ, Kim JW, Kang KC, Choi YR. Bone marrow aspirate concentrate and platelet-rich plasma enhanced bone healing in distraction osteogenesis of the tibia. *Clin Orthop Relat Res.* 2014;472(12):3789–3797.

17. Akram M, Irshad M, Farooqi FM, et al. Role of injecting bone marrow aspiration injection in treating delayed union and non-union. *J Pak Med Assoc.* 2014;64(12 Suppl 2):S154–S158.

18. Sugaya H, Mishima H, Aoto K, et al. Percutaneous autologous concentrated bone marrow grafting in the treatment for nonunion. *Eur J Orthop Surg Traumatol.* 2014;24(5):671–678.

19. Desai P, Hasan SM, Zambrana L, et al. Bone mesenchymal stem cells with growth factors successfully treat nonunions and delayed unions. *HSS J.* 2015;11(2):104–111.

20. Malhotra R, Kumar V, Garg B, et al. Role of autologous platelet-rich plasma in treatment of long-bone nonunions: a prospective study. *Musculoskelet Surg.* 2015;99(3):243–248.

21. Golos J, Walinski T, Piekarczyk P, Kwiatkowski K. Results of the use of platelet rich plasma in the treatment of delayed union of long bones. *Ortop Traumatol Rehabil.* 2014;16(4):397–406.

22. Gunay S, Candan H, Yılmaz R, et al. The efficacy of platelet-rich plasma in the treatment of rib fractures. *Thorac Cardiovasc Surg.* 2016 May 5. [Epub ahead of print].

23. Daif ET. Effect of autologous platelet-rich plasma on bone regeneration in mandibular fractures. *Dent Traumatol.* 2013;29(5):399–403.

24. Le Nail LR, Stanovici J, Fournier J, et al. Percutaneous grafting with bone marrow autologous concentrate for open tibia fractures: analysis of forty three cases and literature review. *Int Orthop.* 2014;38(9):1845–1853.

25. Crass JR, Craig EV, Feinberg SB. The hyperextended internal rotation view in rotator cuff ultrasonography. *J Clin Ultrasound.* 1987;15(6):416–420.

26. Jacobson J. *Fundamentals of musculoskeletal ultrasound.* 2nd ed. Philadelphia, PA: Saunders; 2013.

27. Wesner M, Defreitas T, Bredy H, et al. A pilot study evaluating the effectiveness of platelet-rich plasma therapy for treating degenerative tendinopathies: a randomized control trial with synchronous observational cohort. *PLOS ONE.* 2016;11(2):e0147842.

28. Jo CH, Shin JS, Lee YG, et al. Platelet-rich plasma for arthroscopic repair of large to massive rotator cuff tears: a randomized, single-blind, parallel-group trial. *Am J Sports Med.* 2013;41(10):2240–2248.

29. Vavken P, Sadoghi P, Palmer M, et al. Platelet-rich plasma reduces retear rates after arthroscopic repair of small- and medium-sized rotator cuff tears but is not cost-effective. *Am J Sports Med.* 2015;43(12):3071–3076.

30. Morag Y, Jamadar DA, Miller B, et al. The subscapularis: anatomy, injury, and imaging. *Skeletal Radiol.* 2011;40(3):255–269.

31. Ibrahim VM, Groah SL, Libin A, et al. Use of platelet rich plasma for the treatment of bicipital tendinopathy in spinal cord injury: a pilot study. *Top Spinal Cord Inj Rehabil.* 2012;18(1):77–78.

32. Nazarian LN, McShane JM, Ciccotti MG, et al. Dynamic US of the anterior band of the ulnar collateral ligament of the elbow in asymptomatic major league baseball pitchers. *Radiology.* 2003;227(1):149–154.

33. Battaglia M, Guaraldi F, Vannini F, et al. Efficacy of ultrasound-guided intra-articular injections of platelet-rich plasma versus hyaluronic acid

for hip osteoarthritis. *Orthopedics*. 2013;36(12): e1501–e1508.

34. Sánchez M, Guadilla J, Fiz N, Andia I. Ultrasound-guided platelet-rich plasma injections for the treatment of osteoarthritis of the hip. *Rheumatology (Oxford)*. 2012;51(1):144–150.

35. Dallari D, Stagni C, Rani N, et al. Ultrasound-guided injection of platelet-rich plasma and hyaluronic acid, separately and in combination, for hip osteoarthritis: a randomized controlled study. *Am J Sports Med*. 2016;44(3):664–671.

36. Gordon A, Karam C, Blatz D, et al. administration of platelet rich plasma to hip labral tears reduces pain and improves function. Presented at the Annual Meeting of the Association of Academic Physiatrists on March 12, 2015, March 10–14, 2015.

37. Hauser RA, Orlofsky A. Regenerative injection therapy (prolotherapy) for hip labrum lesions: rational and retrospective study. *The Open Rehab J*. 2013;6:59–68.

38. Robertson WJ, Gardner MJ, Barker JU, et al. Anatomy and dimensions of the gluteus medius tendon insertion. *Arthroscopy*. 2008;24(2): 130–136.

39. Mautner K, Colberg RE, Malanga G, et al. Outcomes after ultrasound-guided platelet-rich plasma injections for chronic tendinopathy: a multicenter, retrospective review. *PM R*. 2013;5(3):169–175.

40. Housner JA, Jacobson JA, Misko R. Sonographically guided percutaneous needle tenotomy for the treatment of chronic tendinosis. *J Ultrasound Med*. 2009;28(9):1187–1192.

41. Curtiss HM, Finnoff JT, Peck E, et al. Accuracy of ultrasound-guided and palpation-guided knee injections by an experienced and less-experienced injector using a superolateral approach: a cadaveric study. *PM&R*. 2011;3(6):507–515.

42. Sibbet WL, Peisajovich A, Michael AA, et al. Does sonographic needle guidance affect the clinical outcome of intraarticular injections. *J Rheum*. 2009; 36(9):1892–1902.

43. Bum Park Y, Ah Choi W, Kim YK, et al. Accuracy of blind versus ultrasound guided suprapatellar bursal injection. *Journal of Clinical Ultrasound*. 2012;40(1):20–25.

44. Xie X, Zhang C, Tuan RS. Biology of platelet-rich plasma and its clinical application in cartilage repair. *Arthritis Res Ther*. 2014;16(1):204. doi:10.1186/ar4493.

45. Filardo G, Kon E, Roffi A, et al. Platelet-rich plasma: why intra-articular? A systematic review of preclinical studies and clinical evidence on PRP for joint degeneration. *Knee Surg Sports Traumatol Arthrosc*. 2015;23(9):2459–2474.

46. Gobbi A, Lad D, Karnatzikos G. The effects of repeated intra-articular PRP injections on clinical outcomes of early knee osteoarthritis of the knee. *Knee Surg Sports Traumatol Arthrosc*. 2015;23(8):2170–2177.

47. Raeissadat SA, Rayegani SM, Hassanabadi H, et al. Knee osteoarthritis injection choices: platelet-rich plasma (PRP) versus hyaluronic acid (A one-year randomized clinical trial). *Clin Med Insights Arthritis Musculoskelet Disord*. 2015;8:1–8.

48. Campbell KA, Saltzman BM, Mascarenhas R, et al. Does intra-articular platelet-rich plasma injection provide clinically superior outcomes compared with other therapies in the treatment of knee osteoarthritis? A systematic review of overlapping meta-analyses. *Arthroscopy*. 2015;31(11):2213–2221.

49. Jackson DW, Evans NA, Thomas BM. Accuracy of needle placement into the intra-articular space of the knee. *J Bone Joint Surg Am*. 2002;84-A(9):1522–1527.

50. Horst J. The efficacy of platelet-rich plasma injection in the treatment of patellar tendinopathy. School of Physician Assistant Studies. Paper 485; 2014.

51. Pascual-Garrido C, Rolón A, Makino A. Treatment of chronic patellar tendinopathy with autologous bone marrow stem cells: a 5-year-followup. *Stem Cells Int*. 2012;2012. doi:10.1155/2012/953510.

52. Murray MM, Spindler KP, Abreu E, et al. Collagen-platelet rich plasma hydrogel enhances primary repair of the porcine anterior cruciate ligament. *J Orthop Res*. 2007;25(1):81–91.

53. Murray MM, Spindler KP, Devin C, et al. Use of a collagen-platelet rich plasma scaffold to stimulate healing of a central defect in the canine ACL. *J Orthop Res*. 2006;24(4):820–830.

54. Fallouh L, Nakagawa K, Sasho T, et al. Effects of autologous platelet-rich plasma on cell viability and collagen synthesis in injured human anterior cruciate ligament. *J Bone Joint Surg Am*. 2010;92(18):2909–2916.

55. Smith J, Hackel JG, Khan U, et al. Sonographically guided anterior cruciate ligament injection: technique and validation. *PM R*. 2015;7(7):736–745.

56. Centeno CJ, Pitts J, Al-Sayegh H, Freeman MD. Anterior cruciate ligament tears treated with percutaneous injection of autologous bone marrow nucleated cells: a case series. *J Pain Res*. 2015;8:437–447.

57. Ishida K, Kuroda R, Miwa M, et al. The regenerative effects of platelet-rich plasma on meniscal cells *in vitro* and its *in vivo* application with biodegradable gelatin hydrogel. *Tissue Eng*. 2007;13(5):1103–1112.

58. Freymann U, Metzlaff S, Krüger JP, et al. Effect of human serum and 2 different types of platelet concentrates on human meniscus cell migration, proliferation, and matrix formation. *Arthroscopy.* 2016;32(6):1106–1116.

59. Gonzales VK, de Mulder EL, de Boer T, et al. Platelet-rich plasma can replace fetal bovine serum in human meniscus cell cultures. *Tissue Eng Part C Methods.* 2013;19(11):892–899.

60. Lee HR, Shon OJ, Park SI, et al. PRP increases the levels of catabolic molecules and cellular dedifferentiation in the meniscus of a rabbit model. *Int J Mol Sci.* 2016;17(1):120. doi:10.3390/ijms17010120.

61. Shin KH, Lee H, Kang S, et al. Effect of leukocyte-rich and platelet-rich plasma on healing of a horizontal medial meniscus tear in a rabbit model. *Biomed Res Int.* 2015;2015:179756. doi:10.1155/2015/179756.

62. Duygulu F, Demirel M, Atalan G, et al. Effects of intra-articular administration of autologous bone-marrow aspirate on healing of full-thickness meniscal tear: an experimental study on sheep. *Acta Orthop Traumatol Turc.* 2012;46(1):61–67.

63. Desando G, Giavaresi G, Cavallo C, et al. Autologous bone-marrow concentrate in a sheep model of osteoarthritis: new perspectives for cartilage and meniscus repair. *Tissue Eng Part C Methods.* 2016;22(6):608–619.

64. Toratani T, Nakase J, Numata H, et al. Scaffold-free tissue-engineered allogenic adipose-derived stem cells promote meniscal healing. *Arthroscopy.* 2017;33(2):346–354.

65. Nordberg RC, Charoenpanich A, Vaughn CE, et al. Enhanced cellular infiltration of human adipose-derived stem cells in allograft menisci using a needle-punch method. *J Orthop Surg Res.* 2016;11(1):132. doi:10.1186/s13018-016-0467-x.

66. González-Fernández ML, Pérez-Castrillo S, Sánchez-Lázaro JA, et al. Assessment of regeneration in meniscal lesions by use of mesenchymal stem cells derived from equine bone marrow and adipose tissue. *Am J Vet Res.* 2016;77(7):779–788.

67. Eirale C, Mauri E, Hamilton B. Use of platelet rich plasma in an isolated complete medial collateral ligament lesion in a professional football (soccer) player: a case report. *Asian J Sports Med.* 2013;4(2):158–162.

68. Yoshioka T, Kanamori A, Washio T, et al. The effects of plasma rich in growth factors (PRGF-Endoret) on healing of medial collateral ligament of the knee. *Knee Surg Sports Traumatol Arthrosc.* 2013;21(8):1763–1769.

69. Hildebrand KA, Woo SL, Smith DW, et al. The effects of platelet-derived growth factor-BB on healing of the rabbit medial collateral ligament. An *in vivo* study. *Am J Sports Med.* 1998;26(4):549–554.

70. Batten ML, Hansen JC, Dahners LE. Influence of dosage and timing of application of platelet-derived growth factor on early healing of the rat medial collateral ligament. *J Orthop Res.* 1996;14(5):736–741.

71. Kim YS, Lee M, Koh YG. Additional mesenchymal stem-cell injection improves the outcomes of marrow stimulation combined with supramalleolar osteotomy in varus ankle osteoarthritis: short-term clinical results with second-look arthroscopic evaluation. *J Exp Orthop.* 2016;3(1):12. doi:10.1186/s40634-016-0048-2.

72. Kim YS, Koh YG. Injection of mesenchymal stem cells as a supplementary strategy of marrow stimulation improves cartilage regeneration after lateral sliding calcaneal osteotomy for varus ankle osteoarthritis: clinical and second-look arthroscopic results. *Arthroscopy.* 2016;32(5):878–889.

73. Buda R, Castagnini F, Cavallo M, et al. "One-step" bone marrow-derived cells transplantation and joint debridement for osteochondral lesions of the talus in ankle osteoarthritis: clinical and radiological outcomes at 36 months. *Arch Orthop Trauma Surg.* 2016;136(1):107–116.

74. Smith J, Finnoff JT, Henning PT, Turner NS. Accuracy of sonographically guided posterior subtalar joint injections: comparison of 3 techniques. *J Ultrasound Med.* 2009;28(11):1549–1557.

75. Monto RR. Platelet rich plasma treatment for chronic Achilles tendinosis. *Foot Ankle Int.* 2012;33(5):379–385.

76. Gaweda K, Tarczynska M, Krzyzanowski W. Treatment of Achilles tendinopathy with platelet-rich plasma. *Int J Sports Med.* 2010;31(8):577–583.

77. Kim E, Lee JH. Autologous platelet-rich plasma versus dextrose prolotherapy for the treatment of chronic recalcitrant plantar fasciitis. *PM R.* 2014;6(2):152–158.

78. Monto RR. Platelet-rich plasma efficacy versus corticosteroid injection treatment for chronic severe plantar fasciitis. *Foot Ankle Int.* 2014;35(4):313–318.

CHAPTER 14

PHYSICAL THERAPY CONSIDERATIONS FOLLOWING REGENERATIVE MEDICINE INTERVENTIONS

Angela T. Gordon and Kwang Han

Regenerative medicine techniques are becoming more common in the treatment of orthopedic conditions. Physical therapy is widely known as an important part of the healing process following any orthopedic injury and is now widely accepted as an integral part of healing postregenerative medicine techniques. Physical therapists need to be up-to-date on the current literature and findings that are supportive of different regenerative medicine procedures such as prolotherapy and platelet-rich plasma (PRP).

A lack of consensus still exists in current literature on the correct parameters for physical therapists to follow post prolotherpay or PRP injection. In actuality, there is not substantial literature on the rehabilitation process for regenerative medicine. Therefore, there is a need for more research and published information on the rehabilitation side for regenerative medicine. Based on the current research findings and our clinical experience, we present the rationale and rehabilitation protocols for various procedures postregenerative medicine techniques in this chapter.

WHAT IS PROLOTHERAPY?

Prolotherapy is defined as the rehabilitation of an incompetent structure by the induced proliferation of new cells. The core component of prolotherapy is the injection of a small volume of solution to painful ligament or tendon sites and adjacent joint spaces over the course of several treatments (1,2). Most types of prolotherapy involve injection of a solution to the fibro-osseous junctions at the point where tendons and ligaments attach to the bone to induce an inflammatory reaction.

Prolotherapy is a method of injection treatment designed to stimulate healing and can be used at multiple painful sites such as ligament and tendon insertions, trigger points, and adjacent joint spaces (3,4). The injection stimulates growth factor production to grow normal cells or tissue. The solution most commonly used is dextrose based, but other solutions have been identified in the literature. Dextrose specifically has been proven to increase cell protein synthesis, DNA synthesis, cell volume, and proliferation. This leads ultimately to increased ligament size and mass, tendon hypertrophy, increased ligament–bone junction strength, and repair of articular cartilage defects. Dextrose has induced healing over a wide range of concentrations.

Prolotherapy causes a temporary inflammatory reaction at the site of injury to trick the body into initiating repair into tissue that has forgotten that there still is an injury. The irritation and needle microtrauma can influence the tissue to start an inflammatory reaction. This will activate fibroblasts and in turn synthesize collagen and connective tissue. Prolotherapy has been shown to be effective in strengthening ligaments and tendons in the treatment of chronic musculoskeletal conditions (1,3–5).

WHAT IS PLATELET-RICH PLASMA?

Platelet-rich plasma (PRP) is a type of prolotherapy that involves the injection of a concentration of plasma into a target tissue. The concentration of plasma has a volume of platelets above baseline and a three- to fivefold increase in growth factor concentration (6–8). The plasma contains proteins, cytokines, and other bioactive molecules that initiate and regulate basic aspect of wound healing (6,9).

PRP overall promotes the enhancement of bone remodeling, proliferation, vessel remodeling, angiogenesis, inflammation, coagulation, and cell differentiation. The cytokines and other bioactive factors released from PRP are also known to affect metabolic processes such as cell proliferation, cell chemotaxis, angiogenesis, cellular differentiation, gene expression, and extracellular matrix production (8,10,11).

Stem Cell Treatments

Since the early 1900s, there has been an interest in the use of "adult stem cells" (3). The use of adult stem cells known as "mesenchymal stem cells" (MSCs), can be used as a proliferating solution. MSC can be found throughout the body and exists to replenish dying cells and regenerate damaged tissues. They are found in bone marrow and adipose tissue. MSCs have the potential to differentiate into a variety of tissues such as bone, cartilage, fat, tendon, muscle, and adipose tissue (3).

SPORTS MEDICINE CONSIDERATION FOR REGENERATIVE MEDICINE

PRP in sports medicine is widely used with variable outcomes. It is most commonly been used in chronic tendinopathies such as elbow lateral epidondylosis, achilles, and patellar tendinopathies (8). It has also been tried in acute injuries; PRP has been used in injuries such as muscle strains and ligament sprains and partial tears. Several studies have noted improved knee stability via revascularization at the osteo-ligamentous interface zone, while other studies have suggested no benefit due to the presence of intra-articular plasmin in a posttraumatic joint (8,12).

STAGES OF HEALING FOR ACUTE AND CHRONIC CONDITIONS

In each phase of healing, there are distinct features that play an integral part in how prolotherapy and PRP work. Target tissues and outcomes are based on the regenerative properties of each tissue. Rehabilitation post injection depends on the target tissue and condition being treated. It is important for the physical therapist to be aware of what the target tissue, condition, and expected outcome is to fully rehabilitate the area. The stage of the condition (acute or chronic) is also another important component to be considered during the rehabilitation process.

Tendon–Tenocytes

Assisting and promoting tendon healing continues to be a challenge to the medical community.

Over the past two decades, there has been a shift in nomenclature of chronic tendon pain from "tendonitis" to "tendonosis" and now to chronic tendinopathy (13,14). Many different attempts have been explored to treat chronic tendinopathy and induce a healing response to the tissue. Other factors to consider when addressing the cause of pain in patients with chronic tendinopathy include the findings of neural sprouting or neoinnervation (13).

Tendon degeneration is an ongoing active process led by many inflammatory mediated responses, such as supbstance P and matrix metalloprotineases (MMPs). Vascular endothelial growth factor (VEGF) is produced by macrophages, and is thought to be responsible for the neovascularity and neoinnervation in chronic tendinopathy.

Tenoblasts and tenocytes constitute 90% to 95% of the cellular elements of tendons, and are cells that are able to proliferate and become metabolically active in response to cytokines and growth factors during the inflammatory phase. Tendons also contain a small percentage of chondrocytes, synovial cells, and vascular cells. Collagen type I constitutes 65% to 80% of the dry mass, and elastin about 2% of the dry mass of tendons (15).

Tendons transmit forces from muscle to bone and absorb external forces to limit muscle damage. The stress strain curve (see Figure 14.1) demonstrates the allowable deformation of the tendon before failure. Forces and rate of loading play a role in the failure of tendons and tendinopathy. Failure to adapt to excessive loads may result in the release of cytokines. Repeated mechanical strain increases levels of cytokines, which induce MMP release that leads to degradation of the extracellular matrix eventually leading to tendinopathy (15).

Recent literature now suggests that the loss of coordinated muscle contractions increases the frequency of the stretch shortening cycle (SSC) of the muscle, which ultimately imposes additional strain on the tendon. The muscles surrounding the tendon complex must be able to function normally and are a key to successful rehabilitation of tendinopathy (16,17).

"Mechanotransduction" refers to the process by which the body converts mechanical loading into cellular responses (18,19). As physical therapists, we understand this concept from the action of bones increasing in size and strength through load, and the process in which our inner ears convert sound waves to an action potential along the acoustic nerve (18–20).

This concept is the basis as to why immobilization of the tendon is not recommended postinjury for an extended period of time. Mechanical stimulus, such as active range of motion (AROM) and exercise, will aid the necessary cellular responses

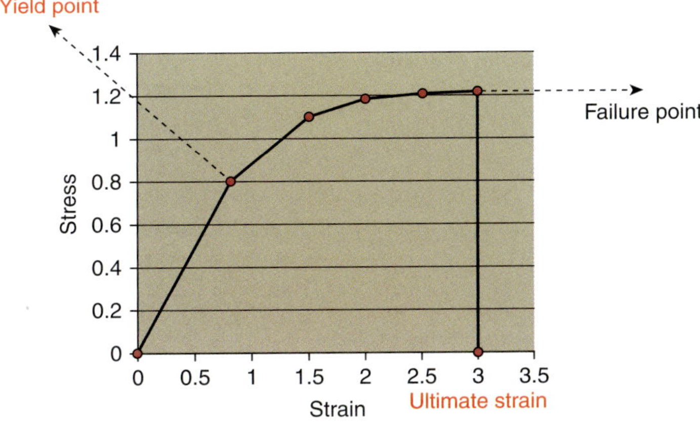

FIGURE 14.1: Stress–strain curve. Tendons and ligaments will first begin to un-crimp in the toe region of the curve, followed by the linear region where the collagen fibers will begin to orient themselves in the direction of mechanical load and begin to stretch, finally reaching the yield point where the tissue is at its physiological limit. If strain continues, then the tissue will reach the failure point and have irreversible plastic deformation.

such as increased protein synthesis for tissue healing. Within the tendon, tenocytes are mechanosensitive and have transcription responses to overloading, physiologic loading, and underloading. Overloading produces an increased expression of proinflammatory cytokines; physiologic loading creates matrix homeostasis with tenocyte proliferation and matrix production. Underloading decreases the expression of several ECM proteins, including collagen (19). Thus, we conclude that frequency, duration, and magnitude of the load create cellular responses that are required for tissue homeostasis and repair (19).

Ligaments-Fibrocytes

Ligaments are dense bands of fibrous connective tissue that join two or more bones of the musculoskeletal system. They can vary in size, shape, orientation, and location. They cross joints that have wide range of motion and function mainly to stabilize joints at rest and during normal range of motion. They are complex pieces of tissue that respond to local and systemic influences. Injuries to ligaments are very common and cause disruptions to the balance between joint mobility and joint stability. Injury to a ligament can also result in damage to other structures in and around the joint complex due to tissue laxity and increased stress (21). In the spine, the mechanoreceptors in the ligaments provide proprioception and kinesthesia and can be disrupted with injury.

Ligaments comprise water, collagen, and amino acids. Primary collagen type I makes up 75% of the dry weight of ligaments. The other 25% is made up of proteoglycans, elastin, and glycoproteins (21). Fibroblasts are located between rows of the collagen fibers and maintain the extracellular matrix of the ligament.

When tension is applied, ligaments deform in a nonlinear manner through recruitment of crimped collagen fibers. As tension increases, the fibers progressively elongate until all fibers are linear. This allows the ligament structure to become increasingly stiff in response to the loads put on it (21). Ligaments follow the same creep principle as tendons (see Figure 14.1).

Spinal ligaments, such as the iliolumbar ligament, do not have a rich supply of blood. The arterol network in the spine is such that nutrient arteries from the anterior vertebral canal travel anteriorly and supply most central vertebral bodies. The larger spinal branches continue as radicular or segmental medullary arteries and supply the nerve roots and spinal cord. The iliolumbar ligament receives its small supply from the lumbosacral trunk and internal iliac arteries. When injury occurs, blood supply and nutrition need to be enhanced to the spinal ligaments to ensure proper healing cascade (22).

When injury occurs to a ligament, it can take months to years for the remodeling phase to end. Continuous tissue synthesis and degradation occur to allow the ligament to adapt and become more functional but also the potential for tissue degradation and failure can happen with applied loads. Remodeled ligament tissue is morphologically and biomechanically inferior to the normal ligament and can result in ligament laxity (21). Injured ligament tissue shows alterations in proteoglycans, collagen, immature collagen cross links, altered cell connections, increased vascularity, altered innervations, and incomplete resolution of matrix.

Prolotherapy with dextrose has been used for a variety of ligament healings. Enhanced inflammatory healing response, involving fibroblastic and capillary proliferation along with growth factor stimulation has been shown with prolotherapy injections. Growth factors such as basic fibroblast growth factor (bFGF) and platelet-derived growth factor (PDGF) mediate the process necessary for ligament healing. Clinical study results of prolotherapy on ligaments show increased strength, mass, and extracellular matrix (21). Prolotherapy treatments have been applied to the treatment of ligaments of the spine, pelvis, and peripheral joints to enhance stability.

Muscle–Myoblasts

Muscle strains are common injuries that account for the most time missed in practice and games in the elite athletic population (6). The most common muscle groups to be injured involve the lower extremities and include: hamstrings, gastrocnemius, and quadriceps. Depending on the severity of the injury, athletes can miss up to 6 weeks of time from sport participation following these injuries.

Muscle injuries follow the same three-phase healing process as the rest of the body and the healing response depends on the vascularity of the tissue. The proliferation and differentiation of muscle cells and the activation of muscle satellite cells characterize skeletal muscle healing. The differentiation of the new precursor muscle cells form myotubles. Many growth factors play a role in muscle regeneration. PDGF is known for regulating myoblast proliferation and increasing myoblasts during muscle regeneration.

PRP has been shown to reduce pain and swelling with muscle injuries and reduce the recovery time by half (9). Other studies have raised concerns about inducing a fibrotic healing response in muscles. This fibrotic healing is a side effect of the elevation of transforming growth factor beta (TGF-β) levels after injection of PRP. This fibrotic healing can raise incidence of reinjury and must be considered prior to performing PRP on a muscle.

Cartliage–Chondrocyte

Articular cartilage damage can be caused by sports injuries, trauma, or aging. It can lead to more serious pathology such as osteoarthritis (OA) and necrosis of subchondral bone tissue. Hyaline articular cartilage has little to no intrinsic capacity for repair due to its lack of blood supply; therefore, even minor insult to a joint can lead to progressive damage or joint degeneration. The degeneration of the cartilage is due mainly to changes in activity of the chondrocytes to catabolic activity. This change in activity causes sclerosis and edema to the subchondral bone and inflammation of the synovium (10,23).

Ultimately, this leads to cartilage loss and increased loads on the subchondral bone which is referred to OA. In OA, different matrix metalloproteinases (MMPs) and cytokines, such as interleukin-1 (IL-1) and tumor necrosis factor (TNF), have been studied in the degenerative process. Results of theses studies demonstrate pro-inflammatory conditions of OA pathology and support the idea that vascularized subchondral region may increase the synthesis of cytokines and MMPs leading to degradation of adjacent cartilage (24). The demonstration of chondrocytes producing IL-1 and TNF within the superficial zones of OA cartilage and the expression of six different MMPs (1, 2, 3, 8, 9, and 13) in similar locations support the concept that cytokine–MMP associations contribute to what appears to be an intrinsic process of cartilage degeneration by resident chondrocytes (25).

PRP plays a role in chondrocyte upregulation and cartilage matrix synthesis by the release of growth factors, in particular TFG-β. Initiating type II collagen synthesis with decreased cartilage degradation, TGF-β is known to be a chondrocyte anabolism in vitro and intra-articular injections help increase bone formation in vitro (10). This growth factor helps promote migration of bone-marrow stromal cells toward the site of injury. TGF β-1 also stimulates proliferation and chondrogenic differentiation, and a sustained release of TGF β-1 is necessary in the process of differentiation into cartilage.

Articular chondrocytes live in a dynamic environment with different forces that specifically regulate genetic responses during physiologic joint loading. Dynamic, cyclic compression, and hydrostatic pressure can upregulate the transcription and translation of ECM proteins, whereas static compression downregulates it. MSCs react to cellular and chemical signals and have the ability to differentiate to lineages of mesenchymal tissue, like chondrocyte, to lead to cartilage repair (26).

Bone–Chondrocytes/Osteoblasts

Fractures and stress fractures are among several types of bone injuries that can occur. Generally, bone healing can take up to 12 weeks for full bone remodeling to occur.

Once a fracture occurs, and broken blood vessels across the fracture line are disrupted, blood runs to the medullary canal between the fractured ends and rapidly coagulates to form a clot and the resulting necrotic material induces an intense inflammatory response. This hematoma serves as a fibrin scaffold and the environment for repair cells to perform their function. MSCs are recruited from activated platelets in the fibrin clot and they differentiate into fibroblasts, chondrocytes, and/or osteoblasts and produce a matrix for fibrous tissue for cartilage or bone (27).

However, in some cases, especially in patients with chronic diseases such as diabetes, the use of PRP with bone healing is shown to affect osteoblasts, osteoclasts, and mesenchymal osteoprogenitor stem cells. The growth factors stimulated via PRP can stimulate the formation of osteoclast-like cells, which will help with bone growth and remodeling (3,15).

REHABILITATION PRINCIPLES

Stages of Healing
In order to properly evaluate and treat patients having regenerative procedures, we must know and understand the three phases of healing (Figure 14.2):

- Phase I Inflammatory/destructive phase
- Phase II Proliferation/repair phase
- Phase III Matrix formation/remodeling/maturation

Inflammation Stage
When injury occurs, the first 3 to 5 days constitute the inflammatory phase. This phase can also be argued to last up to 2 weeks (28). The purpose of the inflammation phase is to localize and eliminate damaged tissue components so the body can heal. The response consists of increased blood flow, increased permeability of blood vessels, and migration of fluid, proteins, and white blood cells.

The four signs of inflammation are: redness, heat, swelling, and pain. Redness results from dilation of small blood vessels, heat results from increased blood flow, swelling is the accumulation of fluid outside the blood vessels, and pain is associated to the distortion of the tissues due to swelling and the release of chemical mediators (bradykinin, histamine, serotonin, and prostaglandins). The plasma is responsible for the release of these mediators plus coagulation factors, complement proteins, and the fibrinolytic system (18).

During this phase of the rehabilitation process, it is important to respect the complex process of healing. Rest to the tissue is important to allow the permeability of fluid exchange to happen. This will bring an influx of macrophages, cell differentiation, and adult stem cells (MSCs) to the area. Phagocytes are cells that are recruited to the area to destroy bacteria and rid the tissue spaces from debris and from dead and dying cells so repair processes can begin. Platelets are also stimulated to aggregate and secrete growth factors, cytokines, and hemostatic factors (29). Histamine and serotonin are released by platelets as well to increase capillary permeability.

A typical healing process in phase I for muscle is as follows: A muscle "tear" occurs—the torn myofibrils become necrotized and the propation of the necrosis is halted by a "fire door" in the tissue—the two ends formed by the contraction band are sealed by the new sarcolemma within a few hours—the ruptured myofibers contract and the gap where the tear lives is filled by the hematoma. This injury induces a brisk inflammatory cell reaction. Platelets, specialized cellular elements suspended in plasma, are one of the first cells at the site of injury, to form a hemostatic plug to stop bleeding (31).

Rehabilitation during the inflammatory phase should be directly correlated to the degree of injury, inflammation, and tissues involved. Respect to the nature of healing and appropriate techniques should be chosen accordingly.

Proliferation Phase
Once the initial inflammatory phase is complete, the proliferation phase begins between days 2 and 5 and can last up to 8 weeks (28). In

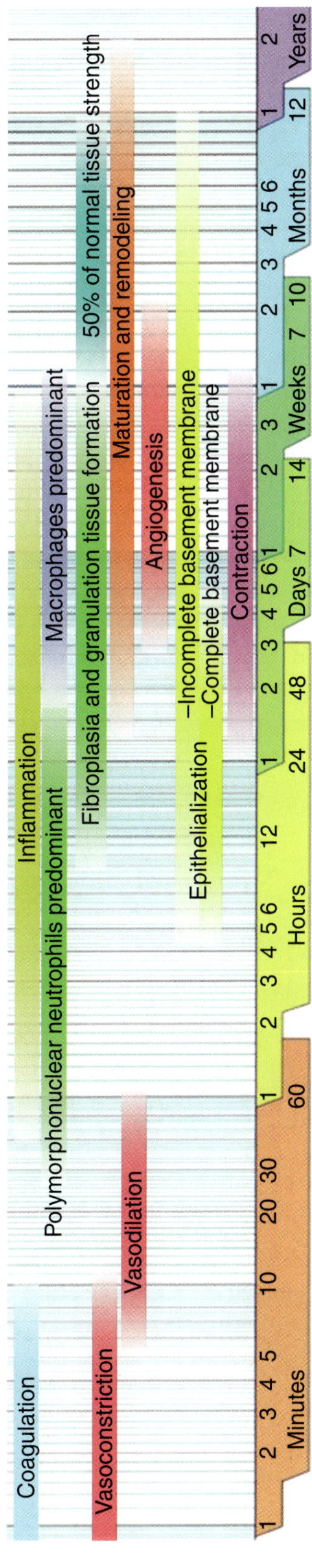

FIGURE 14.2: Stages of healing.

Source: Adapted from Ref. (30). Medical Gallery of Mikael Haggstrom. *WikiJournal of Medicine.* 2014;1(2). doi:10.15347/wjm/2014.008

this phase, any cell capable of proliferation will regenerate. Cells all have different rates and different complexities of regenerating.

Platelets and macrophages are considered the regulatory cells in the repair process, and they trigger the release of bioactive factors that include growth factors that are essential for tissue repair for the cellular and matrix proliferation. These growth factors, such as PDGF, a regulatory protein, recruit fibroblast to the site of injury, and once in the wound fibroblasts synthesize collagen (32). Hence platelets may also contribute significantly to control fibrin deposition, fibroplasia, and angiogenesis for the repair phase of healing.

During this phase, there is new collagen beginning to form. New collagen fibers are laid down in a disorganized manner in the form of a scar (loose framework of connective tissue). This scar formation is compiled of densely packed collagen. Thus, the new tissue is weak and susceptible to disruption by overly aggressive activity. However, according to Davis's law, which is analogous to Wolff's law of

osseous tissue, soft tissue heals according to the manner in which they are mechanically stressed (Figure 14.3). It applies to fibrous collagenous connective tissues, such as ligaments, tendons, and fascia.

In the example of muscle injury: phagocytosis of the necrotized tissue occurs by blood-derived monocytes. The myogenic reserve cells and satellite cells are activated and begin the repair of the breached myofiber (29). First committed satellite cells begin to differentiate into myoblasts; second undifferentiated stem satellite cells begin to proliferate by 24 hours and thereafter contribute to the formation of myoblasts, at the same time providing new satellite cells, by asymmetric cell division, for future needs of regeneration. The myoblasts arising from the committed and stem satellite cells then fuse to form myotubes within a couple of days. Within 5 to 6 days, the necrotized tissue part of the "tear" is replaced by regenerating myofibers. The injury site is also re-vascularized by ingrowing

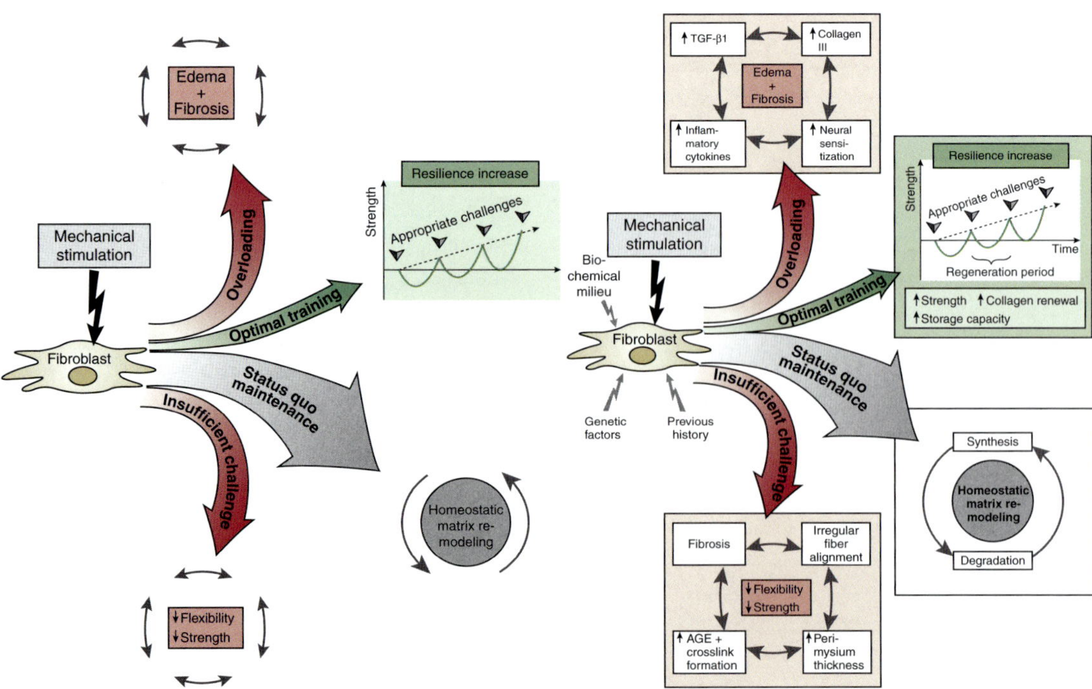

FIGURE 14.3: Davis Law in detail. Overloading as well as insufficient challenge lead to loss of tissue strength. Adequately calibrated tissue challenge can induce an increase of tissue strength.

Source: www.fascialnet.com

capillaries with the first angiogenic capillary sprouts seen 3 days after the injury (31). The satellite cells producing growth factors, insulin-like growth factor 1 (IGF-1), bFGF, epidermal growth factor (EGF), hepatocyte growth factor (HGF), and TGF-β1, may influence the proliferation and differentiation of myoblasts and muscle stem cells (29).

In the proliferation phase of healing, the rehabilitation protocol should take into consideration these principles when selecting the appropriate exercise. Complete rest of the tissue is contraindicated and would only allow disorganized dense scar to continue to form. By allowing the patient to begin active range of motion and progressing to light resistive range of motion at the injured site will allow the collagen to start to remodel and lay down in a more organized fashion. This organized collagen will soon become strong and more analogous to the native tissue. After several weeks, the protocol should progress from concentric to eccentric exercises to start to elongate the new tissue and healing tendon or muscle. Ligamentous tissue surrounding the spine and joint would not be appropriate for eccentric loading as these tissues are generally trying to "shrink" in nature to help support the area of dysfunction.

Remodeling Phase

Tissue continues to remodel, strengthen, and improve its cellular organization. There is less new collagen formation, but increased organization of the collagen fibers, and stronger bonds between them. Gradually, cross linking and shortening of the collagen fibers promote a formation of tight, strong scar (28). Final aggregation, orientation, and arrangement of collagen fibers occur during this phase. Appropriate tension becomes important component because new collagen must orient along the lines of stress to best accommodate the loads required for function. The end of tissue remodeling is unknown and may take months to years for completion.

During this phase of healing, the protocol can begin to take the patient through additional dynamic functional activity, that is, plyometrics

and return to sport programs. The inflammation process, pain, and irritation have now ceased and increased tolerance to activity should be progressed to return the patient back to normal function.

REHABILITATION PROTOCOLS

Regenerative medicine techniques are applied to various tissues and with various outcome expectations. Current literature supplies protocols to use for post PRP injections but does not differentiate between tissues or was developed for one specific tissue only (33–35). Regenerative medicine techniques can involve the use of prolotherpy, PRP, and stem cells for a variety of tissues such as tendon, ligament, muscle, bone, and cartilage. Regenerative treatments are often combined with percutaneous needle tenotomy and scar tissue removal. There are a variety of pathologies that can be treated from acute to chronic conditions with a range of complexity. All of these are factors to consider when a patient presents for rehabilitation. Considerations for each tissue type and an associated protocol for rehabilitation are outlined in this chapter. Because of the lack of evidence-based research on rehabilitation of regenerative medicine, these protocols were developed based on clinical experience and our extensive knowledge of the principles of healing tissue.

Tendon

Several studies have suggested that prolonged immobilization following injury reduces water and proteoglycan content of tendons and increases collagen cross-linking (Table 14.1). This can lead to tendon atrophy, low metabolic rate, and vascularity. Mechanical loads have been shown to greatly influence the tenocyte differentiation and proliferation in tendon healing. However, excessive loading can induce differentiation of tenocytes into adipocytes, chondrocytes, and osteocytes thus inhibiting the healing process of tendons. It

TABLE 14.1 Post-Prolotherapy/PRP Injection Tendon

Overall Goals		
Control pain and inflammation *Regain normal strength and endurance* *Regain normal ROM* *Achieve optimal functional level* *Achieve individual patient goals*		
Clinical applications for: • Epicondylitis • Achilles tendinopathy • Plantar fasciitis • Patellar tendinopathy		
• If percutaneous needle tendinotomy has been performed in conjunction with PRP then non-weight bearing or protected weight bearing may be indicated for the first 3 days		
Inflammatory phase	Days 0–3	Guidelines: • No NSAIDs • Complete rest of tissue—may require immobilization • AROM
Proliferation phase I:	Days 4–14	Guidelines: • Relative rest—progress to full weight bearing • No NSAIDs up to 6 weeks • Increase tolerance to ADLs • Correct biomechanical dysfunctions of all surrounding joints
Goals of proliferation phase I:		
• Control pain and inflammation • Promote healing of tissue • Regain tissue mobility • Educate patient and improve posture • Retard scar tissue formation • Gradual increase from AROM to resisted ROM • Initiate muscle contraction/restore muscular balance • Obtain full ROM • Improve balance and proprioception • Avoid high velocity, intense exercises • Avoid post activity pain		
Treatment	Exercises	
Evaluation (1 week postinjection)	Evaluate kinetic chain	
Manuals	Passive ROM Correct biomechanics of dysfunctions for associated joints Stretches as indicated Mobilizations to joint I/IIs for pain and swelling control after week 2	
Strength	Single plane AROM progressing to resisted ROM Be cautious not to overstress tissue until 2 weeks	
Cardiovascular	Start cardio for opposite body area and vice versa	

(continued)

TABLE 14.1 Post-Prolotherapy/PRP Injection Tendon   (*continued*)

Modalities		As needed to control post injection pain
Proliferation phase II:	Weeks 2–8	Guidelines: • Full weight bearing • No NSAIDs up to 6 weeks • Progressive strength program initiating eccentric activities at week 3–4 • Do no start eccentrics until full ROM is achieved
Treatment		Exercises
Manuals		May begin soft tissue techniques at week 2 Transfer friction massage to affect site Joint mobilization, IIIs/IVs for increased joint mobility and restoring capsular balance, Stretching and PROM as indicated Biomechanical corrections to adjacent joints
Strength		Progressing from concentric resisted exercises to eccentric at weeks 3–4 Progressive increase in weights on concentric activity Balance and proprioception activities initiated after week 2

Progression criteria:

• Full ROM
• No pain postactivity
• Pain-free 5/5 static strength

Remodeling phase:	Begin 6–8 weeks postprocedure	Guidelines: • Return to sport phase • Appointments 1× per week generally

Goals of remodeling phase:

• Demonstrate good eccentric control
• Demonstrate symmetrical proprioception
• Dynamic control in multi-plane activities

Treatment	Exercises
Manuals	As needed for joint arthrokinetmatics Stretching as needed
Strength	All functional activities at this phase, no single plane movements Plyometric training Progressing to high velocity/intensive activity Return to sport program initiation

Clearance to return to sport:

• Pain free
• No soreness that lasts greater than 24 hours
• Demonstrates good dynamic control multi-plane activities
• Physician approval

ADLs, activities of daily living; AROM, active range of motion; NSAIDs, nonsteroidal anti-inflammatory drugs; PRP, platelet-rich plasma; ROM, range of motion.

is important to understand the concept of progressive loading to allow the enhancement of fibroblast proliferation, collagen synthesis, and collagen realignment in order to improve tendon strength and accelerate healing (8).

After the acute inflammatory phase of healing, controlled stretching and early range of motion increase collagen synthesis, improving fiber alignment, which leads to higher tensile strength. During the proliferation and remodeling phases, if collagen remains unstressed, it will become haphazard in organization and weaker than collagen that was properly stressed. DNA content, protein synthesis, and cellular proliferation have been seen with repetitive motion during this phase.

In tendon healing postregenerative treatments, 3 to 5 days of rest and protection of the tendon are recommended to allow for incorporation of the injected graft or injectate. In general, immobilization is discouraged. Beyond several days, early mobilization and motion are recommended to start the process of healing and collagen synthesis. Repetitive load to the tissue is necessary to allow for proper organization of new collagen tissue and proper strength of tissue to form after the initial inflammatory phase. Care should be taken to avoid tissue OVERload. Nonsteroidal anti-inflammatory drugs (NSAIDs) should also be avoided for up to 6 weeks as they have been shown, in the literature, to have deleterious effects on long-term tendon healing (15).

After the initial inflammatory phase, rehabilitation should progress to incorporate the Davis's Law principle. Low-load mechanical stress can be applied by isometric, then concentric, and ultimately eccentric activity. Care should be taken to progress per tolerance of the tissue and patient. Eccentric loading is crucial for tendon healing and remodeling of the new tissue (14,16). Eccentric loading should be applied prior to attempting plyometric and sport-specific training. Eccentric activity should be used with caution prior to the 4- to 6-week mark postinjection due to the healing and tissue remodeling principles. Early eccentric activity will cause a disruption in the healing process and negate any potential outcomes of the regenerative treatments.

Once the eccentric strength phase begins, it is recommended to perform 3 × 15 repetitions, one to two times per day, for up to 12 weeks to allow adequate changes in the tissue (14). Debate still exists in the literature as to the mechanism behind how eccentric exercises improve tendinopathy. Current literature suggests changes in neuromuscular output, increased muscle tendon unit (MTU) stiffness, and increases in muscle strength that shifts the length tension curve. There is also clinical suggestion that improper muscle function leads to altered strain on the tendon and that associated muscular rehabilitation is imperative with eccentric exercises (16).

During the eccentric movement, muscles lengthen toward the end of their range. Muscle lengthening then ceases and the tendon undergoes a stretch shortening cycle (SSC). If the muscle is weak or poorly coordinated, the muscle appears to undergo a stop start eccentric type of contraction, identified by Rees et al. as "force fluctuations." The force fluctuations expose the tendon to more frequent SSCs during a given action. The neuromuscular coordination issues may expose the tendon to repeated SSCs during a single functional movement, that is, walking or running. The greater frequency of the SSC exposures is likely to influence the tendon's rate of wear and ultimately its ability to repair. This potentially links to the development and perpetuation of tendinopathy (16).

General guidelines for tendon rehabilitation are:

- Initial protection phase 0 to 7 days

- Initial strength phase isometrics 3 to 7 days

- Concentric strength phase 7 days to 2 to 4 weeks (will vary depending on procedure and physician)

- Eccentric phase 2 to 4 weeks to 6 weeks (will vary depending on procedure and patient tolerance)

- Plyometric/return to sport phase 6 to 8 weeks

Prior to return to sports, physical therapists should coordinate with the physician on a return to sport testing protocol for full clearance. There are several options for functional testing: the Functional Movement Screen (FMS), Selective Functional Movement Assessment (SFMA), Athletic Movement Index (AMI), Hop testing and the Landing Error Scoring System (LESS). There are many options to use from general full kinetic chain assessment to specific localized assessment. It is always wise to have a functional measure to assess especially athletes to clear for full activity.

Important components of healing tendons:

- Inflammatory phase (3 to 5 days post-injection)
    - o Erythrocytes and neutrophils enter site of injury
    - o Monocytes and macrophages predominate phagocytosis of necrotic materials
    - o Tenocytes migrate to the site and type III collagen synthesis initiates
- Proliferation phase
    - o Synthesis of type III collagen peaks
    - o Water content and glycosaminoglycan remain high
- Remodeling phase (6 weeks)
    - o Decreased cellularity and decreased collagen and glyocosaminoglycan synthesis
    - o Tenocyte metabolism remains high with tenocytes and collagen fibers become aligned in the direction of stress
    - o Type I collagen is synthesized
    - o Gradual change of fibrous tissue to scar-like tendon over the course of a year

Ligaments

For many ligaments, healing begins after the injury or stress is removed. Some ligaments, due to their native environment, have minimal potential for healing, for example, anterior cruciate ligament (Table 14.2). Generally, ligament healing follows the same three-phase healing process as tendons. Immobilization of a joint with a ligament injury leads to synovial adhesion,

increase in collagen degradation with decreased collagen synthesis, and a greater percentage of disorganized collagen fibrils. Therefore immobilization is discouraged. Decreased loading of ligament tissue alters matrix turnover. Newly synthesized matrix becomes less organized leading to a decline in tissue stiffness and strength. Prolonged immobilization decreases water content and glycosaminoglycans in the ligament. Overall less mass and strength occur when decreased loading of the ligament is present (21).

Therefore, for most ligament injuries, the affected joint is protected to shield the ligament from forces with some type of bracing, which allows for controlled range of motion.

Early controlled resumption of activity on the injured soft tissue has been shown to have beneficial outcomes. Increased cellular activity, increased tissue mass, improved matrix organization, and more normalized collagen content occur in tissue that is moved during the early phases postinjury.

Important components of healing ligaments:

- Acute inflammatory phase:
    - o Blood collects at injury site
    - o Platelets interact with matrix to form clot
    - o Platelet-rich fibrin clot releases growth factors
    - o Neutrophils, monocytes, and other immune cells migrate to area
    - o Fibroblasts are recruited to the injured area
- Proliferation phase
    - o Immune cells release various growth factors and cytokines
    - o Fibroblasts begin laying down various collagen tissue
    - o Disorganized scar forms with blood vessels, fat cells, fibroblasts, and inflammatory cells
    - o Collagen becomes aligned
- Remodeling phase
    - o Collagen maturation
    - o Tissue matrix starts to resemble normal ligament tissue
    - o Can last up to a year

TABLE 14.2 Post-Prolotherapy/PRP Injection Ligament

Overall Goals		
• Control pain and inflammation *• Regain normal strength and endurance* *• Regain normal ROM* *• Achieve optimal functional level* *• Achieve individual patient goals*		
Clinical applications for: • Peripheral joint ligaments • Insertional areas to bone		
Inflammatory phase	Days 0–3	Guidelines: • No NSAIDs • Complete rest of tissue • AROM
Proliferation phase I:	Days 4–14	Guidelines: • Educate patient and restore posture • No NSAIDs 4–6 weeks • Increase tolerance to ADLs • Correct biomechanical dysfunctions of all surrounding joints
Goals of proliferation phase I:		
• Control pain and inflammation • Promote healing of tissue • Regain tissue mobility • Gradual increase from AROM to resisted ROM • Initiate muscle contraction/restore muscular balance		
Treatment	Exercises	
Evaluation (within 1 week post injection)	Evaluate kinetic chain	
Manuals	Passive ROM Joint mobilizations I/IIs for pain and swelling control, IIIs/IVs to restore joint mobility Correct biomechanical errors for associated joints Stretches as indicated	
Strength	Single plane AROM progressing to resisted ROM after week 2 Be cautious not to overstress tissue until 2 weeks	
Cardiovascular	Start cardio for opposite body area and vice versa	
Modalities	As needed to control postinjection pain	
Proliferation phase II:	Weeks 2–8	Guidelines: • Full weight bearing • No NSAIDs up to 4–6 weeks • Progressive strength program initiating proprioceptive activities and joint compressive loading at week 3

(continued)

TABLE 14.2 Post-Prolotherapy/PRP Injection Ligament   (*continued*)

Goals of proliferation phase II:	
• Obtain full ROM • Improve balance and proprioception • Avoid high velocity, intense exercises • Avoid post-activity pain	
Treatment	**Exercises**
Manuals	May begin soft tissue techniques at week 2 Transfer friction massage to affected site Joint mobilization IIIs, IVs for increased joint mobility Stretching and PROM as indicated Biomechanical corrections to adjacent joints
Strength	Progressing concentric resisted exercises Proprioception activities and closed kinetic chain activity at week 3 Progressive increase in weights on concentric activity Balance and proprioception activities initiated after week 2

Progression criteria:		
• Full ROM • No pain postactivity • Pain-free 5/5 static strength		
Remodeling phase:	Begin 6–8 weeks post procedure	Guidelines: • Return to sport phase • Appointments 1× per week generally

Goals of remodeling phase:	
• Demonstrate good eccentric control • Demonstrate symmetrical proprioception • Dynamic control in multi-plane activities	
Treatment	**Exercises**
Manuals	As needed for joint arthrokinematics Stretching as needed
Strength	All functional activities at this phase, no single plane movements Plyometric training Progressing to high velocity/intensive activity Return to sport program initiation

Clearance to return to sport:
• Pain free • No soreness that lasts greater than 24 hours • Demonstrates good dynamic control multi-plane activities • Physician approval

ADLs, activities of daily living; AROM, active range of motion; NSAIDs, nonsteroidal anti-inflammatory drugs; ROM, range of motion.

Muscle

Muscle injury is broken down into three grades: Grade I tear of few muscle fibers with minimal swelling and minimal loss of strength; Grade II constitutes a greater amount of damage to the muscle with partial loss of strength and limitation of movement; Grade III is a full tear across a section of muscle and loss of muscle function (Table 14.3). Skeletal muscle regeneration is characterized by proliferation and differentiation of precursor cells. Growth factors play a significant role in the muscle regeneration process. There is still questionable evidence about whether or not muscle tissue is fully restored to its previous level due to the competing processes of healing and fibrosis (6,9).

When rehabilitating a muscle tissue post regenerative injection, the stage of the injury must be a critical component to consider. If prolotherapy or PRP is administered to a chronic muscular pathology, then the protocol is considerably shorter and accelerated more quickly. If prolotherapy or PRP is administered during the acute phase of the original injury, then a conservative approach to rehabilitation should be considered. This is due to the extensive healing process the muscle tissue will undergo during the acute phases of the healing process. Care must be given to not overstress the new tissue formation during the acute and proliferation phases balanced by maintaining motion to avoid scar formation. During remodeling phase at 3 to 4 weeks postinjury, increased stress can be applied to the healing tissue to help remodel and align the collagen fibers in an organized fashion. Full muscle length and extensibility should be a goal of the clinician to regain as much of the original muscle tissue strength (9).

For most lower extremity muscle injuries, eccentric training will be an integral part of the rehabilitation process. Eccentric loading has been shown to be effective in tissue remodeling, collagen reorganization, increased rate of collagen synthesis, and improved coordination of muscle contractions (16,17,36).

At 4 weeks, in most cases, eccentric training can begin. Soreness in the tissue during this phase can be expected and care should be taken by the physical therapist to perform eccentric training in a slow progressive loading fashion. Eccentric exercises allow for improved muscular strength and should be performed prior to plyometric/sport-specific activity. Full length of the muscle tissue should be achieved before beginning the eccentric exercises.

Important components of healing muscle:

- Inflammation phase:
  - o Blood clot formation
  - o Local degranulation of platelets
  - o Pain, swelling, redness, and increased local temperature
  - o Recruitment of satellite muscle cells and stem
- Proliferation phase:
  - o Fibroblasts synthesize scar tissue
  - o Capillary neoformation
- Remodeling phase:
  - o Collagen remodeling
  - o Muscle tissue regeneration

Cartilage: Stem Cell Treatments

In the early 1990s, existence of adult MSCs, described as "non-committed progenitor cells," was discovered to have an active role in connective tissue repair (Table 14.4). These cells were first labeled by Caplan in 1991 as "mesenchymal" stem cells (MSCs) because of the ability to differentiate to lineages of mesenchymal tissue, and were recognized to be an essential component of the tissue repair process (37). There are two kinds of stem cells, embryonic (prenatal) and adult (postnatal). Stem cells can be located in adipose tissue and bone marrow. Recent studies indicate that adipose-derived stem cells show identical structure

TABLE 14.3 Post-Prolotherapy/PRP Injection Muscle

Overall Goals		
Control pain and inflammation *Regain normal strength and endurance* *Regain normal ROM* *Achieve optimal functional level* *Achieve individual patient goals*		
Clinical applications for: • Muscular conditions		
Inflammatory phase I	Up to 1 week	Guidelines: • No NSAIDs • Complete rest of tissue but no immobilization
Proliferation phase II:	Weeks 1–8	Guidelines: • No NSAIDs up to 4–6 weeks • Increase tolerance to ADLs • Correct biomechanical dysfunctions of all surrounding joints • Avoid high velocity, intense exercises • Avoid postactivity pain
Goals of proliferation phase II:		
• Control pain and inflammation • Promote healing of tissue • Regain tissue mobility/extensibility • Educate patient and improve posture • Retard scar tissue formation • Gradual increase from AROM to resisted ROM • Initiate muscle contraction/restore muscular balance • Initiate eccentric muscle contraction for tissue remodeling at week 3 • Improve balance and proprioception		
Treatment	Exercises	
Evaluation (1 week postinjection)	Evaluate kinetic chain	
Manuals	Passive ROM Stretching Joint mobilization as needed in associated joints Correct biomechanical errors for associated joints	
Strength	Single plane AROM progressing to resisted ROM after week 2 Isometrics week 1–2 Be cautious not to overstress tissue until 2 weeks Begin eccentrics at week 3 if full ROM is achieved	
Cardiovascular	Start cardio for opposite body area and vice versa	
Modalities	As needed to control post injection pain	

(continued)

TABLE 14.3 Post-Prolotherapy/PRP Injection Muscle   (*continued*)

Progression criteria:		
• Full ROM • No pain postactivity • Pain-free 5/5 static strength		
Remodeling phase III:	Begin 8 weeks postprocedure	Guidelines: • Return to sport phase • Appointments 1x per week generally
Goals of remodeling phase III:		
• Demonstrate good eccentric control • Demonstrate symmetrical proprioception • Dynamic control in multi-plane activities		
Treatment	Exercises	
Manuals	As needed for joint arthrokinetmatics Stretching as needed	
Strength	All functional activities at this phase, no single plane movements Plyometric training Progressing to high velocity/intensive activity Return to sport program initiation	
Clearance to return to sport:		
• Pain free • No soreness that lasts greater than 24 hours • Demonstrates good dynamic control multi-plane activities • Physician approval		

ADLs, activities of daily living; AROM, active range of motion; NSAIDs, nonsteroidal anti-inflammatory drugs; ROM, range of motion.

and differentiation capabilities as bone marrow stem cells. Adipose tissue, however, has greater quantities and is less invasive to harvest (38).

MSCs, along with other cells within the adipose stroma, react to cellular and chemical signals, and have been shown to differentiate to assist in healing for a wide variety of cellular types. This includes cartilage repair, OA, tendon defects, ligament tissue, and intervertebral disc degeneration.

With stem cell prolotherapy, a stem cell niche is moved from one tissue in which these niches are abundant, adipose, into one where they are scarce, a non-repairing connective tissue. The ability of adipose-derived stem/stromal cells (AD-SC) to support and serve as a cell reservoir

for connective tissue and joint repair is the basic theory of stem cell prolotherapy. AD-SCs have been shown, in multiple studies, to produce growth factors, cytokines, stimulate fibroblast proliferation, migration, and collagen secretion (4,37). Studies have also demonstrated improvements with adult stem cell therapy by the successful regeneration of osteoarthritic damage and articular cartilage defects (8,37).

Regenerative medicine physicians have started to utilize the potential of AD-SC within nonmanipulated fat graft scaffolding, combined with high-density PRP concentrates (HD-PRP) to provide a potent therapeutic combination. HD-PRP is able to enhance musculoskeletal healing and stimulate local microenvironmental

TABLE 14.4 Post-Stem Cell Injection Cartilage

Overall Goals		
• *Control pain and inflammation* • *Protect the injected area* • *Regain normal strength and endurance* • *Regain normal ROM* • *Achieve optimal functional level* • *Achieve individual patient goals*		
Clinical applications for: • Osteoarthritis • Cartilage degeneration/defects • Disc degeneration		
Inflammatory phase	Days 0–3	Guidelines: • No NSAIDs • Complete rest of tissue • AROM
Proliferation phase I:	Days 4–14	Guidelines: • Relative rest; progress to full weight bearing • No NSAIDs up to 4–6 weeks • Increase tolerance to ADLs • Correct biomechanical dysfunctions of all surrounding joints
Goals of proliferation phase I:		
• Control pain and inflammation • Promote healing of tissue • Protect tissue scaffold created by stem cell injection • Educate patient • Gradual increase from PROM to AROM to resisted ROM		
Treatment	Exercises	
Evaluation (1–2 weeks postinjection)	Evaluate kinetic chain	
Manuals	Passive ROM Joint mobilizations I/IIs for pain and swelling Correct biomechanical errors for associated joints Stretches as indicated	
Strength	Single plane AROM progressing to resisted ROM after week 2 Be cautious not to overstress tissue until weeks 3–4	
Cardiovascular	Start cardio for opposite body area and vice versa at end of 2 weeks	
Modalities	As needed to control post injection pain	
Proliferation phase II:	Weeks 2–8	Guidelines: • Full weight bearing • No NSAIDs up to 4–6 weeks • Progressive strength program initiating eccentric activities at weeks 4–6

(continued)

TABLE 14.4 Post-Stem Cell Injection Cartilage (*continued*)

Goals of proliferation phase II:	
<ul><li>Obtain full ROM</li><li>Initiate eccentric program at weeks 4–6</li><li>Improve balance and proprioception</li><li>Avoid high velocity, intense exercises</li><li>Avoid postactivity pain</li></ul>	
Treatment	**Exercises**
Manuals	May begin soft tissue techniques at week 2 Joint mobilization IIIs/IVs for joint mobility Stretching and PROM as indicated Biomechanical corrections to adjacent joints
Strength	Progressing from concentric resisted exercises to eccentric at week 3 Progressive increase in weights on concentric activity Balance and proprioception activities initiated after week 2

Progression criteria:		
<ul><li>Full ROM</li><li>No pain postactivity</li><li>Pain-free 5/5 static strength</li></ul>		
Remodeling phase:	Begin 6–8 weeks post procedure	Guidelines:<ul><li>Return to sport phase</li><li>Appointments 1x per week generally</li></ul>

Goals of remodeling phase:	
<ul><li>Demonstrate good eccentric control</li><li>Demonstrate symmetrical proprioception</li><li>Dynamic control in multiplane activities</li></ul>	
Treatment	**Exercises**
Manuals	As needed for joint arthrokinematics Stretching as needed
Strength	All functional activities at this phase, no single plane movements Plyometric training Progressing to high velocity/intensive activity Return to sport program initiation

Clearance to return to sport:
<ul><li>Pain free</li><li>No soreness that lasts greater than 24 hours</li><li>Demonstrates good dynamic control multi-plane activities</li><li>Physician approval</li></ul>

ADLs, activities of daily living; AROM, active range of motion; NSAIDs, nonsteroidal anti-inflammatory drugs; ROM, range of motion.

regenerative capabilities especially during the early phase of tendon healing. Proliferation and differentiation of AD-SCs are directly related to the platelet concentration. HD-PRP releases large quantities of growth factors which, when activated, significantly enhance stem–stromal cell proliferation and enhance the survival of the fat scaffolding (37).

When rehabilitating a patient who has had stem cell prolotherapy, there are several factors to be aware of. First, when an AD-SC scaffold is injected into the target tissue, care must be taken not to overstress the specific tissue until the scaffold links to the existing tissue and starts to differentiate. This will be a rest period between when the patient has the injection and when he or she starts physical therapy. On initiating physical therapy, a kinetic chain evaluation should be completed and PROM to affected areas can begin. Although loss of range of motion is not a concern postinjection, PROM and grades I, II joint mobilizations will assist in blood flow to the healing tissue.

Second consideration to have in mind when rehabilitating stem cell patients is the proper progression of resistive exercises. As the cells start to differentiate and collagen remodels from type III to type I, proper stress of the tissue is crucial. Tissue overload will disrupt the cell regeneration process. It is wise to be more conservative than aggressive in your rehabilitation plan. Starting at week 2, isometrics can be initiated, then move to concentric isotonic exercises. Between weeks 4 and 6, under guidance of the physician, progression to eccentric exercises can be initiated. Ultimately return to activity progresses at 6 to 8 weeks post injection.

Important components of stem cell rehabilitation:

- MSC differentiation during three phases of healing
- Osetogenesis to osteoblast to osteocyte to bone
- Chondrogenesis to chondrocyte to hypertophy chondrocyte to cartilage
- Myogenesis to myoblast to myotube to muscle
- Tendogenesis/ligamentagenesis to fibroblast to tendon/ligament (26)

Spinal Conditions

Osseous or soft tissue injury of the spine, predispose the joint to premature painful degenerative changes (Table 14.5). Intersegmental laxity or instability can be a result of the poor healing response to an injury or chronic postural adaptations and degenerative changes especially in the cervical spine. Facet joints are richly innervated, but have poor blood supply which leads to a poor healing response to even low impact forces. Spinal discs, once injured, can lose their water content and their jelly-like center. Over time, the disc will reduce in height and degenerate. Although the disc may not be painful once degenerated, surrounding tissues will likely become affected due to the decreased height of the spinal complex. Increased wear on the surrounding tissues will lead to pain and instability (33).

Spinal instability is defined as the vertebral column's loss of ability to support physiological loads in order to maintain the relationship between vertebrae, as well as to prevent nerve root damage or irritation (39). Signs of instability include loss of stiffness, disk height reduction, ligament and facet capsule laxity, and degeneration of facet joints. Over time, the ligament loses its ability to restrain the limits of motion and can lead to involvement of the sympathetic system. Scar tissue around the joint capsule and spinal ligaments forms over time with repetitive stress to the joint capsule due to the ligament's laxity. This also leads to muscular tightness, spasm, and myofascial pain. Both the intervertebral discs and facet joints have a limited blood supply leading to a poor healing response and tissue remodeling and ultimately further degeneration of the intervertebral segments. Muscle

TABLE 14.5 **Post-Prolotherapy Spinal Injection**

Overall Goals		
• Control pain and inflammation *• Regain normal strength and endurance* *• Regain normal ROM* *• Achieve optimal functional level* *• Achieve individual patient goals*		
Clinical applications for: • Spinal instability/hypermobility		
Inflammatory phase I:	Days 0–3 up to week 1	Guidelines: • No NSAIDs • AROM and normal ADLs
Proliferation phase II:	Weeks 1–8	Guidelines: • No NSAIDs up to 4–6 weeks • Increase tolerance to ADLs • Educate patient and improve posture • Correct biomechanical dysfunctions of all surrounding joints
Goals of proliferation phase II:		
• Control pain and inflammation • Promote healing of tissue • Regain tissue mobility and obtain full ROM • Gradual increase from AROM to resisted ROM • Initiate spinal stabilization program • Improve spinal proprioception • Avoid high velocity, intense exercises • Avoid post-activity pain		

Treatment	Exercises
Evaluation	Evaluate kinetic chain
Manuals	May begin soft tissue techniques at week 2 Passive ROM Joint mobilizations to adjacent hypomobile segments (protect hypermobile segments and injected vertebral segments) Correct biomechanical errors for associated joints
Mobility strength	Mobility exercises to achieve proper spinal curves with AROM Spinal mobility before spinal stability Spinal stabilization—activation of erector spinae and co-contraction of abdominal muscles Proprioception activities to improve joint awareness
Cardiovascular	Start cardio for opposite body area and vice versa
Modalities	As needed to control postinjection pain

Progression criteria:
• Full ROM • No pain postactivity • Pain-free 5/5 static strength

(*continued*)

TABLE 14.5 Post-Prolotherapy Spinal Injection   (*continued*)

Remodeling phase III:	Begins 6–8 weeks postprocedure	Guidelines: • Return to sport phase • Appointments 1× per week generally
Goals of remodeling phase III:		
• Demonstrate good control • Demonstrate symmetrical proprioception • Dynamic control in multiplane activities		
Treatment	Exercises	
Manuals	As needed for joint arthrokinetmatics Stretching as needed for tissue extensibility	
Strength	All functional activities at this phase, no single plane movements Plyometric training Progressing to high velocity/intensive activity Return to sport program initiation	
Clearance to return to sport:		
• Pain free • No soreness that lasts greater than 24 hours • Demonstrates good dynamic control multi-plane activities • Physician approval		

ADLs, activities of daily living; AROM, active range of motion; NSAIDs, nonsteroidal anti-inflammatory drugs; ROM, range of motion.

protective mechanisms and spasm often occur in response to the spinal instability and loss of mechanical integrity. Studies have indicated that the erector spinae muscles are in close proximity to the facet joint capsule and have fibrous insertions into the capsule to provide dynamic control of the joint.

Prolotherapy injections into the zygapophysial joints show improved pain and function, by addressing not only the symptoms but also the underlying pathology of the ligament and facet degeneration. This in turn improves the ligamentous strength and stabilizing effects of the joint. Prolotherapy injections can be given on a weekly basis for up to three to six times or over a span of several months. Solutions range from 5% to 25% and can be mixed with a variety of other solutions including lidocaine (39).

Rehabilitation following prolotherapy in the spinal segments with dextrose is outlined in the protocol. It should be noted the overall goal of rehabilitation after spinal injections is to promote stability and regain joint proprioception. Overstressing the spinals segments is discouraged, as mechanical overload and ligament laxity are the underlying causes of the joint pathology. Biomechanical correction of any hypomobile segments is advised to decrease the adjacent stress of the hypermobile segment and reduce facilitation of the hypermobile segments. Currently, many pain management treatments of facet and disc pathology include the use of corticosteroid injections and/or denervation procedures, that is, radiofrequency ablation. There are many concerns that have been raised regarding the potential complications and limited effectiveness of these long-used treatments. Therefore, regenerative treatments are used with increasing evidence of efficacy (40).

Spinal ligaments surrounding the vertebral segments are often overlooked as a source of pain and disability in the patient suffering from back pain. Ligamentous tissue contains afferent nerve endings where vertebral discs do not. Therefore, if the patient has a degenerative disc condition, pain is more likely coming from the surrounding soft tissues that are being overstressed due to the loss of disc height. The iliolumbar ligament is a great example of pain source in the patient with a combined degenerative disc at L5/S1 and a sacroiliac instability. The iliolumbar ligament is a strong ligament that arises from the tip of the transverse process of the fifth lumbar vertebra and inserts on to the posterior part of the inner lip of the iliac crest. Traditional treatments that can reduce pain arising from this ligament include transverse friction massage, joint stabilization, and joint mobilization. However, in the presence of true sacroiliac instability, prolotherapy has been shown to be an effective treatment to regain ligament cross-sectional area stiffness and increase stability to the sacroiliac joint complex (41,42).

Important components of the rehabilitation of spinal ligaments:

- Acute inflammatory phase:
  - Blood collects at injury site
  - Platelets interact with matrix to form clot
  - Platelet-rich fibrin clot releases growth factors
  - Neutrophils, monocytes, and other immune cells migrate to area
  - Fibroblasts are recruited to the injured area
- Proliferation phase
  - Immune cells release various growth factors and cytokines
  - Fibroblasts begin laying down various collagen tissue
  - Disorganized scar forms with blood vessels, fat cells, fibroblasts, and inflammatory cells

  - Collagen becomes aligned
- Remodeling phase
  - Collagen maturation
  - Tissue matrix starts to resemble normal ligament tissue
  - Can last up to a year

CONCLUSION

Physical therapy is a vital component to the recovery of chronic soft tissue injury. A variety of injuries can be treated with regenerative medicine. Techniques such as prolotherapy, PRP, and stem cell therapy are among these treatments. An appropriate course of rehabilitation can be instrumental in ensuring that these treatments are maximally effective. To date, rehabilitative protocols for regenerative medicine are an area lacking evidence-based practice. As musculoskeletal specialists, physical therapists should understand in detail the healing process and the process by which these various regenerative treatments affect tendon, ligaments, muscle, and cartilage in order to better guide rehabilitation of patients during their recovery from these procedures.

REFERENCES

1.   Hauser RA, Maddela HS, Alderman D, et al. Journal of Prolotherapy International Medical Editorial Board Consensus Statement on the use of prolotherapy for musculoskeletal pain. *J Prolother.* 2011;3(4):744–764.

2.   Rabago D, Slattengren A, Zgierska A. Prolotherapy in primary care practice. *Prim Care.* 2010;37(1):65–80.

3.   Alderman D. The new age of prolotherapy. *Pract Pain Manag.* 2010;10(4):54–72.

4.   Hauser RA, Hauswer MA, et al. Evidence-based use of dextrose prolotherapy for musculoskeletal pain: a scientific literature review. *J Prolother.* 2011;3(4):765–789.

5.   Hauser RA, Sprague IS. Outcomes of prolotherapy in chondromalacia patella patients: improvements

in pain level and function. *Clin Med Insights Arthritis Musculoskelet Disord*. 2014;7:13–20.

6. Foster TE, Puskas BL, Mandelbaum BR, et al. Platelet-rich plasma: from basic science to clinical applications. *Am J Sports Med*. 2009;37(11):2259–2272.

7. Marx RE. Platelet-rich plasma (PRP): what is PRP and what is not PRP? *Implant Dent*. 2001;10(4):225–228.

8. Yuan T, Zhang CQ, Wang JH. Augmenting tendon and ligament repair with platelet-rich plasma (PRP). *Muscles Ligaments Tendons J*. 2013;3(3):139–149.

9. Borrione P, Gianfrancesco AD, Pereira MT, et al. Platelet-rich plasma in muscle healing. *Am J Phys Med Rehabil*. 2010;89(10):854–861.

10. Zhu Y, Yuan M, Meng HY, et al. Basic science and clinical application of platelet-rich plasma for cartilage defects and osteoarthritis: a review. *Osteoarthr Cartil*. 2013;21(11):1627–1637.

11. Charousset C, Zaoui A, Bellaiche L, et al. Are multiple platelet-rich plasma injections useful for treatment of chronic patellar tendinopathy in athletes? A prospective study. *Am J Sports Med*. 2014;42(4):906–911.

12. World Anti-Doping Agency. WADA 2011 prohibited list now published, 2010. www.wada-ama.org/en/media/news/2010-09/wada-2011-prohibited-list-now-published

13. Rees JD, Stride M, Scott A, et al. Tendons—time to revisit inflammation. *Br J Sports Med*. 2012;1–7.

14. Murtaugh B, Ihm JM. Eccentric training for the treatment of tendinopathies. *Curr Sports Med Rep*. 2013;12(3):175–182.

15. Sharma P, Maffulli N. Tendon injury and tendinopathy: healing and repair. *J Bone Joint Surg Am*. 2005;87(1):187–202.

16. O'Neill S, Watson PJ, Barry S. Why are eccentric exercises effective for Achilles tendinopathy? *Int J Sports Phys Ther*. 2015;10(4):552–562.

17. Rees JD, Wolman RL, Wilson A. Eccentric exercises; why do they work, what are the problems and how can we improve them? *Br J Sports Med*. 2009;43(4):242–246.

18. Khan KM, Scott A. Mechanotherapy: how physical therapists' prescription of exercise promotes tissue repair. *Br J Sports Med*. 2009;43(4):247–252.

19. Dunn SL, Olmedo ML. Mechanotransduction: relevance to physical therapist practice: understanding our ability to affect genetic expression through mechanical forces. *Phys Ther*. 2016;96(5):712–721.

20. Gillespie PG, Müller U. Mechanotransduction by hair cells: models, molecules, and mechanisms. *Cell*. 2009;139(1):33–44.

21. Hauser RA, Dolan EE, Phillips HJ, et al. Ligament injury and healing: a review of current clinical diagnostics and therapeutics. *Open Rehabilit J*. 2013;6:1–20.

22. Bogduk N. *Clinical and Radiological Anatomy of the Lumbar Spine*. Churchill: Livingstone, Elsevier (2nd edition); 2005.

23. Yamaguchi S, Aoyama T, Ito A, et al. The effects of exercise on the early stages of mesenchymal stromal cell-induced cartilage repair in a rat osteochondral defect model. *PLOS ONE*. 2016;11(3):1–10.

24. Hulejová H, Baresová V, Klézl Z, et al. Increased level of cytokines and matrix metalloproteinases in osteoarthritic subchondral bone. *Cytokine*. 2007;38(3):151–156.

25. Tetlow LC, Adlam DJ, Woolley DE. Matrix metalloproteinase and proinflammatory cytokine production by chondrocytes of human osteoarthritic cartilage: associations with degenerative changes. *Arthritis Rheum*. 2001;44(3):585–594.

26. Alderman DD, Alexander RW, Harris GR, et al. Stem cell prolotherapy in regenerative medicine: background, theory and protocols. *J Prolotherapy*. 2011;3(3):689–708.

27. Echeverri LF, Herrero MA, Lopez JM, et al. Early stages of bone fracture healing: formation of a fibrin-collagen scaffold in the fracture hematoma. *Bull Math Biol*. 2015;77(1):156–183.

28. McCulloch JM, Kloth LC, Feeder JA. *Wound healing in alternatives in management*. Philadelphia: F.A. Davis Company; 1995:3–43.

29. Prisk V, Huard J. Muscle injuries and repair: the role of prostaglandins and inflammation. *Histol Histopathol*. 2003;18(4):1243–1256.

30. Medical Gallery of Mikael Haggstrom. *Wiki Journal of Medicine*. 2014;1(2). DOI:10.15347/wjm/2014.008. ISSN 2002-4436. Public Domain.

31. Järvinen TA, Järvinen M, Kalimo H. Regeneration of injured skeletal muscle after the injury. *Muscles Ligaments Tendons J*. 2013;3(4):337–345.

32. Middleton KK, Barro V, Muller B, et al. Evaluation of the effects of platelet-rich plasma (PRP) therapy involved in the healing of sports-related soft tissue injuries. *Iowa Orthop J*. 2012;32:150–163.

33. Krogman K, Sherry M, Wilson J, et al. Platelet-rich plasma rehabilitation guidelines. 2014. PDF File. www.uwsportsmedicine.org

34. Kaux JF, Forthomme B, Namurois MH, et al. Description of a standardized rehabilitation program based on sub-maximal eccentric following a platelet-rich plasma infiltration for jumper's

knee. *Muscles Ligaments Tendons J.* 2014;4(1): 85–89.

35. Dolgin E. Cellular rehab: physical therapy and exercise are critical to the success of cell therapies approaching the clinic. *The Scientist.* 2015; 12:1–8.

36. Rees JD, Lichtwark GA, Wolman RL, et al. The mechanism for efficacy of eccentric loading in Achilles tendon injury; an *in vivo* study in humans. *Rheumatology (Oxford).* 2008;47(10):1493–1497.

37. Alderman DD, Alexander RW, Harris GR, et al. Stem cell prolotherapy in regenerative medicine. *J Prolother.* 2011;3(3):689–708.

38. Zuk PA. The adipose-derived stem cell: looking back and looking ahead. *Mol Biol Cell.* 2010;21(11): 1783–1787.

39. Hauser RA, Steilen DR, Fisher, P. Upper cervical instability of traumatic origin treated with dextrose prolotherapy: a case report. *J Prolother.* 2015;7:932–936.

40. Landa J, Kim Y. Outcomes of interlaminar and transforminal spinal injections. *Bull NYU Hosp Joint Diseases.* 2012;70(1):6–10.

41. Auburn A, Benjamin S, Bechtel PT, et al. Increase in cross sectional area of the iliolumbar ligament using prolotherapy agents: an ultrasonic case study. *J Prolother.* 2009;1(3):156–162.

42. Auburn A, Benjamin S, Bechtel R. Prolotherapy for pelvic ligament pain: a case report. *J Prolother.* 2009;1(2):89–95.

Index